Food and Western Disease

Health and Nutrition from an Evolutionary Perspective

Staffan Lindeberg

MD, PhD, Associate Professor
Center for Primary Health Care Research, Lund University
Sankt Lars Primary Health Care Centre, 22185 Lund
Sweden

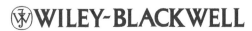

WILEY-BLACKWELL

A John Wiley & Sons, Ltd., Publication

This edition first published 2010
© 2010 Staffan Lindeberg

Blackwell Publishing was acquired by John Wiley & Sons in February 2007. Blackwell's publishing programme has been merged with Wiley's global Scientific, Technical, and Medical business to form Wiley-Blackwell.

Registered office
John Wiley & Sons Ltd, The Atrium, Southern Gate, Chichester, West Sussex, PO19 8SQ, United Kingdom

Editorial offices
9600 Garsington Road, Oxford, OX4 2DQ, United Kingdom
2121 State Avenue, Ames, Iowa 50014-8300, USA

For details of our global editorial offices, for customer services and for information about how to apply for permission to reuse the copyright material in this book please see our website at www.wiley.com/wiley-blackwell.

The right of the author to be identified as the author of this work has been asserted in accordance with the Copyright, Designs and Patents Act 1988.

Library of Congress Cataloging-in-Publication Data

Lindeberg, Staffan, 1950–
  [Maten och folksjukdomarna. English]
  Food and western disease : health and nutrition from an evolutionary perspective / Staffan Lindeberg.
     p. ; cm.
  Includes bibliographical references and index.
  ISBN 978-1-4051-9771-7 (pbk. : alk. paper) 1. Nutritionally induced diseases.
2. Human evolution.   3. Diet in disease.   4. Prehistoric peoples–Food.   I. Title.
  [DNLM: 1. Nutritional Physiological Phenomena.   2. Chronic Disease.   3. Dietetics.
QU 145 L743f 2010a]
  RA645.N87L5613 2010
  362.196′39–dc22
                                                                    2009035246

A catalogue record for this book is available from the British Library.

Set in 10/12.5 pt Sabon by Aptara® Inc., New Delhi, India
1   2010

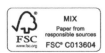

Contents

Foreword by *Loren Cordain*   vii
Preface   xi

1 Introduction   **1**
　1.1 Why do we get sick?   1
　1.2 We are changing at pace with the continental drift   3
　1.3 Are we adapted for milk and bread?   5

2 Expanding our perspective   **8**
　2.1 The perspective of academic medicine   8
　2.2 The concept of normality   11
　2.3 Genetics   12
　2.4 Dietary guidelines   13
　　　　Problems and limitations in nutritional research   14
　　　　Old and new concepts of healthy diets   21

3 Ancestral human diets   **30**
　3.1 Available food   30
　3.2 Nutritional composition   34
　　　　Minerals, trace elements   35
　　　　Common salt   36
　　　　Vitamins   37
　　　　Protein content   40
　　　　Protein quality   41
　　　　Fat content   42
　　　　Saturated fat   45
　　　　Polyunsaturated fat   45
　　　　Trans fatty acids   48
　　　　Monounsaturated fat   48
　　　　Cholesterol content   48

Carbohydrate content	49
Carbohydrate quality	49
Energy density	51
Total energy intake	52
pH	52
Fibre	52
Phytochemicals	52

4   Modern diseases   **56**

4.1   Ischaemic heart disease (coronary heart disease)   57
  Incidence studies   57
  The Kitava study, Trobriand Islands   58
  Effects of urbanisation   63
  Relevant dietary factors   63
  Tobacco smoking   83
  Physical activity   84
4.2   Stroke   84
  Incidence studies   85
  Relevant dietary factors   89
4.3   Atherosclerosis   90
  Prevalence studies   92
  Appearance in animals   93
  Regression studies   94
  Relevant dietary factors   95
4.4   Type 2 diabetes   101
  Prevalence studies   102
  Preventive/causative dietary factors   104
  Diet in established type 2 diabetes   111
4.5   Overweight and obesity   115
  Prevalence studies   115
  Potential consequences   119
  Relevant dietary factors   126
  William Banting   131
4.6   Insulin resistance   133
  Prevalence studies   133
  Attempts to explain   135
  Associated abnormalities   139
  Relevant dietary factors   152
4.7   Hypertension (high blood pressure)   156
  Prevalence studies   157
  Effects of urbanisation   159
  Risks with hypertension   161
  Relevant dietary factors   161
4.8   Dyslipidaemia (blood lipid disorders)   166
  Prevalence studies   167
  Effects of urbanisation   170
  Risks with dyslipidaemia   174
  Relevant dietary factors   176

4.9	Heart failure	178
	Prevalence studies	179
	Primary prevention	180
	Secondary prevention	181
4.10	Dementia	183
	Prevalence studies	183
	Relevant dietary factors	184
4.11	Cancer	185
	Prevalence studies	185
	Prehistoric skeletal remains	186
	Relevant dietary factors	187
	Future research	191
4.12	Osteoporosis	192
	Prevalence studies	193
	Prehistoric skeletal remains	194
	Relevant dietary factors	196
4.13	Rickets	204
	Rickets in osteological material	204
	Rickets in medical literature	204
	Relevant dietary factors	205
4.14	Iron deficiency	208
	Prevalence studies	208
	Prehistoric	208
	Relevant dietary factors	209
4.15	Autoimmune diseases	210
	Relevant mechanisms	210
	Relevant diseases	212
	Palaeolithic elimination diet	215

5	**Risks with the Palaeolithic diet**	**216**
5.1	Haemochromatosis	216
5.2	Iodine deficiency	217
5.3	Exaggerated drug effects	219
	Hypotension (abnormally low blood pressure)	219
	Low blood sugar	219
	Warfarin-induced bleeding	219

6	**Viewpoint summary**	**221**
6.1	Evolutionary medicine instead of vegetarianism?	221
6.2	Traditional populations are spared from overweight and cardiovascular disease	222
6.3	Insulin resistance is more than abdominal obesity and diabetes	222
6.4	Non-Europeans are affected the hardest	223
6.5	'Foreign' proteins in the food	223
6.6	Effects of an ancestral diet	223
6.7	The ancestral diet: a new concept	224

7   Healthy eating   **225**
   7.1   Non-recommended foods?   225
       Grains   225
       Dairy products   226
       Refined fats   226
       Sugar   226
       Beans   226
   7.2   Recommended foods   227
       Lean meat   227
       Fish   228
       Vegetables   228
       Fruit   228
       Root vegetables   228
       Tap water   228
       Nuts   228
   7.3   Variation   229
   7.4   Compromises   229

Glossary   231
References   250
Index   345

Foreword

I consider it an honour to have the privilege to be one of the first people to read this masterpiece on optimal human diet by Dr Staffan Lindeberg. Throughout my life, I have always had an interest in health, fitness and diet starting from my early years as a university track and field athlete in the late 1960s, and then later as a beach lifeguard in the 1970s and finally as I began my career as a university professor in the early 1980s. In those halcyon days, people, including myself, who exercised regularly and attempted to eat healthy diets were dubbed 'health nuts'. At the time, many physicians, health professionals and nutritionists considered vegetarian diets based upon legumes and whole grains to be the healthiest diet one could eat. As a young man, I was swayed by popular vegetarian diet books such as *Diet for a Small Planet* and attempted many times to adopt such diets, but my attempts invariably ended in failure. As a young university professor, I was influenced by the popular low-fat, high-carbohydrate, plant-based diets that were universally being recommended by governmental agencies and nutritional authorities. Finally in about 1987, when I got around to reading Boyd Eaton's now classic paper ('Paleolithic nutrition: a consideration of its nature and current implications') published in the prestigious *New England Journal of Medicine*, a light suddenly came on. From the void of nutritional chaos concerning what one should and should not eat to optimise health, I now realised a rational pathway existed to organise all of the seemingly contradictory and conflicting ideas on human diet. At the time, I did not realise that another person on this planet had also read this pioneering paper by Dr Eaton and was far ahead of my thoughts, as he was already planning scientific expeditions to the remote island of Kitava to study indigenous people consuming non-Westernised diets. This person, of course, is my scientific colleague, Dr Staffan Lindeberg, and the author of this enlightening and groundbreaking book – a book that represents a paradigm shift in how modern medicine is beginning to understand the link between diet and disease. As I read this book it occurred to me that Dr Lindeberg had not only provided me with the specifics of how the Western diet was implicated in virtually every single chronic disease that afflicts us, but he had also eloquently delineated the ultimate basis for the link between nutrition and disease. Let me characterise my impressions of Dr Lindeberg's message.

Although humanity has been interested in diet and health for thousands of years, the organised, scientific study of nutrition has a relatively recent past. For instance, the world's first scientific journal devoted entirely to diet and nutrition, *The Journal of Nutrition*, only began publication in 1928. Other well-known nutrition journals have a more recent history still: *The British Journal of Nutrition* (1947), *The American Journal of Clinical Nutrition* (1954) and *The European Journal of Clinical Nutrition* (1988). The first vitamin was 'discovered' in 1912 and the last vitamin (B$_{12}$) was identified in 1948[1]. The scientific notion that omega-3 fatty acids have beneficial health effects dates back only to the late 1970s[2], and the characterisation of the glycaemic index of foods only began in 1981[3].

Nutritional science is not only a newly established discipline, but also a highly fractionated, contentious field with constantly changing viewpoints on both major and minor issues that impact public health. For example, in 1996 a task force of experts from the American Society for Clinical Nutrition (ASCN) and the American Institute of Nutrition (AIN) came out with an official position paper on trans fatty acids stating:

> *We cannot conclude that the intake of trans fatty acids is a risk factor for coronary heart disease*[4].

Fast forward six short years to 2002 and the National Academy of Sciences, Institute of Medicine's report on trans fatty acids[5] stating:

> *Because there is a positive linear trend between trans fatty acid intake and total and LDL ('bad') cholesterol concentration, and therefore increased risk of cardiovascular heart disease, the Food and Nutrition Board recommends that trans fatty acid consumption be as low as possible while consuming a nutritionally adequate diet.*

These kinds of complete turnabouts and divergence of opinion regarding diet and health are commonplace in the scientific, governmental and medical communities. The official US governmental recommendations for healthy eating are outlined in the 'My Pyramid' program (www.mypyramid.gov/), which recently replaced the 'Food Pyramid' – both of which have been loudly condemned for nutritional shortcomings by scientists from the Harvard School of Public Health[6]. Dietary advice by the American Heart Association (AHA) to reduce the risk of coronary heart disease (CHD) is to limit total fat intake to 30% of total energy, to limit saturated fat to <10% of energy and cholesterol to <300 mg/day while eating at least 2 servings of fish per week[7]. Although similar recommendations are proffered in the United States Department of Agriculture's 'MyPyramid', weekly fish consumption is not recommended because the authors of these guidelines feel there is only 'limited' information regarding the role of omega-3 fatty acids in preventing cardiovascular disease (www.mypyramid.gov/). Surprisingly, the personnel make-up of both scientific advisory boards is almost identical. At least 30 million Americans have followed Dr Atkin's advice to eat more fat and meat to lose weight[8]. In utter contrast, Dean Ornish tells us fat and meat cause cancer, heart disease and obesity, and that we would all be a lot healthier if we were strict vegetarians[9]. Who's right and who's wrong? How in the world can anyone make any sense out of this apparent disarray of conflicting facts, opinions and ideas?

In mature and well-developed scientific disciplines, there are universal paradigms that guide scientists to fruitful endpoints as they design their experiments and hypotheses. For instance, in cosmology (the study of the universe) the guiding paradigm is the 'Big Bang' concept showing that the universe began with an enormous explosion and has been expanding ever since. In geology, the 'Continental Drift' model established that all of the current continents at one time formed a continuous landmass that eventually drifted apart to form the present-day continents. These central concepts are not theories for each discipline, but rather are indisputable facts that serve as orientation points for all other inquiry within each discipline. Scientists do not know everything about the nature of the universe, but it is absolutely unquestionable that it has been and is expanding. This central knowledge then serves as a guiding template which allows scientists to make much more accurate and informed hypotheses about factors yet to be discovered.

The study of human nutrition remains an immature science because it is young and because it lacks a universally acknowledged unifying paradigm[10]. Without an overarching and guiding template, it is not surprising that there is such seeming chaos, disagreement and confusion in the discipline. The renowned Russian geneticist Theodosius Dobzhansky (1900–1975) said, '*Nothing in biology makes sense except in the light of evolution*'[11]. Indeed, much in nutrition does not seem to make sense because most nutritionists have little or no formal training in evolutionary theory, much less human evolution. Nutritionists face the same problem as anyone who is not using an evolutionary model to evaluate biology: fragmented information and no coherent way to interpret the data.

All human nutritional requirements like those of all living organisms are ultimately genetically determined. Most nutritionists are aware of this basic concept; what they have little appreciation for is the process (natural selection) which uniquely shaped our species nutritional requirements. By carefully examining the ancient environment under which our genome arose, it is possible to gain insight into our present-day nutritional requirements and the range of foods and diets to which we are genetically adapted via natural selection[12–16]. In his book Dr Lindeberg shows us how this insight can then be employed as a template to organise and make sense out of experimental and epidemiological studies of human biology and nutrition. Finally, he provides us with the practical knowledge to implement contemporary diets that comply with the fundamental nutritional characteristics that shaped the human genome.

Loren Cordain, PhD
Professor, Colorado State University

References

1. Bogert, L.J., Briggs, G.M., Calloway, D.H. (1973) *Nutrition and physical fitness*, 9th ed. W.B. Sanders Company, Philadelphia, PA.
2. Dyerberg, J., Bang, H.O. (1982) A hypothesis on the development of acute myocardial infarction in Greenlanders. Scand *J Clin Lab Invest Suppl*, **161**, 7–13.
3. Jenkins, D.J., Wolever, T.M., Taylor, R.H., *et al.* (1981) Glycemic index of foods: a physiological basis for carbohydrate exchange. *Am J Clin Nutr* **34**(3), 362–6.
4. No authors listed (1996) Position paper on trans fatty acids. ASCN/AIN Task Force on Trans Fatty Acids. American Society for Clinical Nutrition and American Institute of Nutrition. *Am J Clin Nutr* **63** (5), 663–70.
5. National Academy of Sciences, Institute of Medicine. Letter Report on Dietary Reference Intakes for Trans Fatty Acids, 2002. http://www.iom.edu/ CMS/5410.aspx.
6. Willett, W.C., Stampfer, M.J. (2003) Rebuilding the food pyramid. *Sci Am* **288** (1), 64–71.
7. Krauss, R.M., Eckel, R.H., Howard, B., *et al.* (2000) Dietary guidelines: revision 2000. A statement for healthcare professionals from the Nutrition Committee of the American Heart Association. *Circulation* **102** (18), 2284–99.
8. Blanck, H.M., Gillespie, C., Serdula, M.K., Khan, L.K., Galusk, D.A., Ainsworth, B.E. (2006) Use of low-carbohydrate, high-protein diets among Americans: correlates, duration, and weight loss. *Med Gen Med* **8** (2),5.
9. Ornish, D. (1990) *Dr. Dean Ornish's Program for reversing heart disease: the only system scientifically proven to reverse heart disease without drugs or surgery.* New York, Random House.
10. Nesse, R.M., Stearns, S.C., Omenn, G.S. (2006) Medicine needs evolution. *Science* **311**, 1071.
11. Dobzhansky, T. (1973) Nothing in biology makes sense except in the light of evolution. *Am Biol Teacher* **35**, 125–9.
12. Cordain, L., Eaton, S.B., Sebastian, A., *et al.* (2005) Origins and evolution of the Western diet: health implications for the 21st century. *Am J Clin Nutr* **81** (2), 341–54.
13. Lindeberg, S., Jönsson, T., Granfeldt, Y., *et al.* (2007) A Palaeolithic diet improves glucose tolerance more than a Mediterranean-like diet in individuals with ischaemic heart disease. *Diabetologia* **50** (9),1795–1807.
14. Lindeberg, S., Berntorp, E., Nilsson-Ehle, P., Terént, A., Vessby, B. (1997) Age relations of cardiovascular risk factors in a traditional Melanesian society: the Kitava Study. *Am J Clin Nutr* **66** (4), 845–52.
15. Lindeberg, S., Lundh, B. (1993) Apparent absence of stroke and ischaemic heart disease in a traditional Melanesian island: a clinical study in Kitava. *J Intern Med* **233** (3), 269–75.
16. Lindeberg, S., Cordain, L., Eaton, S.B. (2003) Biological and clinical potential of a Palaeolithic diet. *J Nutr Environ Med* **13** (3), 149–60.

Preface

When I was a young physician, I was not particularly interested in nutrition. I was eager to help my patients with everyday health problems, including avoiding serious diseases in the future. I was an acquiescent member of the medical community. Although my teachers, colleagues and I were aware that diet could have a great impact on common diseases, as briefly stated in the textbooks, we did not think much about it.

Instead, we focused on medications and technical solutions. And when the scientific community discovered a new receptor that seemed to be triggered in some common disease, we all shared the hope for a new drug that would block the receptor. It hardly occurred to us that food components could cause the disease by binding to the same receptor.

I knew, of course, that there was a world of nutrition research. There were even medically trained professors of nutrition. In Sweden, all of them were biochemists with limited clinical experience. They focused on nutrients and calories, later also on dietary fibre. We thought that their focus had little to do with atherosclerotic disease, if we thought of it at all.

At some point I started to wonder. Why did atherosclerosis affect everybody? Why were 'age-related' diseases, such as hypertension, dyslipidaemia and osteoporosis, so common and so difficult to distinguish from normal ageing? At the time, hypertension was defined as the level of blood pressure above which drug treatment was better than placebo for the prevention of cardiovascular disease. Any other criterion was dubious.

Then I stumbled upon Boyd Eaton's paper about foods that were consumed during human evolution, including a brief note on the absence of Western disease among hunter-gatherers (Eaton, S.B., Konner, M. (1985) Paleolithic nutrition – a consideration of its nature and current implications. *N Engl J Med* **312**, 283–9). One of the things I found striking was that meat was part of the ancestral diet, so I mentioned it to my neighbour who was a vegetarian. She objected and claimed that the human gut is designed for plant foods. I went to the library and found that this and many other widespread myths were based on stories with no or little scientific foundation. To my surprise, I later found that most nutritional scientists were reluctant to apply evolutionary theory to nutritious food, thus acting very different from experts in animal nutrition. It gradually dawned on me that John Harvey Kellogg, a vegetarian zealot, had more influence on dietary advice than Charles Darwin had.

Now I was hooked for real. I began to read scientific papers systematically. After a while, I cut grains, dairy, salt and processed food from my own diet, and my blood pressure, weight and blood lipids went from normal to low. I could see no obvious risk with a diet mainly based on meat, fish, root vegetables, vegetables, eggs, fruits and nuts. I informed my patients who were usually interested and often surprised of the results.

I phoned Göran Burenhult, an archaeologist who had also read Eaton's paper and who had visited the traditional horticulturalists of the Trobriand Islands, Papua New Guinea. He convinced me to organise a clinical study there, due to the significant proportion of elderly and their ancestral dietary pattern. This is the Kitava study, mentioned here and there in the text.

And I started writing this textbook. The book is an attempt to provide an overview of the state of research within a very large subject area. It is also a policy statement, a new way of gathering information and conducting research about healthy foods from the perspective of evolutionary medicine. The basic premise is that human internal organs function best with the foods that have been available during human development. On the other hand, we should be more restrictive in terms of recently introduced foods that nature has not given us sufficient means to handle, including plant constituents that are part of the herbivore defence system.

Up to now, there has been no overarching theoretical structure for optimal human nutrition, surprising as it may seem. Instead, various models have built on uncertain epidemiological observations and molecular biology, and the impact of economic interests and belief systems has been substantial. The inability or refusal to apply evolution's basic principles when interpreting dietary studies, 150 years after the publication of Darwin's *The Origin Of Species*, is astounding.

This book is primarily aimed at physicians, nurses, dietitians, biology teachers and health promotion professionals, but it may also be an interesting read for anybody interested in the subject. Certain sections have particular relevance for cardiology, stroke care, diabetic medicine, nephrology, oncology, geriatrics, paediatrics, cell biology, physiology, biology, plant ecology, comparative zoophysiology, zooecology, human ecology, archaeology, osteology and biological anthropology. The book summarises close to 25 years of systematic reading of scientific literature (up to April 2009) in terms of the role of diet in preventing and treating our most common and serious diseases. My approach has been to regularly read the most respected and relevant journals in the fields of nutrition, clinical medicine, epidemiology and molecular biology, and to conduct systematic computer-based literature searches regarding specific issues of particular importance. These searches included natural science articles outside the field of medicine and nutrition. For roughly the first 5 years, I followed professional journals in the field of biological anthropology and archaeology, but in later years I relied on summary articles regarding the composition of food prior to the development of agriculture.

Some of my conclusions may be considered rather radical. However, they are quite reasonable for people who want to understand why our most common diseases are missing in ethnic populations with ancestral-like dietary habits. Almost all Westerners suffer from atherosclerosis from an early age, but most things seem to indicate that this disease is not biologically normal. We have to search for the background causes in our lifestyle in a more thorough way than previously. Quitting smoking, daily walks, extra vegetables and fruits, Mediterranean-like food choices, as well as reducing our consumption of energy-dense foods and salt are one step on the path, but it is evidently not enough.

The book addresses each disease group in an individual chapter, where the current state of research is critically reviewed. Particular emphasis is given, whenever possible, to controlled studies of the effect on clinically significant outcomes, such as death or new event of serious disease. Considerable effort has been put into the arguments for and against the more controversial health statements, for example, that meat is wholesome or whole-grain bread is less healthy than vegetables. The possible risks of a high protein intake and a low intake of calcium are addressed in particular.

Term definitions are provided at the end of the book to help readers without an academic background in medicine. Most readers, regardless of their background, will probably have to look up a few words due to the interdisciplinary nature of the book.

During the many years of writing this book, I have been helped and inspired by many more persons than I can recall. I am immensely grateful to all of them. I am more indebted to my wife, Eva Lindsten, than to any other person. She has been my intellectual and emotional coach and much more. Additionally, the ones I can remember at this moment are John Agabu, Bo Ahrén, Michael Alpers, Joseph Anang, Henrik Andersson, Kjell Asplund, Mette Axelsen, Nigel Balmforth, Thorbjörn Berge, Göran Berglund, Erik Berntorp, Emma Borgstrand, Jennie Brand-Miller, Göran Burenhult, Carl Carlsson, Sigrid Carlsson, Loren Cordain, Susanne Danielsson, Boyd Eaton, Champion and Rosalyn Elliot, David Freed, Johan Frostegård, Yvonne Granfeldt, Bo Gräslund, Leif Göransson, Marie Henschen, Michael Hermanussen, Anders Hernborg, Lena Hulthén, Björn Isaksson, Per-Axel Janzon, Peter Johansson, Horst Jüptner[†], Tommy Jönsson, Hasse Karlsson, Ingrid Karlsson, Sören Kerslow, Anita Laser Reuterswärd, Quiming Liao, Björn Lundh[†], Amar Nalla, Åke Nilsson, Peter Nilsson-Ehle, Stig Norder, Kate Nuttall, Kerin O'Dea, Stefan Olsson, Tommy Olsson, Paddy Osborne, Leif Pierre, Chief Philemon and many other Kitavans, Paramount Chief Pulayasi of Omarakana, Brittmarie Sandström[†], Bengt Scherstén[†], Wulf Schiefenhövel, Peter Sinnett, Sverre Sjölander, Trygve Sjöberg, Kit Sjöström, Jerry Soffman, Stig Steen,

---

[†] Deceased.

Frank Sundler, Andreas Terént, Dag Thelle, Lars-Olof Tobiasson, Stewart Truswell, Martin Ugander, Bengt Vessby, Knut Westlund, Björn Weström, Anders Wirfält, Arvids Zamuelis[†], Bo Zachrisson, Torbjörn Åkerfeldt and Hans Öhlin. Thank you all for your support.

Staffan Lindeberg
Lund, September 2009

1 Introduction

In his theory of evolution, Charles Darwin gave a simple and logical explanation for the diversity and adaptability of species[372,1165]. Everything that used to be a mess of riddles and contradictions suddenly became comprehensible and coherent. The results of Darwin's theory were enormous and have had a dramatic effect on theoretical developments within the field of biology. The theory of evolution has subsequently been applied to an increasing number of disciplines.

Evolution occurs because there are differences in the hereditary characteristics of different individuals within a species, created through mutation and the transfer of genes, and because selection may or may not favour these different traits. The individuals who do best in a certain environment, i.e. produce the most offspring, are those who subsequently outcompete others in that species. The genetic traits of these successful and well-adapted individuals become increasingly common within the species while others gradually disappear. This process is called natural selection. Hence, evolution depends on elimination.

Natural selection benefits those that have more offspring than others. While carnivores become better hunters during evolution, their prey become better at fleeing. Bacteria attack animals that, in turn, develop defence mechanisms, which the bacteria then outsmart, and so forth. Plants develop toxins and other bioactive substances that are harmful to animals that feed off them. Evolution is an eternal, escalating struggle that continues to this day.

1.1 Why do we get sick?

Evolutionary theory has been applied sporadically within the field of medicine since the early twentieth century. The activation of the sympathetic nervous system during stressful periods has long been considered a part of the 'fight-or-flight response', and pain has been seen to encourage healing by forcing that part of the body to relax. Later, the appearance of microorganisms with resistance to antibiotics led to

Table 1.1 Mechanistic and evolutionary causes of diseases or symptoms.

	Mechanistic explanation	Evolutionary explanation
Breakdown of the immune system in AIDS	HIV binds to the CD4 molecule on the surface of helper T cells to invade and gradually destroy them	Attack: spread of HIV fostered at the expense of the host organism
Fever	Pyrogenes stimulate the synthesis of prostaglandin E2	Defence: increased body temperature appears to make cell division difficult in the microorganism
Myopia (nearsightedness)	Abnormal growth of the eye ball mediated by local growth factors	Lack of adaptability to new environment: we have left the life of hunting and gathering
Choking on pieces of meat	Inhalation during swallowing	Design error: airway and gastrointestinal systems are crossed

an understanding of how this resistance develops according to the laws of natural selection. The relative protection against malaria among heterozygous carriers of sickle cell anaemia has been thoroughly discussed. However, only recently has evolutionary thinking emerged as a wide-ranging discipline in medical science in the form of evolutionary medicine[1286,1716,1809].

Evolutionary medicine looks at health and illness from an evolutionary perspective and generally focuses on what is typical rather than what is the exception, more on evolutionary (ultimate) rather than mechanistic (proximate) explanations for disease (Table 1.1).

A proximate explanation for disease is therefore synonymous with pathogenesis, which provides a detailed, often physiological or biochemical, description of the origin of the disease. Evolutionary explanations for diseases or symptoms try to explain who or what benefits from the process and in what way. To the extent that something can be done in terms of environmental factors, this is of great interest.

Roughly speaking, evolutionary explanations for disease can be divided into four categories: attack, defence, lack of adaptation to unfavourable environments and design errors. Attack is thought to benefit the attacker, while defence benefits the person attacked. The methods can vary from the bite and scratch of an animal or the invasion of microorganisms to the pricks and poisons of plants. For hundreds of millions of years, in an escalating struggle for survival, both attack and defence have been strategies in the evolutionary history of the animals. This process is still going on, and no animal can be said with certainty to be the 'winner' in the game of survival of the fittest.

Humans with a tendency for anxiety may potentially create a more secure environment for their offspring than those who are clueless or foolhardy[1286]. It has been suggested that fever also has an evolutionary purpose by impeding the growth of bacteria[925].

However, diabetes can hardly be said to have a purpose, and therefore, it lands in the category of lack of adaptation. The fact that this lifestyle disease has affected an increasing percentage of the earth's population in the last few decades shows that genetics is not the only cause, since the timescale of genetic change is very much slower. In general, heredity has a great impact on individual resistance to a Western lifestyle but is rarely the sole explanation. These ideas are explained further in Section 4.6.

An even clearer example of a lack of adaptability to new eating habits is the loss of lactase activity during childhood, which leads to an inability to digest lactose in the adult. Such a loss is the rule in most ethnic groups, like in other animals. During human evolution, when cow's milk was not part of the diet, there was no advantage in maintaining lactase activity after childhood. On the contrary, natural selection benefited those groups that did not spend resources on an enzymatic activity that would not be used – in this case, that of lactase.

A design error can often be seen as the best design of the given alternatives, in contrast to the best theoretically imaginable design. The problem with choking on pieces of meat could have been avoided by separating the respiratory tract from the digestive apparatus. But we all descend from an ancestor with crossed systems[557] and now it is too late. Evolution cannot go backwards, and any species that might by chance develop the rudiments of a better system would, for other reasons, have been outcompeted.

Certain hereditary diseases can be seen as the result of design errors, but often one or more environmental factors are required for a disease to appear. Heredity therefore does not preclude environmental influence.

Past scientific discussion can sometimes give one the impression that the diseases of the Western world are caused by design flaws that can only be corrected with the help of pharmaceuticals or other medical procedures. I consider this book an argument for the case that this is a misunderstanding.

1.2   We are changing at pace with the continental drift

During the unbelievably slow process we call 'evolution', changes through natural selection have led to the appearance of our own species[1165]. These changes occur sometimes in great strides and sometimes more gradually in many small steps. Often there is no change in a certain trait across millions of years, when natural selection favours stability, say for the metabolism of glucose. Microevolution involves a slow process of adaptation within the species and the development of new species, which are relatively similar to the original. However, macroevolution involves the appearance of radically new strains and thereby new groups at a higher level than their relatives.

One way of clarifying how much time has passed from the first vertebrates to live on land until the appearance of humans is displayed in the 'evolutionary calendar' in Table 1.2. For the sake of simplicity, we will assume that the first vertebrate life forms to walk on land lived 365 million years ago, and then we can allow 1 day in the calendar to represent 1 million years in reality.

Table 1.2   The last 365 million years converted to a calendar year.

Time	Event
January 1	Amphibian ancestor
March 5	Reptile ancestor
June 10	Early mammal
July 20	'America' starts to separate from 'Europe' and 'Africa'
October 28	Primate ancestor
Christmas Eve	Bipedal ancestor (hominid)
New Years Eve	
19:30:00	*Homo sapiens* (modern humans)
21:30:00	Some of us leave Africa
22:45:00	Some go to New Guinea
23:00:00	Some of us go to Europe
23:40:00	And even to Scandinavia
23:45:00	Agriculture starts in Middle East
23:52:00	Agriculture starts in Scandinavia
23:53:00	The Ice Man dies in the Alps
23:59:00	The Black Death (the European pandemic of plague)
23:59:50	Cardiovascular disease

Note: 1 day = 1 million years, 1 hour = 41,700 years, 1 minute = 694 years.

The changes that occurred since one of our ancestors left the fish stage more than 400 million years ago primarily concerned size and form, temperature regulation and the methods for reproduction and obtaining food. We have stopped laying eggs, we have lost our tail and we no longer carry fur. We use tools to obtain food and obviously look different from our mammalian relatives.

But despite the enormous amount of time that has passed since our first amphibian ancestor crawled up onto land, there are still more similarities than differences between the current descendants in the chain of development. The cells of different mammals are essentially built up by the same protein-based information systems, regulated by the same DNA-based genetic language. Food is chewed and broken down in very similar ways by various types of animals. The few exceptions include the fact that mammals can move their lower jawbone sideways in relation to their upper jawbone, and that ruminants have bacteria in their digestive tract that can break down cellulose and 'disarm' some plant defences. Curiously, few changes in our ancestors' long history have occurred in terms of how our food is processed once it has been absorbed by the organism. Consequently, the metabolism between different mammals that are used in research is very similar to each other, despite the fact that their common ancestors may have lived 100 million years ago. It is thanks to this close similarity that we can perform experiments on animals to understand human biochemistry. We have obtained most of our knowledge of our own biochemistry from studies on rats and other types of animals.

For millions of years, species have been fine-tuning how they use the available food substances in the most beneficial manner possible. Notice the word 'available'; this process has not been able to change our bodies to handle food that did not appear during evolution, e.g. salted food or cheese sandwiches.

However, adapting to available food has not been problem-free. Most plants protect themselves from being eaten by mammals, insects and fungi by synthesising toxins and a host of antinutritional bioactive substances[721]. These include plant lectins, alkylresorcinols, protease inhibitors, tannins and polyphenols. Evolution has forced plant-eating animals (herbivores) to develop sophisticated defence systems, including variation of plants eaten in order to minimise the dose of each individual substance. Animal species that support themselves exclusively on one particular plant have been forced to develop defence mechanisms to minimise the damaging effects of its phytochemicals. One example is the ability of some herbivores to consume large quantities of cyanide-forming (cyanogenic) plants[596].

From this perspective, the term 'natural' somehow gets a new meaning. Naturally occurring substances in the plant kingdom are not necessarily as benign or as useful as we often imagine. Somewhat drastically, you could say that it is completely natural to die of mushroom poisoning, that this is part of the mushroom's natural strategy to make short work of its enemies. Today, it is natural to die of a myocardial infarction (heart attack), which is a natural consequence of the Western lifestyle. In the light of this, herbal medicines are given credit that is not truly justified. The fact that these medications have their origin in the plant world does not mean that they are safer than drugs that are manufactured synthetically.

Our primate ancestors have been consuming fruit, vegetables, nuts and insects for 50 million years or more. Meat was successively added, with a probable increase around 2 million years ago. Underground storage organs (roots, tubers, bulbs, corms) possibly become staple foods 1–2 million years ago (see Section 3.1)[1971]. The variability was large; single plant foods were rarely available in excess. Modern staple foods such as grains, milk, refined fats and sugar, and salt were not available, but are now providing the bulk of calories in most countries.

1.3   Are we adapted for milk and bread?

If milk and bread are capable of causing illnesses that would have reduced fitness in early agriculturalists, would not have Europeans been able to adapt to these items over the past 10 000 years? If that were the case, it would have been a result of the gradual elimination of people who suffered from early death or low fertility caused by such foods, and we, who are the descendants of the survivors, would accordingly be created differently. This is a multifaceted question[831]. First, it depends on which adaptations you look at. Genetic adaptation to a deadly threat in childhood, in certain cases, can apparently occur in less than 50 generations (which may correspond to less than 1200 years), starting at the time when 1% of the population carry the protective trait and ending at the time when the large majority, say more than 90%, are carriers. However, the necessary time from complete absence of the trait to its first appearance in an individual carrier may be very long, and is actually mathematically impossible to calculate. In addition, it may take several thousand generations for the prevalence to increase from 0 to 1%.

The timescale of genetic adaptation can be illustrated by the observed change in colour of the peppered moth (a winged insect) in the area of Manchester during the 1800s. In the 1700s, almost all of these moths were speckled grey and were therefore perfectly camouflaged against the lichen covering English birch trees. By chance, however, a small founder population of moths were black and therefore easier to be spotted by birds. This could have caused their elimination if an unexpected saviour had not appeared, namely industrialism. The soot from Manchester's smoke stacks blackened the area's birch trees so severely that suddenly it was the grey speckled individuals that were at the greatest risk of being eaten by the birds. Just 50 generations later – after 50 years in their case – the result was that almost all peppered moths in the area were black. This process of natural selection went unusually fast, but the danger was also very significant in the first day of life for those that had the wrong colour.

Now assume in our case that people in a downright barren Europe 10 000 years ago were forced to drink milk to survive the harsh winters after the hoofed mammals had been hunted down to near extinction by humans. Lactose intolerance, the hitherto normal condition for adult humans (and animals), would then be a serious threat to survival; i.e. the inability to thrive on milk would exert a strong negative selection pressure. Assuming also the presence of a large enough founder population, after a few hundred generations it is highly possible that most lactose intolerant families had been eliminated, which also seems to have been the case among the Scandinavian people[239].

Assume further that milk caused atherosclerosis (see Section 4.2), stroke and myocardial infarctions in most people in their 50s, apart from some individuals who were genetically resistant and did not develop these conditions before the age of 80. If such a resistance-promoting gene would be passed on to their children, how quickly can it spread in the population; i.e. how big of an advantage do these resistant relatives have despite drinking milk? Do they have more children? Barely, if a heart attack at age 50 years or later is the sole result. Do the children fare better? Perhaps, but the difference is marginal. When a mother is 50 years old, the children often deal quite well without her help. Other populations, by and large, can just as easily propagate their offspring, and the roughly 10 000 years since the dawn of agriculture is very unlikely enough time for the majority of Europe's population to belong to this resistant group. However, grandmothers could have had a certain amount of significance during evolution (which would explain the long time a woman can live after menopause). Adult children's independence of their elder parents became most apparent in civilised society, where competence and knowledge could be spread to a larger number of people than in hunter-gatherer societies.

However, a few thousand years may be enough if fertility is strongly and negatively affected. The relation between Western dietary habits and insulin resistance (a precursor to type 2 diabetes and hypothetically a partial cause of cardiovascular disease), as well as reduced fertility, is therefore an important issue that will be addressed in Section 4.6 on insulin resistance. In that section, the relatively low prevalence of type 2 diabetes in people of European descent, as compared to most other ethnic groups, will also be discussed.

While cow's milk is relatively easy to dismiss as optimal human food from the perspective of genetic adaptation, seeds (including beans) are slightly more complicated. Grass seeds from the Poaceae family, which includes wheat, rye, barley, oat, rice and maize, have not been staple foods before the advent of agriculture. In contrast, fatty seeds from various African plant species probably have been part of our ancestors' diets for millions of years. We know that seeds have high concentrations of phytochemicals[721]. Hence, if African fatty seeds were regularly consumed during human evolution there may have been some adaptation to these particular species, whereas grass seeds are just as recent as milk in the human diet. In addition, a narrow range of seeds are now consumed every day as staple foods, a very recent phenomenon in evolutionary terms.

The question of root vegetables is even more complex. As outlined in Section 3.1, humans may be highly adapted to a high intake of root vegetables. Such an adaptation would mainly pertain to the particular phytochemicals that are present in African roots, including those found in some species of *Dioscorea* or *Ipomoea*. However, the potato, which originates from South America, may contain bioactive substances that are too foreign for us to cope with. For example, the potato lectin (Solanum tuberosum agglutinin or Solanum tuberosum lectin) activates tyrosine kinase receptors not necessarily affected by lectins from more distantly related plant tubers[558]. Considering the amounts of potato consumed in Western countries, a higher degree of adaptation would have been preferable.

2 Expanding our perspective

2.1 The perspective of academic medicine

Prevention is an important part of today's health care work in order to delay, prevent or detect the onset or recurrence of any of the widespread public illnesses in modern society. The potential benefits for public health are great[1082]. Today's diseases, primarily cardiovascular diseases, cancer, osteoporosis and some autoimmune diseases, are the most common causes of disability and premature death in Europe (see Tables 2.1–2.3). Each year, more than 10% of the population over 65 years of age is treated in hospitals for cardiovascular diseases, which are also the most common causes of death. One out of five Europeans dies from cancer, which is the second most common cause of death. Every second Swedish woman will break one or several bones due to osteoporosis[871], and the estimated worldwide incidence (occurrence) of osteoporotic fractures was 9 million in the year 2000[836]. Each of the autoimmune diseases is relatively uncommon, but as a group, they make up a large portion of the diseases in the Western world. One of the most common autoimmune diseases is rheumatoid arthritis

The largest group of preventable diseases is cardiovascular disease: ischaemic heart disease (myocardial infarction, sudden cardiac death and angina pectoris), heart failure, stroke and certain forms of dementia. Prior to becoming ill, often for several years, a large percentage of the patients show warning signals such as increased waist circumference, hypertension (high blood pressure), diabetes or high serum cholesterol. Watching for these warning signals during individual meetings between patient and doctor, regardless of the reason for the visit, is an increasingly high priority in European health care.

Along with the increased awareness of the need for preventive measures, scientific methods have been increasingly applied within the field of academic medicine, especially in the form of randomised controlled trials (comparative studies with two or more randomly selected groups where one receives a control treatment).

Table 2.1   The ten leading causes of death worldwide, 2001[1083].

	Deaths (millions)	Percentage of total deaths
Low- and middle-income countries		
Ischaemic heart disease	5.7	11.8
Cerebrovascular disease	4.6	9.5
Lower respiratory infections	3.4	7.0
HIV/AIDS	2.6	5.3
Perinatal conditions	2.5	5.1
Chronic obstructive pulmonary disease	2.4	4.9
Diarrhoeal disease	1.8	3.7
Tuberculosis	1.6	3.3
Malaria	1.2	2.5
Road traffic accidents	1.1	2.2
High-income countries		
Ischaemic heart disease	1.4	17.3
Cerebrovascular disease	0.8	9.9
Trachea, bronchus, lung cancers	0.5	5.8
Lower respiratory infections	0.3	4.4
Chronic obstructive pulmonary disease	0.3	3.8
Colorectal cancers	0.3	3.3
Alzheimer's disease and other dementias	0.2	2.6
Diabetes mellitus	0.2	2.6
Breast cancer	0.2	2.0
Stomach cancer	0.2	1.9

Table 2.2   Two different ways to indicate cause of death in Sweden in 1998[4].

	Percentage of deaths in total	Percentage of deaths under 65 years of age
Cardiovascular disease		
Men	47	30
Women	49	17
Tumours		
Men	25	28
Women	22	52
Injuries		
Women	6	20
Women	3	12
Other		
Men	22	21
Women	26	19

Note: Of the total number of deaths, 17.3% occurred among men and 10.3% among women under the age of 65 years.

Table 2.3   The ten diseases/injuries (in order of priority) that contribute to the most DALYs (disability adjusted life years) in Sweden in 1998[4]

Men	Percentage of DALYs	Women	Percentage of DALYs
Ischaemic heart disease	19.2	Ischaemic heart disease	13.7
Depression and neurosis	6.6	Depression and neurosis	10.9
Stroke	5.8	Stroke	6.9
Alcoholism	4.5	Dementia	6.3
Self-inflicted injuries	4.2	Breast cancer	3.1
Dementia	3.1	Chronic obstructive pulmonary disease	2.8
Chronic obstructive pulmonary disease	2.8	Psychosis (schizophrenia excluded)	2.6
Lung cancer	2.7	Back and neck illnesses	2.3
Traffic accidents	2.3	Respiratory infections	2.1
Psychosis (schizophrenia excluded)	2.3	Gynaecological cancer	2.0

Note: A DALY is a year of healthy living that is lost due to illness or death.

These studies are then evaluated in terms of important clinical events such as death or serious illness, and not only in terms of changed risk factor levels[1551]. Many experts believe that epidemiological and molecular biological studies do not provide a sufficient basis for lifestyle recommendations or drug treatment of obesity and high blood sugar.

This new approach, which is called evidence-based medicine, is revealing a number of gaps in treatment and a strong need for more effective prevention. Preventive pharmaceutical treatments for established heart diseases (secondary prevention), e.g. using statins or acetylsalicylic acid (aspirin) after a myocardial infarction, or beta-blockers and angiotensin-converting enzyme inhibitors in the event of heart failure, have displayed an unequivocal effect, with a 15–30% reduction or more in the risk for serious diseases in the future. However, when it comes to primary prevention (prevention before the real disease appears), the effect of medication is not always as obvious. In the case of moderate hypertension in middle age, blood pressure medication only appears to be warranted in the case of a markedly increased risk for cardiovascular disease[597,1948]. In the case of drug-resistant hypertension, further treatment with additional antihypertensive drugs has no proven extra benefit, beyond what is achieved with one single drug[665], and the widespread belief in such a benefit is based on observational studies, not randomised controlled trials[251]. Pharmacological blood sugar regulation in type 2 diabetes apparently has no or little effect on complications associated with atherosclerosis, such as myocardial infarction, stroke and heart failure[442,582,749,1394], despite strong relationships in observational studies[1620,1734].

When health care professionals receive their initial training and continued education regarding prevention, priority is traditionally given to the use of pharmaceuticals, while relatively little room is allotted to the strong scientific support that

---

Case report: a rather typical case of sudden death.

David was about to turn 65 years old. He had been looking forward to a quiet retirement together with his wife. He was somewhat careful about his health, never smoked, walked the dog almost every day, and drank the way most people do – a glass of wine with dinner, once or twice a week.

The week before he turned 65, he went in for his last annual check-up at the health centre. Over the course of the year, his blood pressure was around 140/85; for a short period 10 years earlier, it had temporarily risen to 150/95. All of the tests were normal and the ECG did not show any signs of illness. Nobody at the health centre had reason to comment on his somewhat round belly (he weighed 15 kg more than he did in his adolescence).

The 65-year-old appeared to be lucky at his celebration party. David was in good shape and danced for half the night. Therefore, there was a lot of shock and confusion when he suddenly died 3 weeks later during a walk through the woods. The autopsy showed serious atherosclerosis in several coronary arteries of the heart and a blood clot adjacent to a ruptured plaque. The probable cause of death was cardiac arrest due to myocardial infarction. Advanced atherosclerosis was noted in a number of blood vessels in the internal organs.

A few of his friends thought that it was nice for David to die so suddenly in such vigour, but his wife was deeply depressed for a long time. His eldest son has become very eager to find out the truth about Western disease.

---

currently exists, highlighting the importance of a person's lifestyle for the development of atherosclerosis, diabetes, obesity, hypertension, dyslipidaemia (e.g. high cholesterol) and several forms of cancer.

2.2   The concept of normality

The term 'normal' is frequently used in discussions between doctors and patients, e.g. in statements like 'blood pressure is normal'. This means that blood pressure is on an average or low level for that population, and that it is not so high that drug treatment is required. The truth, however, is more complicated. Since the risk of cardiovascular disease increases continuously with rising blood pressure, it is safer to have low than average blood pressure, but not very much, and even those Westerners with low blood pressure are at significant risk (see Section 4.7).

Hence, a clearer answer would be: 'Your blood pressure is normal, which means you are at a normal level of risk for heart attack and stroke.' Normal risk then means the average risk of the population (Figure 2.1). Furthermore, increasing evidence favours the notion that most healthy elderly Westerners could benefit from medication for blood pressure and serum cholesterol[382].

It is not unusual to view typical Western ageing as synonymous with normal ageing. The fact that body weight and blood pressure increase with age may then by some authorities even be regarded as part of normal biology, while traditional populations who do not show these same signs of ageing are seen as unexplainable

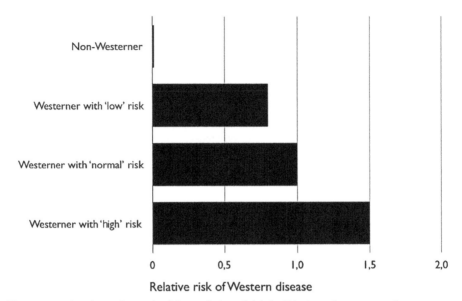

Figure 2.1   A schematic graph of the variation of risk for Western diseases, such as cardiovascular disease, depending on risk factor levels, such as serum cholesterol. A Westerner at average risk has been set as the reference. 'Low'-risk Westerners have a markedly higher risk than non-Westerners.

exceptions that tend to get forgotten in the discussion[1043]. In migrant studies, a couple of years after transition to an urbanised lifestyle, virtually everyone has higher blood pressure and blood sugar than non-migrants of the same ethnic origin[350,1437]. The fact that virtually all Westerners will develop pronounced atherosclerosis in the coronary arteries of the heart with age, while other free-living mammals apparently go free of this problem (see Section 4.3) is not often discussed today.

The late Geoffrey Rose, a highly respected epidemiologist, talked about healthy and sick populations[1532]. If a person belongs to a sick population, they are at risk for myocardial infarction even if they have a blood pressure that is normal for this population. This reasoning is often overlooked when the focus is only on how the disease and risk factors correlate *within* the individual population. Even trained scientists fall into the trap of using the 'low-risk' group as a true reference group.

If the majority of people with a modern lifestyle need treatment for their 'normal' cardiovascular risk factors, then we truly have a problem. I can only see one radical solution: to search for the biologically normal.

2.3   Genetics

It is important to comment on a common misunderstanding of the role of genetics. A genetic predisposition for an illness typically does not mean that the disease is independent of a person's lifestyle. One example is lactose intolerance: If you do not drink milk, you do not develop diarrhoea, even if you carry this hereditary 'defect'. Correspondingly, coeliac disease (intestinal disease of gluten intolerance) develops among those people with a hereditary predisposition if, and only if, they eat grains containing gluten.

Most widespread Western diseases seem to have a significant hereditary component. For type 2 diabetes and cardiovascular diseases, we do inherit a certain amount of resistance, which means that two people with the exact same lifestyle are at varyingly high degrees of becoming ill. But all evidence suggests that if both these people had lived as hunter-gatherers, neither of them would have been affected, as outlined in this book. Furthermore, if people with a predisposition for type 2 diabetes would revert to an original hunter-gatherer lifestyle, they would actually be expected to do better than other people because of a better capacity to reproduce on a meat-based diet. Their inborn insulin resistance seems to minimise the risk for low blood sugar after an extremely high meat intake (see Section 4.6).

It is also of interest to distinguish between genetics at the individual/familial level and genetically determined ethnic characteristics. In both cases, if you have the 'wrong' parents, you have to be more careful than other people about your lifestyle. But there is some comfort for you; if you use preventive measures, you can reduce your risk to a point below that of people without a genetic predisposition (if those other persons continue to live an unhealthy lifestyle).

Hence, it is not contradictory that most modern diseases are genetically conditioned, and, at the same time, that they depend on a person's lifestyle (to manifest themselves). It involves heredity *and* environment – not either/or. Or, in the words of Geoffrey Rose, the answer to 'Why does this particular individual in this population get this disease?' is not necessarily the same as the answer to 'Why does this population have so much disease?'[1532]. The new science of nutrigenomics usually deals with the first question[341]. This book mainly explores the second, and also a third one: why are most modern humans afflicted with Western disease?

2.4 Dietary guidelines

Nutritional recommendations formulated by national or international bodies are designed to provide information for planning a diet, which at the group level, will ensure people's primary physiological needs for growth and function (the nutritional goal), and provide the basis for general good health (the public health goal). Roughly stated, the nutritional goal is the prevention of symptoms of acute deficiencies (scurvy, pellagra, etc.), while the public health goal is largely to prevent diet-related diseases (cardiovascular diseases, cancer, osteoporosis, etc.).

In terms of the intake of protein, minerals and vitamins, the recommendations are based on the estimated minimum requirements plus a margin of safety (often two standard deviations above the average for the population) in order to cover both individual variations and an increased need during stress. Based on this, the risk for deficiency symptoms is considered to be low among most individuals whose intake is just under the recommendations.

For many nutrients, the estimated minimum requirement is not fully known, and the recommended intake is based largely on data about the population's intake when obvious deficiency symptoms are absent. The recommended energy intake is based on the current intake among healthy subjects. For fibre, sodium and alcohol, as well as protein, fat and carbohydrates, the recommendations are based on an 'overall assessment' of current knowledge of food's importance for health.

While knowledge of the minimum requirements to avoid deficiency symptoms may be considered good, there is significant uncertainty in terms of what the optimal nutritional intake for preventing widespread Western diseases should be. The key reason for this is that estimation methods that are available have serious limitations.

Problems and limitations in nutritional research

Problems with epidemiology

Epidemiological (observational) research investigates the distribution of diseases in relation to lifestyle and other characteristics. One type of epidemiological study is the ecological study, which typically compares nations or regions at one particular time, while prospective cohort studies (or cohort studies for short) assess a large group (cohort) of people who are followed over a period of time. In case–control studies, individuals already diagnosed with a disease ('cases') are compared with healthy individuals ('controls').

The biggest problem with epidemiological studies consists of 'confounders' or confounding factors, i.e. when the suspected dietary factor being examined is associated with one or multiple other factors that are not being taken into considerations, or that cannot be fully adjusted for residual confounding[45,1000]. For example, assume that a group of people are asked how much wine they drink, and then they are monitored for a number of years with respect to developing disease. If there is a negative relation between wine consumption and mortality due to myocardial infarction, it could be assumed that this is due to a protective factor in the wine, or that drinking wine correlates with some other factors that are the real reasons for the relationship. One of several such confounding factors, particularly in ecological studies within Europe, might be milk: The more wine, the less milk[1248,1614].

Antioxidant vitamins and cardiovascular health constitute another example of confounding. Despite strong and consistent evidence from observational studies, no benefit has been seen in randomised controlled trials[467,1175].

If the findings from one study are repeated in subsequent studies, this may be due to the fact that the same confounders tend to reoccur simply because many modern populations have similar conceptions. One population's opinion of the health benefits of a particular food or supplement is naturally often shared by other populations. Each new study that finds a connection, and which is broadcast by the media, may actually reinforce the source of the error.

Likewise, the failure of medication that lowers blood sugar to prevent cardiovascular disease in diabetes[442,582,749,1394], despite a decreased risk with lower blood sugar in observational studies[1620,1734], clearly shows the tenuous basis of epidemiology.

Studies that are based on food questionnaires contain another source of errors due to a lack of reliability, in terms of the answers to questions about eating habits and the inferences that can be drawn from them. For example, if the reported colour of the usually consumed bread (brown or white) is used to estimate glycaemic index, as in the influential Nurses' Health Study (http://www.channing.harvard.edu/nhs/), there is a risk of overestimating the role of this dietary factor, since glycaemic index is barely associated with the colour of bread[88]. Furthermore, the consumption of unhealthy food is often underestimated. Another difficulty is that the variation of dietary habits in the population being studied may be too small to allow for demonstration of a possible relationship with health. Salt consumption among a particular ethnic group may not show much variation, and the majority has an intake that is much higher than what was practically feasible during evolution. This problem can be compared to studying the importance of smoking for myocardial infarction without having access to non-smokers. (In the case of smoking, often no relation is apparent in epidemiological studies.)

Underreporting is a very significant problem in observational studies based on self-reported food intake. It has been suggested that as much as 25% of the energy consumed is not reported[1497], although the underlying assumption that basic caloric needs are independent of food choice has not been proven.

Often a large number of people are missed, i.e. many of those who were asked to participate in the study refused to do so. Sometimes these people are considerably different from the participants in important respects. Furthermore, in many studies accuracy is low because the incidence of disease or death (i.e. the clinical endpoints) in each group is limited. Therefore, it is appropriate not only to consider the relative risks between the groups, but also the confidence intervals of the differences, i.e. the interval, within a certain range of probability, where the true difference is located. Normally, a confidence interval of 95% is indicated. If a study shows a relative risk of myocardial infarction among smokers (compared with non-smokers) of 1.4 with a 95% confidence interval of 1.05–2.6, this means that there is a 95% probability that the actual relative risk lies between 1.05 and 2.6. (A relative risk of 1.0 would mean that there is no increased risk compared to non-smokers.)

In epidemiological studies of the incidence of disease in relation to a variable, such as consumption of a food, consideration should be given to the size of R^2 (the determination coefficient, which is the correlation coefficient squared). If $R^2 = 0.23$, then 23% of the variation in the incidence of disease is explained by the variation of the variable being examined. If R^2 is less than 0.10, more than 90% is explained by something else, a fact that is often not mentioned by the researchers.

In ecological studies comparing several different countries, where the number of people who become ill or die from a certain disease is recorded over a longer period of time, there is a risk that the diagnostic criteria will vary between some of the countries. If a cause of death is found to be unusual in a certain country, this can be due to under-diagnosis rather than a truly low incidence. This problem is particularly significant for studies of long-term time trends.

The uncertainty in epidemiological studies is so great that the results should be interpreted with considerably greater caution than what is normally the case[1169] (Box 2.1).

Box 2.1   The basis of our opinion on diets.

Science

Epidemiology
Physiology, molecular biology
Randomised controlled trials (RCTs)
Evolutionary biology

Other influences

Belief systems
Alliances, group dynamics, funding etc.

Problems with molecular biology

The methodological limitations of molecular biology and physiological studies are to some extent quite different from those described above. The number of substances involved is unimaginably large, and new substances are constantly being discovered. A vast number of yet undiscovered molecules are expected to have a large impact on human physiology. Mechanistic models in textbooks are strongly oversimplified and thereby potentially misleading. Most laboratory experiments are performed on laboratory animals, which increases the uncertainty.

For a long time, beta-blocking antihypertensive drugs were considered to be dangerous in patients with heart failure, on the basis of the prevailing mechanistic models, but today we know that they actually prolong life in such patients. Lidocaine infusions were thought to improve survival in patients with multiple ventricular extrasystoles during myocardial infarction, but today we know that this type of treatment worsens survival.

Hypotheses regarding lifestyle are even more uncertain since they cannot be tested in double-blind studies, where no one knows who changed what until after the study. A myriad of intricate networks with thousands of enzymes, coenzymes, receptors and transcription factors, many of which have yet to be discovered, are included in those parts of the metabolic system (the construction, utilisation and breakdown of substances) that are thought to affect the development of cardiovascular disease. Once food is broken down and absorbed, its later metabolic fate is largely unknown, which is why its role in chronic disease is highly uncertain. Therefore, it is impossible to draw firm conclusions regarding causal relationships based on knowledge of metabolic processes, especially when it comes to the long-term effects of diet. Moreover, the concept of 'biological plausibility', one of Bradford Hill's criteria of causation (as opposed to confounding), is rarely applied to associations in nutritional epidemiology.

Problems with intervention studies

The ideal situation would be to conduct a randomised controlled trial where the intervention consisted of a group of people who altered their diet in a predetermined way, but not in any other way. The problem is that the test subjects (the intervention group) often simultaneously improve their lifestyle in other respects. It is also well known that subjects in the control group, more or less consciously, alter their lifestyle in accordance with what they know or believe are the goals of the study, or simply because they become inspired to improve their health, or because they are worried about the lifestyle they were allocated to follow. Unlike drugs, most lifestyle changes cannot be studied in a double-blind manner. It is also theoretically impossible to adjust the intake of energy-supplying food without changing the consumption of other energy-supplying nutrients or the total energy consumption at the same time. It can later get difficult to determine the cause of the effects that were found – or not found.

If the scientists succeed to perform the perfect trial, they may still have the problem of limited external validity, i.e. an uncertainty of how the results should be applied in the general population, as opposed to the particular people studied and the settings and procedures of the study.

Large-scale dietary intervention studies on a societal basis are even more difficult to interpret. If you achieve the desired effect, it is usually very hard to say exactly what it was due to or if lifestyle had any impact at all.

In animal experiments, the fact that the control group may have been fed a type of food that the animal in question is not genetically adapted for is often forgotten. This creates the risk of ignoring adverse effects of the supposedly neutral control diet. One example is casein (from cow's milk), which apparently is highly bioactive despite its widespread use as a 'neutral' protein in animal feeding experiments.

Publication bias

Another potential source of errors can arise if studies with positive effects are published to a greater extent than those with absent or negative effects, making the intervention in question appear unduly positive (publication bias). The primary reason seems to be negligence to write and submit manuscripts, rather than an unwillingness by journal editors to publish them[1352]. This is often discussed in terms of medications, but less often in terms of lifestyle. One study analysed financial sponsorship, or lack thereof, with regard to research articles on the health effects of soft drinks, juice and milk in order to determine how sponsorship affects published conclusions[1019]. A total of 206 articles were included in the study, of which 111 declared financial sponsorship. Of these, 22% had all industry funding, 47% had no industry funding, and 32% had mixed funding. Funding source was significantly related to conclusions when considering all article types ($P = 0.037$). For interventional studies, the proportion with unfavourable conclusions was 0% for all industry funding versus 37% for no industry funding ($P = 0.009$). Thus,

100% of industry-sponsored studies came to the conclusion that the beverage under investigation was beneficial or not adverse to health.

The risk of publication bias is probably highest for short-term studies with a small number of test subjects and lowest for long-term studies with clinically important events such as death or serious disease, since the latter studies are more often known within the scientific community before they are completed. Requirements for mandatory registration in connection with the application to an ethics committee have been suggested in order to minimise this problem. Currently, the largest such database of clinical trials is the web-based ClinicalTrials.gov.

In terms of controlled trials, publication bias is sometimes uncovered through meta-analysis (compiling all the studies) using a so-called funnel plot, a graph where each study's odds ratio (an estimate of relative risk in case–control studies), such as measurements of the intervention's effect, are set in relation to the number of clinical endpoints[475,1723]. Studies with few endpoints may randomly appear relatively far from the true odds ratio, while larger trials are clustered around the true ratio. In the case of publication bias, an asymmetric funnel plot is achieved. In dietary intervention studies, the number of clinical endpoints, unfortunately, is often so small that the studies are at the bottom of the pyramid, so to speak, where this method is of little help.

The first really large controlled study of intravenous magnesium treatment in acute myocardial infarction was published in 1995, and to the surprise of many experts, there was no effect on survival[803]. Previously, several smaller intervention studies were published, the majority of which showed a markedly reduced mortality. Funnel plots published later suggest the presence of publication bias[475].

Citation bias

Very few readers of scientific papers have the time required to follow all the published studies in a certain area. It is therefore problematic that, in some cases, studies lending support to commonly held notions are cited more often than contradictory studies. It seems obvious that reviews without strict criteria for inclusion of studies more often conclude that a certain relation exists or a certain treatment is beneficial, as compared to high quality reviews based on systematic screening of every available study irrespective of where (or even if) they were published.

The apparent overestimation of omega-3 fatty acids in the prevention of ischaemic heart disease may to some extent be due to citation bias[756] and the same could possibly be true for the health benefits of a low intake of saturated fat[755,1475]. Another example is genistein, a hormone from soya, whose proposed benefit in my experience is claimed more often in nutritional science (in journals and at conferences) than among experts of plant ecology or toxicology. A third example may be the uncertain effect of dairy products in fracture prevention[981,1921,1957].

Dietary intervention studies often get less attention than pharmacological studies. A striking example was the Lyon Diet Heart study that demonstrated reduced total mortality through dietary change after myocardial infarction[386,388]. Despite the fact that the results were published in one of the top ranked medical journals, *The*

Lancet, it did not, for the first years, achieve by far the same breakthrough as drug studies of similar clinical importance. Drug trials of similar importance generally spread within hours across the medical community.

Preconceived ideas

The impact of financial interest is difficult to assess. Deliberately withholding facts is hopefully uncommon, but subconscious preconceived opinions can likely be reinforced by the employer's wishes. The researchers' interpretations of their own randomised studies are thought to be influenced by how these are financed, a problem which is well acknowledged in the pharmaceutical science[919]. It has become common to declare any potential connections to the pharmaceutical industry (financed projects, etc.), and the same requirements are reasonably placed on authorities involved in nutritional research. One obvious problem that can be highlighted is camaraderie: Repeated social interactions with food industry representatives, even if there are no strict financial ties, can cause an expert to possibly develop a more positive attitude to certain food products than if such relations were avoided. It should be noted that the opposite could also occur – that the industry can become less biased than the so-called independent experts.

Some concepts are less prone to find sponsors than others. For obvious reasons, much more money is invested in technologically advanced production of functional foods than in old-fashioned foods of basic origin. There is a risk that research on profitable foodstuffs that have only marginal health effects is overemphasised at the expense of studies on the effects of unprocessed meat, fish, fruits and vegetables, for example. The fact that the fibre hypothesis has been backed by the cereal industry since it was launched by nutritional scientists around 1970 is undeniable, and it is possible that this has had an impact on nutritional recommendations to some extent. The scientific support for health effects of cereal fibre, in particular wheat fibre, is remarkably weak, except in epidemiological studies (see Sections 4.1, 4.8 and 4.11). In addition, the sources for fibre in the often cited East African populations did not consist of wheat, but rather of vegetable, corn and millet, which may be very significant[827]. A partial explanation of the enthusiastic acceptance of the fibre hypothesis may have been a long tradition to regard constipation as the prime disease of civilisation[1935].

An important source of inspiration for researchers themselves is the hope that their own hypotheses will be confirmed. It has long been known that this hope can affect the interpretation of study results, and early philosophers like Descartes and Bacon embraced doubt and critical examination. For the same reason, the philosopher of science Karl Popper felt that each researcher should try to discredit their own hypotheses[1432]. In 1877, Charles Peirce, whom Popper considered one of the greatest philosophers of all time, had already written that, 'the state of belief ... is a calm and satisfactory state which we do not wish to avoid, or to change to a belief in anything else' [http://www.peirce.org/writings/p107.html#note2].

Ideas are strongly linked to stories or analogies. The power of stories in human culture can be enormous and academia is no exception. Once you start to think

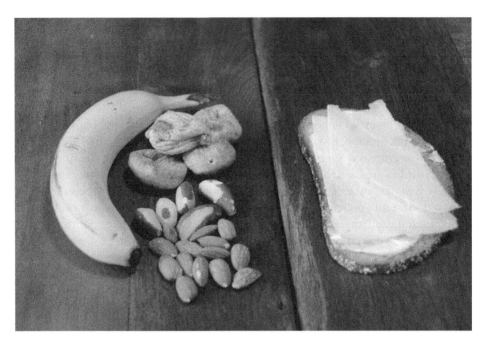

Figure 2.2 Fat and carbohydrates – both to the left and to the right.

about it, you find experts telling tales everywhere. Analogies help us to understand new thoughts, but our sense of 'knowing' is thereby easily overestimated[579].

One common effect of preconceived ideas is their tendency to direct the scientist's focus towards those dietary aspects that are considered interesting in a trial, such as the proportion of fat versus carbohydrate or the amount of some micronutrient (Figure 2.2). An intervention diet based on lean meat, fish, vegetables and fruit may, depending on your particular belief system, be described as low glycaemic index, low carbohydrate, low starch, high protein, high omega-3, Mediterranean-like, low fat, high potassium, low casein, high folate, low lectin, low gluten, or numerous other designations.

Thus, there is a considerable amount of room for personal interpretation when viewing previously completed studies, an interpretation that may be a potential source of errors. All of us interpret the results of dietary studies based on our own personal ideas of what constitutes wholesome food. A common preconceived notion, which is based on generations' understanding of the benefits of vegetarian cooking, is that meat is less healthy than vegetables.

Another common idea is that substances that come from nature are healthier than synthetic substances. Research reports on the effects of phytoestrogen are often infused with an exaggerated enthusiasm for 'natural' hormones, without any apparent understanding that the 'aim' of the plant in producing these hormones is to injure anyone who tries to eat it[1976]. One example of injury is infertility in sheep after consuming clover with a high phytoestrogen content[1064].

Each country has their traditional dietary customs. These affect the dietary recommendations from experts on every level, something which seldom appears in writing. Unofficially, it is acknowledged that certain dietary advice is adapted to what people usually eat. The national dietary recommendations for Papua New Guinea highlight this issue. The fact that the urban population there receives recommendations for less healthy food than the rural population does, e.g. two large biscuits with peanut butter for breakfast for adults[402], may be seen as a form of 'realpolitik'" It is obviously not because the nutritional needs of the two groups are actually different.

Lack of time

The significance of a lack of time appears substantial. Many thousand articles related to nutrition are published annually, and still more publications concern nutrition although this may not be explicitly stated. Therefore, it is difficult for nutritional experts to get a complete overview and they need to rely on each other when forming their concepts of healthy diets. Important studies on the effects of dietary changes on cardiovascular diseases are often presented in clinically oriented journals and conferences, and are not always read by those who actually make the nutritional recommendations. Systematic literature surveys (meta-analyses) according to the principles of evidence-based medicine are particularly complicated when it comes to food, due to difficulties of delimiting and defining a certain dietary intervention.

Reports in the mass media about the importance of diet apparently influence even the most knowledgeable authorities. Many of these reports are, for various reasons, highly selected and do not always reflect current knowledge. There is also a tendency to report findings from epidemiological studies without proper regard for potential sources of errors, as outlined above[123].

Conclusions

Nutritional science is intrinsically biased because epidemiology is confounded, physiology is complicated and randomised trials usually cannot be placebo-controlled. As a consequence, non-scientific influence may play a substantial role in shaping the concepts of diet–health relationships.

Old and new concepts of healthy diets

During the last 50 years there has been much debate on the optimal dietary advice for improving long-term health in the general population, as well as in patients with established cardiovascular disease, diabetes, high blood pressure, overweight, osteoporosis and other problems related to the Western lifestyle. Various concepts have emerged, but none of them is supported by strong and consistent evidence. Six concepts, most of which are overlapping, are more widely accepted by mainstream authorities: low-fat high-fibre diets, fruits and vegetables, calorie restriction, Mediterranean-style diets, omega-3-enriched diets and sodium restriction. A number of additional concepts exist, such as enrichment with vitamins and minerals, low glycaemic index, carbohydrate restriction and red wine. A brief review is given below; for more details see Sections 4.1–4.12.

Low-fat, high-fibre diets

Restriction of dietary fat, in particular saturated fat, has been promoted since the mid-twentieth century in order mainly to prevent atherosclerotic disease and overweight, which became increasingly common during the first half of the century[951]. The benefits of dietary fibre were proclaimed around 1970 although proponents of 'coarse food' have been heard long before. The latter idea largely emerged from belief systems concerning disturbed bowel function, bloating and 'autointoxication' in the nineteenth and early twentieth centuries[1935]. The popularity of the hypothesis increased dramatically around 1970 when Hugh Trowell, an internist, and Denis Burkitt, a surgeon, launched the idea that dietary fibre would prevent certain age-related, degenerative diseases[240,1814]. For more than 20 years, working at clinics in Kenya and Uganda, they noted what seemed obvious to any foreign doctor: that Western diseases were largely non-existent among the native population. Burkitt, above all, had the greatest success positing the fibre hypothesis. He was a good speaker and also the first to characterise the type of lymphoma that later carried his name, which gave extra weight to his credibility.

The notion that fat is unhealthy essentially emerged from epidemiological studies, in particular the ecological Seven Countries Study[902]. In this study, 12 095 men aged 40–59 were followed for 10 years starting around 1960. The incidence of ischaemic heart disease was positively associated with total and saturated fat intakes, which, respectively, explained 25 and 70% of the disease rates among the study populations.

However, despite widespread consensus among nutrition experts today, there is no solid evidence of fat enrichment or (cereal) fibre depletion being important causes of Western disease. In the Seven Countries Study, US men had more than 100-fold higher incidence of ischaemic heart disease than Cretan men despite identical fat intake, i.e. 40% of dietary energy (E%)[902]. In one large randomised controlled study of nearly 49 000 US women, the Women's Health Initiative Dietary Modification Trial, no beneficial effect was seen on cardiovascular disease, cancer or total mortality during 8 years' follow-up by a low-fat, high-fibre diet[768]. For the 3.4% of women with diagnosed cardiovascular disease at the start of the trial, a statistically significant *increased* risk of worsening of cardiovascular disease was seen in the intervention group (relative risk 1.26; 95% confidence interval 1.03–1.54). Diet changes at 6 years after study start (evaluated from food frequency questionnaires), in the intervention group as compared with the control group, were as follows: fruits/vegetables +30%, grains +11%, fibre +16%, total fat −8%, trans fat −22%, saturated fat −23%, monounsaturated fat −23% and carbohydrate +18%. The intervention and control groups differed with regard to intensity of dietary education but not with regard to type of dietary advice.

In contrast to these disappointing findings, in two other studies, subjects with impaired glucose tolerance had a lower risk of being diagnosed with diabetes during 3 years after being adviced to eat a low fat, high fibre diet and to increase their physical activity[928,1828]. The study design precludes any strong opinion about the independent roles of diet and exercise, but post-hoc analysis of one of the studies suggests that increased leisure-time physical activity was more important than dietary changes[968]. In a meta-analysis of randomised controlled trials in humans, restriction of total and saturated fat apparently had no positive overall effect on total mortality or cardiovascular disease[755]. However, in trials with at least 2 years' follow-up, a 24% reduction of premature death or cardiovascular events was seen (relative risk 0.76; 95% confidence interval 0.65–0.90), although no effect on total mortality was found. In published studies of changing fat intake in the treatment of overweight or obesity, fat restriction does not seem more effective than energy restriction for long-term weight loss[86,371,446,818,1321,1415,1422,1552,1628].

However, studies in animals have shown high-fat diets to be a partial cause of both atherosclerosis[952] and insulin resistance[276,907]. In some of these studies, a very moderate increase in dietary fat has caused abdominal obesity and insulin resistance, one of the main culprits in Western disease[907]. Moreover, this effect has been independent of total caloric intake[907]. In other animal experiments, a high-fat diet has led to intracellular fat accumulation, which is suspected of leading to long-term loss of cell function by way of lipotoxicity[1386,1927]. This disturbance is closely related to insulin resistance and the metabolic syndrome (see Section 4.6)[1838].

With regard to dietary fibre, the evidence from intervention studies is even less convincing. The only published randomised controlled study of increased fibre intake, mainly from whole grain cereals, resulted in *increased* risk of death from heart disease among patients who were already affected by heart disease at study start, a non-significant effect[242] which became significant after adjustment for possible confounding factors such as health state and medication[1285] (see Section 4.1). In several prospective epidemiological studies, people who prefer whole grain cereals to more refined ones have a lower risk of cardiovascular disease[1816], but this may possibly represent confounding by other lifestyle factors, rather than a direct effect of dietary fibre. Not even the long held notion that colon cancer is prevented by dietary fibre is supported by available evidence[75,1222,1388].

In summary, these and other studies suggest that low-fat diets are slightly better than the average Western diet, while there is less convincing evidence in support of a high fibre diet, at least one based on grains.

Fruits and vegetables

For people on a Western diet, fruits and vegetables may provide an important source of essential vitamins, minerals and trace elements. However, once nutrient requirements are met it is uncertain whether these foods are important for long-term health in the prevention of Western disease. The high water content of fruits and vegetables is expected to prevent obesity by way of satiation[982]. Several studies found beneficial effects on health-related variables of lifestyle or dietary advice, which included increased amounts of fruits and vegetables[1973]. In the successful Lyon Diet Heart Trial, fruits and vegetables were some of the foods recommended to the intervention group, which conceivably explained some of the reduced mortality in that group[386]. Epidemiological prospective studies suggest a slightly reduced risk of cardiovascular disease and several types of cancer.

However, no randomised controlled trial has specifically addressed the independent effects of fruits and/or vegetables on the incidence of death or serious disease such as cardiovascular disease or cancer. In a study on males with angina pectoris, Burr and co-workers found no effect on total mortality or cardiovascular disease of advice to eat 4–5 portions of fruit and vegetables and drink at least one glass of natural orange juice daily, and also increase the intake of oats[241]. Hence, there is as yet no strong evidence that a low intake of fruits or vegetables is an independent cause of Western disease.

Calorie restriction

In animal experiments, restriction of dietary energy has been found to increase lifespan in dogs, rats, mice, fish, worms, yeast and fruit flies, but not (yet) in primates[528,707]. In controlled trials in non-human primates, calorie restriction has not been shown to retard atherosclerosis or prolong life, but markedly beneficial effects have been noted on cardiovascular risk factors[189,274]. A study on rhesus monkeys (8 calorie-restricted and 109 controls) starting in 1977 found a relative risk of death of 0.42 (95% CI 0.1–1.4) during the first 25 years in the calorie-restricted group. Recently, in a similar trial in Rhesus monkeys, a reduced total mortality nearly reached statistical significance (P=0.16), and diabetes was clearly prevented[2014].

An observational study in 18 middle-aged rigorously calorie-restricted humans suggests that the atherosclerotic process can be attenuated[529]. At age 50 years, after an average of 6 years of calorie restriction, the thickness of the intima-media part of the carotid artery (the large neck artery) was 0.5 ± 0.1 mm compared to 0.8 ± 0.1 mm in 18 comparison subjects. Cardiovascular risk factor levels were excellent, including C-reactive protein at 0.3±0.2 μg/mL in the calorie restricted group compared to 1.6 ± 2.2 in the comparison group.

However, interpretations of these studies are not straightforward, since people on rigorous calorie restriction also change their food choices. In the mentioned study, calorie restricted subjects strictly avoided processed foods, such as refined carbohydrates, desserts, snacks and soft drinks[529]. Furthermore, one prospective cohort study in the general Swedish population found that moderately high caloric intake was associated with *lower* total mortality in women, and a similar trend in men[1015]. In addition, most observational studies do not support the idea that weight loss is beneficial (see Section 4.5). It is therefore premature to state that eating less without altering food choices is healthy.

In spite of these controversies, calorie restriction is widely believed to promote health for the average Westerner, and a common conception is that they do so independently of which foods are consumed. Energy intakes in excess of expenditures are often thought to be the sole explanation of the high rates of overweight in Western populations. The first law of thermodynamics is then often cited, the one saying that energy is constant and cannot disappear. However, it also states that energy can take various forms, including heat, and that conversion from one form of energy to another is more or less efficient. Two foods with identical caloric content do not necessarily transfer equal amounts of energy between different systems. If one of them yields more work for biochemical reactions and muscle contractions than the other, then less heat is produced per calorie. Highly relevant in this context is the finding in animal experiments of decreased body temperature on a low-calorie diet[980].

The emerging notion that calorie restriction is not independent of food composition finds additional support from findings in the fruit fly *Drosophila*, one of the most extensively studied species in this context[1112,1679]. In these experiments, reduction of either dietary yeast or sucrose reduced mortality and extended life span, but to an extent that was independent of the calorie content of the food, and with yeast having a much greater effect per calorie than sucrose. Some experiments with caloric restriction in rats suggest that protein intake should be maintained at reasonably high levels in order to improve mitochondrial cell function and prevent loss of muscle mass (sarcopenia)[1998].

To summarise, calorie restriction, in accordance with the guidelines of The Calorie Restriction (CR) Society (www.calorierestriction.org), has several apparent benefits, but only counting calories may sometimes be misleading. Reduction of waist circumference and fat mass is preferable to crude weight loss. If overweight persons restrict their food intake they should be advised to concomitantly change their consumption patterns. Substituting fruits, vegetables, root vegetables and lean meat for bread, pasta and other Western staple foods generally leads to decreased energy intake despite increased or unaltered amounts of food.

Mediterranean-style diets

International comparisons from the second half of the twentieth century have found lower rates of ischaemic heart disease, most notably before the age of 65, in Mediterranean countries like Greece, Italy, Spain and former Yugoslavia. In the Seven Countries Study, Crete had the lowest incidence of ischaemic heart disease at follow-up after 10 years[902] and after 20 years[1206]. After 25 years, total mortality was lowest in the Cretan men, although ischaemic heart disease mortality now had slightly surpassed the two Japanese groups[1204]. For this reason, the Cretan diet has become a standard model for Mediterranean-style diets[859]. In 1948, 12 years before the beginning of the Seven Countries Study, the major sources of energy in the Cretan diet were cereals (mainly sourdough bread), nuts, pulses, olives, olive oil, vegetables and fruits, together with limited quantities of goat meat and milk, game and fish[38]. Wine was consumed regularly. The intake of β-casein A1, a protein in milk which has been proposed to cause ischaemic heart disease, was particularly low, less than 0.5 g/day[989].

The Lyon Diet Heart Study found reduced mortality and morbidity (non-fatal disease) of ischaemic heart disease after advice to follow a Mediterranean-style diet[386]. However, the Mediterranean group was given more intense lifestyle education than the control group, who received 'usual care', posing a possible bias to the study. In addition, the Mediterranean group was provided with a margarine based on rapeseed oil, enriched with α-linolenic acid (plant-based omega-3 fat).

Today, type 2 diabetes and possibly ischaemic heart disease, are apparently common in Crete[1058]. Hypertension and stroke have been prevalent for many years in Mediterranean populations, including the Cretans[511,1205].

In conclusion, Mediterranean diets are apparently a step in the right direction for many people, but they may not be the best choice for long-term human health.

Omega-3-enriched diets

One of the strongest beliefs held about healthy food is that fatty fish prevents heart disease and that omega-3 polyunsaturated fatty acids are the main reason[382,1688]. However, the evidence is not by far as solid as it may seem. In 2004, a Cochrane (see Glossary) meta-analysis of randomised controlled trials found no net benefit on cardiovascular disease, total mortality or cancer[756]. A shorter report of this meta-analysis was later published in the *British Medical Journal*[757]. Criticism of these findings has largely focused on the fact that exclusion of one trial, DART-2[241], seems to change the results in favour of omega-3[1252,1457]. However, DART-2 is not the only trial showing negative effects of omega-3 fat in patients with ischaemic heart disease[230]. Furthermore, the results of the Cochrane review suggest the presence of publication bias, such that large trials do not show a positive effect[756]. Much of the criticism of the short report is taken into account in the long one[756] (http://www.bmj.com/cgi/content/abstract/332/7544/752). The debate will most certainly continue.

Even the statement that cardiovascular disease was uncommon in the Greenland Eskimos, as long as they pursued their traditional lifestyle, has been questioned[177]. In a review of twentieth-century clinical and autopsy studies and mortality statistics from Greenland, Canada and Alaska, atherosclerosis and cardiovascular disease were not found to be lower among the Eskimos than among white comparison populations.

Sodium restriction

A starting point for discussions about salt and health was a French experiment 100 years ago showing raised blood pressure after high salt intake[47]. Considerable evidence now suggests that restriction of dietary sodium below 100 mmol Na/day (<6 g sodium chloride or <2.4 g sodium per day) will reduce blood pressure and prevent cardiovascular disease in people with hypertension[1948]. Since only a minority of middle-aged and elderly Westerners have optimal blood pressure (< 120/80 mm Hg), and since low levels are more healthy than average or high levels, most people would seem to benefit from a low salt intake. Several studies suggest that dietary salt is a contributing factor in the development of stroke and heart failure, particularly among overweight people, and possibly independently of blood pressure (see Sections 4.2 and 4.9). A correlation between sodium intake and stroke has also been noted among Europeans[1411], as well as in China and Japan[1833]. The influence of dietary salt on ischaemic heart disease is more controversial, but here, again, the risks with high salt intake may be highest for overweight subjects (see Section 4.1).

Vitamins and minerals

Ever since the discovery of human being's dependence on vitamins and minerals, and the abundance of such substances in fruits and vegetables, there has been much interest in their role for human health. Deficient intakes of many vitamins and minerals, including a number of trace elements, have been suggested as underlying causes of Western disease, as will be noted in the following chapters. Much of the evidence comes from epidemiological studies. However, when these nutrients later have been given in large-scale randomised double-blind controlled trials, essentially no beneficial effects have been seen[174,467,1175]. A recent Cochrane meta-analysis found that supplementation with vitamins A and E may actually increase mortality, while the impact of vitamin C and selenium was thought to need further study[175]. A later randomised controlled trial of selenium supplementation found an increased risk of diabetes in the selenium supplement group[1733].

Low glycaemic index foods and carbohydrate restriction

In the year 1825, Brillat-Savarin, the influential French writer on food, cooking and nutrition, suggested that high-starch foods were a major cause of corpulence in his book *The Physiology of Taste* (http://www.gutenberg.org/etext/5434). His authority reached a few of the medical practitioners in France and England, and in 1862 in London, the now famous William Banting was advised by his physician to '...abstain as much as possible from bread, butter, milk, sugar, beer, and potatoes ...', and lost 21 kg in the following 12 months (see Section 4.6). By tradition, this often cited diet has been described as a low-carbohydrate diet rather than one based on meat, fish, fruits and vegetables, which it was. The proceeding history of carbohydrate restriction includes proponents such as Stefansson in the 1920s, Pennington, Cleave and Mackarness in the 1950s, Donaldson and Lutz in the 1960s, Atkins in the 1970s (and again in the 1990s), and more recently dietary programs such as the Zone, the Carbohydrate Addict's Diet, Protein Power, South Beach Diet, Sugar Busters and many others.

A low glycaemic index food is one that, despite being rich in carbohydrates, does not increase blood sugar as much as another food with the same amount of carbohydrate. Carbohydrate restriction refers to reduction of the amount of carbohydrate in the food without necessarily changing the glycaemic index. If you multiply the glycaemic index by the absolute amount of carbohydrate, you get the glycaemic load[88]. The rationale behind low glycaemic index and restriction of carbohydrates is to reduce the rise in blood sugar and insulin secretion after a meal, which in turn is intended to prevent insulin resistance, overweight, glucose intolerance, type 2 diabetes, dyslipidaemia and the metabolic syndrome[208]. A recent meta-analysis of 37 observational cohort studies found an increased risk of ischaemic heart disease, type 2 diabetes and gall bladder (gallstone) disease in people who consumed high glycaemic index or glycaemic load foods[113].

However, an independent beneficial effect, irrespective of food source, on these variables is not unequivocally supported by available evidence[86,207,371,565,892,1312,1480,1876,2015]. In people with diabetes, avoiding excess increases in blood sugar after meals is in some sense undeniably beneficial, but exchanging carbohydrate for fat may sometimes pose other long term threats. In overweight or obese subjects, initial weight loss in the first few months is usually more pronounced on a very, very low-carbohydrate diet such as the Atkins diet, but energy intake and adherence seem to be more important than choice of dietary program for long-term (>1 year) weight maintenance[86,371,446,572,1321,1552,1628]. Generally, serum triglycerides are reduced, while low density lipoprotein (LDL) cholesterol is slightly increased[1876]. Although triglycerides usually decrease more than LDL increases, the net health benefit of this is uncertain[1766]. Exclusively changing the glycaemic index seems to have little impact on body weight (see Section 4.5) or cardiovascular risk factor levels[889].

The long primate history of fruit eating[185], the high activity of human salivary amylase for efficient starch digestion[1564] and some other features of human mouth physiology[1087], as well as the absence of Western disease among starch-eating traditional populations[1050,1669] suggest that humans are well prepared for a high carbohydrate intake from non-grain food sources. Although restriction of all types of carbohydrates may provide some benefit for subjects with type 2 diabetes, it seems unlikely that dietary carbohydrate is a primary cause of Western disease.

Red wine

The claimed benefits of red wine are so often reported that they may seem to be a proven fact, and the critical voices do not get much attention. As usual for notions based on observational studies, we have a possible bias in the form of confounders (see Problems with epidemiology under Section 2.4). Furthermore, in order to get a true protection against cardiovascular disease you may need to drink so much every week that your brain and liver are damaged[813]. In epidemiological studies, the difference in mortality between people who drink two glasses of wine per day and those who drink once a month is negligible or non-existent. Enthusiastic reports about resveratrol, a substance in red wine which prolongs life in mice that are fed high-fat/sucrose diets, sometimes forget to mention that the doses used correspond to more than 700 bottles of wine per day[131].

Other concepts

There are a large number of additional philosophies about diet and health, many of which will appear throughout this book. The idea that *soya foods* are healthy is largely based on the *vegetarian* tradition, and both have had considerable impact on nutritional science despite inconsistent research findings. *Red meat* is basically an epidemiological story without strong evidence from other research areas[1950]. The *antioxidant* story mainly emerged from intriguing hypotheses in molecular biology, but randomised double-blind controlled trials with antioxidants have essentially failed to show any benefit[325,1175].

Conclusions

Foods that are generally perceived as healthy, most notably fruits and vegetables, are apparently a better choice than foods that are not perceived as healthy. Nevertheless, many of the prevailing concepts are not firmly based on good evidence. Nutritional recommendations for public health are resting on such unstable ground that evolutionary medicine may provide an important complement to traditional scientific methods[460,463]. Reading the scientific literature through the lens of evolutionary biology can sometimes make it easier to understand the extremely complex relationships between diet and health.

Dietary advice to prevent and treat common Western diseases should be designed in accordance with human biological heritage as much as possible. Foods that have been part of the human staple diet for less than 10 000 years should be critically examined before they are recommended as staple food. Even the risks with foods that were available during the Palaeolithic era (Old Stone Age, approximately 2.5 million–10 000 years ago), but which may contain antinutritional substances, should be carefully examined, in particular, foods that are consumed in large quantities on a daily basis.

3 Ancestral human diets

3.1 Available food

What did humans eat in their original environment? A simple answer is: Food that was available and that provided dietary energy with a reasonable amount of effort, such as fruits, vegetables, nuts, insects, larvae, wild game meat, fish, shellfish and root vegetables. However, it is difficult to define what we mean by 'original environment', since most of the shaping of human digestion and metabolism took place long before we become human-like and started to walk on two legs, approximately 6 million years ago. Hence, it could be argued that the Miocene vegetarian-like habitats, from 23 to 5 million years ago, provide a proper reference for human nutrition[822]. In contrast, others argue that later habitats exerted such strong selection pressures that humans became adapted to a high intake of meat[206]. However, neither position excludes the other. We may be adapted to any kind of food without necessarily being dependent on it for high reproductive success.

The latest period of fine-tuning of human physiology dates back the 2.5 million years or so, leading up to the emergence of fully modern humans in Africa approximately 200 000 years ago, i.e. the Palaeolithic[203,613]. The habitats occupied less than 100 000 years should rarely be considered in the context of optimal foods for all living humans, since these habitats occurred after the divergence into different ethnic groups[1737] and since nutrient requirements are essentially the same worldwide.

In addition to the problem of defining 'original human habitats', it is often impossible to determine, for any particular habitat, the percentage of food that came from each of the available foodstuffs. Hence, the staple food items typically consumed by our bipedal ancestors in Africa is a matter of debate, but the principal food available included sweet and ripe fruits and berries, shoots, flowers, buds and young leaves, meat, bone marrow, organ meats, fish, shellfish, insects, larvae, eggs, roots, bulbs, nuts and non-grass seeds. In principle, this was the only type of food that was available during human evolution, but now only provides one quarter or less of the caloric intake for the average European or American. In contrast, we currently get most of our energy from cereal grains (grass seeds), dairy products, refined fats and sugar, and legumes. In addition, we have extremely little variation among plant foods today.

Obviously, dairy products, refined fats and refined sugar were absent from the original menus of humans. Wild seeds were available from various plants, but not from the grass family (Poaceae), which includes today's wheat, rice and maize, and rarely or never from one plant species every day. Seeds from legumes (beans, peas, lentils) apparently became staple foods during the emergence of agriculture, as evidenced by gradual changes in their form and quality in consequence of domestication[155,2013]. Contemporary hunter-gatherers, in particular those living in arid, hot, marginal environments (Australian Aborigines, Kalahari Bushmen), often include large, fatty seeds in their diet, but these account for a relatively small part of the diet, and each of them not by far as much as is now provided by wheat, rice or maize among modern humans[335,1005,1330].

Attempts to determine food patterns of prehistoric hunter-gathers are fraught with considerable methodological problems. There is already great uncertainty in terms of which dominant edible animals and plants were present in the ecological niches in Africa where *Homo sapiens* evolved from 2 to 0.2 million years ago[198,1485,1881]. The total number of skeletal remains from African Palaeolithic humans is very small[532], and it is unclear how representative these findings are[1282,1581]. Furthermore, archaeological reconstructions of past diets from morphological characteristics of bones and teeth, analyses of remaining tools and measurements of bone chemistry do not provide strong evidence in a particular direction, except that we were omnivores[1503]. With regard to contemporary hunter-gatherers, these are not in every respect representative of their Palaeolithic counterparts.

Our primate ancestors probably consumed large amounts of fruit regularly during 50 million years until they became bipedal around 6 million years ago[185,613]. Today, fruit makes up more than 75% of the diet for chimpanzees, bonobos and orangutans[1709]. During the long period of primate evolution, the foragers and their prey gradually changed in close coevolution, where seed dispersal was highly dependent on fruit consumption by primates (and birds)[721]. As fruits became rich in colour to signal ripeness, their consumers developed colour vision. As the flesh of ripe fruits became sweeter, primates became increasingly fond of sugar. The fruit seeds, on the other hand, became bitter-tasting, slippery and deeply embedded in the centre. Furthermore, ripe fruits generally have low contents of bioactive substances, since there is no benefit of inflicting damage on the animals as long as they do not destroy the seeds. The optimal scenario for the plant is that the seeds are swallowed and later buried and fertilised on the ground. Interestingly, it has been suggested that some fruits enhance intestinal motility in order for the seeds to be deposited not too far from the habitat which was suitable for the parent[1976].

Human preference for sweet food clearly suggests that our ancestors would have savoured one exquisite choice: honey. It may have been a major source of concentrated sweetness, and for several contemporary hunter-gatherers the intake has been considerable during the honey season[43].

Increasing evidence suggests that large starchy underground storage organs (roots, tubers, bulbs and corms), which plants form in dry climates, were staple foods 1–2 million years ago[1971]. There are at least three arguments in favour of this notion. Firstly, in contrast to most other animals including non-human primates, humans have an exceptional capacity to produce salivary amylase in order to begin hydrolysis of starch in the mouth. The underlying change in copy number of the gene coding for salivary amylase may have occurred approximately 1 million years ago[1564]. Root vegetables are rich in starch, while carbohydrates in other vegetables (leafy greens, most other vegetables) and fruits are dominated by simple sugars (mono- or disaccharides). Apparently, human populations with a recent history of high-starch consumption have, compared with other human populations, on average a slightly higher copy number of the gene coding for salivary amylase, a number which explains about 35% of the variation of salivary amylase concentration[1410]. Although this suggests some degree of ongoing positive selection, the fact that 'low-starch' human populations have an almost threefold higher copy number than chimpanzees ('high-starch' humans are slightly above threefold)[1410] indicates significant adaptation to high-starch root vegetables among hominins.

Secondly, roots often need to be prepared under high temperature in order for its starch to be available for digestion and for its bioactive or toxic substances to be neutralised[1971]. There are many indications of Palaeolithic humans using fire for cooking, and one of the most common cooking methods for plant foods was probably the so-called earth oven, where food wrapped in large leaves is placed in a covered pit with hot stones or glowing coals. Thirdly, human tooth morphology, including incisal orientation, seems to be well designed for chewing root vegetables[1087].

An adaptation to root vegetables may have started several million years back. It has been suggested that the early hominids became dependent on underground storage organs as fallback foods from about 6 million years ago[970]. During periods of repeatedly dry and cool climates, plants with large underground storage organs are thought to have become more common. Our bipedal ancestors were apparently less efficient hunters than many carnivorous animals and less efficient fruit-foragers than the arboreal primates. In order to increase the caloric yield per workload ('optimal foraging strategy'), root vegetables may often have been an optimal dietary choice. An illustrative example is the Machiguenga tribe of the Amazon, among whom one woman can dig up enough root vegetables in one hour to feed 25 adults for one day[837]. The excellent health status among this and other starch-eating ethnic groups, including our own study population in Papua New Guinea (see Section 4.1), contradicts the popular notion that such foods are a cause of obesity and type 2 diabetes.

Another food which could provide a high-energy yield is meat. The chimpanzee, our closest relative among primates, eats considerable amounts of meat[1709]. In one observational study, adult chimpanzees consumed an average of 65 g meat per day in the dry season[1710]. For humans, available archaeological evidence is consistent with, but does not prove, regular high meat intake in the last 2 million years[1503]. Contemporary hunter-gatherers have generally been able to eat large amounts of meat or fish, although the figures are based on rather imprecise ethnographic data[338,1377]. Of the 229 hunter-gatherer populations studied during the twentieth century, the majority (73%) were estimated to get more than half their caloric intake from meat, fish and shellfish[338]. Among those five African populations, for which more exact, quantitative data were available, meat and/or fish constituted on average 26, 33, 44, 48 and 68% of the food[332]. Although Palaeolithic humans cannot in every aspect be represented by contemporary hunter-gatherers, particularly not the ones living in sub-Arctic or Arctic climates, the findings strongly suggest that humans are well adapted for a high intake of meat. Nevertheless, even the most dedicated meat eaters in ancient times most probably had an intake of healthy plant foods that sharply exceeded that of most modern humans. As a matter of fact, today's vegetarians do not usually eat a lot of vegetables; rather they consume large amounts of grains, dairy foods, refined fats and sugar.

In some habitats, Palaeolithic humans may have lived by the shores of lakes and rivers where they could catch fish and shellfish and venture inland for hunting small and large animals and gathering insects, plants and eggs. However, dependence on marine food seems to have emerged essentially after humans left Africa, and less than 100 000 years ago[1503]. It should be noted that this issue is not related to the question of whether bipedalism emerged near water some 6 million years ago[1240]. For long periods of time thereafter, our ancestors were apparently not dependent on marine food sources.

In most habitats, the consumption of insects and larvae may have been substantial and would have provided an important source of protein and fat. Western society has long resisted such food, but other cultures in the world often value them highly[394], and they are regularly consumed by non-human primates[128].

Nuts are a complicated issue. Many of them are not actually nuts in a botanical sense (e.g. peanuts). Nuts are energy-dense often provide a relatively high amount of energy for the amount of work involved, and may have made up an essential part of the diet during certain time periods. However, they are obviously critical for the mother plant to be able to spread its genes. Therefore, it is logical to find that nuts that are protected by very hard shells have a lower content of phytochemicals than other nuts[721]. Nevertheless, many stone fruits and seeds may have tasted worse – and been more poisonous – during the Palaeolithic era than today[414]. Almonds at that time are thought to have been more bitter than sweet. At the beginning of agriculture, our ancestors supposedly prioritised the sweetest types of almonds, an early example of plant breeding.

The extent to which alcohol was a part of human's original environment, such that we adapted to it genetically, is a matter of debate. Some of the oldest archaeological evidence for beer and wine comes from the Middle East, and the word alcohol is of Arabic origin (al'kohol, originally meaning a powdered essence)[420]. If storage vessels were made of leather or plants in earlier prehistoric times, they have long since disappeared without a trace. Our current genotypic intelligence is more than 100 000 years old, and consequently the ability to figure out how to brew alcohol is at least as old as that. The attraction of light intoxication is evident in most ethnic groups in the world and seems to be independent of the effect of culture[1685]. Even without deliberate production of alcoholic beverages, a low-level dietary exposure to ethanol via ingestion of fermenting fruit may have characterised our lineage of humans and human-like ancestors for about 40 million years[444].

Published studies in the area of human physiology do not provide solid evidence of which dietary habits humans are best adapted for[1044]. One reason is scarcity of research: we are only beginning to understand the complex relationships of molecular biology, nutritional physiology and food-related disorders. In addition, selection pressures may have been low when the relevant foods and nutrients were consumed in suboptimal amounts. Commonly, physiological traits that are specific for a certain species can mirror food patterns of ancestors many million years earlier.

To summarise the evidence from different fields of science, humans are apparently omnivores who are well adapted for a diet based either on animal or plant foods, the relative proportions of which have been highly variable depending on habitat. The discussion about human's ancient diets is often misdirected to a debate on meat versus plant foods. Thereby, the main point is missed: most of the calories in Western countries are provided by foods that were practically unavailable during human evolution.

3.2 Nutritional composition

Compared with the average European or American diet, Palaeolithic diets and other ancestral human diets were characterised by a high concentration of minerals, vitamins and trace elements (micronutrients). The absence of refined fats and sugar is the primary reason for this, but even cereals tilt the balance in the direction of a number of nutritional deficiencies. Moreover, today's nitrate fertilisers cause an increase in grain volume, which forces the plant to prioritise the development of proteins and biomass at the expense of secondary metabolites, many of which could probably be considered nutrients.

An example of a nutritional deficiency in today's food is folic acid: If vegetables and fruit were staple foods in the Western world, folic acid supplementation would never be an issue. In addition to being a rich source of nutrients, Palaeolithic food contains a lot of water, fibre and protein, which makes it satiating (filling) at a low calorie intake. The high water content of certain food items results in a relatively low content of minerals and vitamins, expressed per unit of weight (mg/kg), while the nutrient density, expressed per unit of energy (mg/kJ), is very high, with few exceptions. However, the content of individual antinutritional factors is generally low. The characteristics in terms of types and proportions of fats, carbohydrates and proteins are discussed below. Notes on the relevant health effects will in most cases be saved for later chapters.

The quantities given in the tables should be taken with caution. They are generally based on Swedish food composition tables which typically show nutrient contents in Swedish or Scandinavian food, which may differ from food bought in other countries[474,1471]. For domestic meat, the fat content can vary tremendously between countries. For fruit, the amount of sunlight can influence nutrient levels, the soil can affect trace element levels and so forth. In addition, there may be large variations even within countries between different varieties of food and different times and places. Thus, the comparisons below only give hints.

Minerals, trace elements

Palaeolithic food is rich in minerals such as potassium and magnesium from vegetables, as well as trace elements like iron and zinc from meat and fish. The mineral density of these foods (calculated per unit of energy) is high compared with cereals, but not always higher than low-fat dairy products. Vegetables thus provide high levels of potassium, assuming that they are consumed in large amounts (Table 3.1; see Table 3.2 for recommended nutrient densities). The potassium density in a banana (1 g/MJ) is well below that of most vegetables, and the reason that it is often considered to be particularly rich in potassium is that the water content is relatively low, which is why the potassium content is high when calculated by weight. An average banana (100 g, edible part) provides as much potassium as 90 g of broccoli, but roughly 4 times as many calories.

In the best case, calcium consumption can be quite high from a Palaeolithic diet due to the high calcium density in vegetables. However, since vegetables are also rich in water, large amounts must be consumed to achieve the recommended calcium intake (see Section 4.12 for comments on calcium recommendations). The calcium density in spinach is actually higher than in skim milk, which may be surprising (Table 3.3). For the average Westerner, roughly one-fourth of their energy intake is provided by food that is lacking in calcium (primarily oil, margarine and sugar). Cereals, which provide an additional 25%, contain relatively little calcium. Hence, it should come as no surprise that the calcium intake among many hunter-gatherer societies is estimated to have been higher than among modern Westerners[461].

Table 3.1 Potassium content (g/MJ) in selected food groups.

Food group	25th percentile	Median	75th percentile
Vegetables	1.7	2.8	3.9
Fruits	0.6	0.9	1.3
Fish	0.6	0.8	0.9
Meat	0.4	0.5	0.7
Nuts	0.2	0.3	0.3
Dairy products	0.1	0.5	0.8
Cereals	0.1	0.2	0.3
Sausages	0.1	0.1	0.2

Note: Adapted from food composition tables, Swedish National Food Administration, 2006; www.slv.se. The 25th and 75th percentiles refer to the value below which 25 and 75% of foods have in that group. Recommended intake is 0.4 g/MJ.

Table 3.2 Recommended nutrient density intended for meal planning for groups of people 6–60 years of age with a heterogeneous age and sex distribution.

	Content per MJ
Vitamin A, retinol equivalents (RE)	80
Vitamin D, µg	1.0
Vitamin E, alfa-TE	0.9
Thiamine, mg	0.12
Riboflavin, mg	0.14
Niacin, NE	1.6
Vitamin B_6, mg	0.13
Folate, µg	45
Vitamin B_{12}, µg	0.2
Vitamin C, mg	8
Calcium, mg	100
Phosphorus, mg	80
Potassium, g	0.35
Magnesium, mg	35
Iron, mg	1.6
Zinc, mg	1.1
Iodine, µg	17
Selenium, µg	4

Note: The values are adapted to individuals with the highest requirements.

Whole grain cereals and beans are rich in phytates, which impair the intestines' ability to absorb iron, calcium, zinc and magnesium[259,542,668,1243,1535,1571,1572,1703]. Because the Palaeolithic diet does not include these foods, it provides an additional defence against mineral deficiencies. In addition, the diet improves iron absorption due to the large amounts of vitamin C in vegetables and fruits, and because iron in meat is very efficiently absorbed. When meat or fish were abundant during the Palaeolithic, iron intake was particularly high, along with zinc and selenium.

Since iodised salt and dairy products were not available to our Palaeolithic ancestors, only those with high regular access to fish or shellfish would be expected to have reached the currently recommended intake of iodine (Table 3.4). There is insufficient data to suggest that humans, by way of natural selection, would have become completely dependent on marine food sources. Therefore, it is highly possible that human requirements for iodine are currently increased by some modern lifestyle factors and that less was enough for ancient humans. These factors theoretically include goitrogens (goitre-inducing substances) in certain roots, vegetables, beans and seeds. For further discussion, see Section 5.2.

Common salt

Consumption of salt (sodium chloride, NaCl) was most likely low during human evolution, similar to what was the case during the evolutionary history of land animals. An average Westerner consumes 150–200 mmol/day (9–12 g salt/day),

Table 3.3 Calcium content in selected foods.

	Calcium	
	mg/MJ	mg/100 g
Spinach	1517	93
Skim milk	838	120
Cheese, 17% fat	696	860
Cheese, 28% fat	479	740
Cabbage	470	45
Broccoli	428	48
Milk, 3% fat	422	106
Cauliflower	218	23
Cottage cheese, 4% fat	165	68
Wheat bran	77	76
Whole grain bread	60	57
Cod	51	16
Apple	27	6
Chicken, breast	25	11
Wheat flour	15	22
Potato	13	4
Butter	6	18
Oil	0	0

Note: The foods above the dotted line facilitate and those below make it more difficult to meet the suggested requirement of calcium (110 mg/MJ), assuming that the total energy intake is maintained constant.
Source: Adapted from food composition tables, Swedish National Food Administration, 2006; www.slv.se.

which can be compared with an estimated intake of less than 30 mmol/day among prehistoric hunter-gatherers[459] and 1 mmol/day among the Yanomamo Indians in the Amazon rainforest[1132]. Note that not just sodium, but also the chloride intake, was originally very low[29]. In modern times, the balance between both sodium and potassium, as well as between chloride and bicarbonate, has shifted strongly in favour of sodium and chloride[541].

The physiological need for sodium has been estimated to be less than 0.6 mmol/kg of body weight/day[1221]. Since the intake among the Yanomamo Indians fell below this level, the actual requirement is probably considerably lower[1350]. Real sodium deficiency in the tropics occurs because of rapid salt depletion among people who are used to a high salt intake. Salt supplements are therefore only required in the initial 10–15 days, until the sweat glands reset their salt secretion patterns[912].

Vitamins

Humans differ from most other animals in that vitamin C (ascorbic acid) cannot be synthesised and must be obtained from the food[1310]. Our early primate ancestors lost this ability, probably 40–50 million years ago, but this was apparently no

Table 3.4 Iodine content in selected food items.

	N	Iodine content (µg/100 g)	Median (range) (µg/MJ)
Fish, raw	25	25 (7–85)	48 (16–222)
Shellfish, raw	3	180 (60–700)	409 (188–1912)
Meat, raw	22	1 (0–6)	1.5 (0–13)
Thyroid gland	1	50 000	
Other organ meats	18	3 (0–8)	5 (0–19)
Vegetables, raw	26	1 (0–6)	9 (0–132)
Root vegetables, raw	7	1 (0.3–3)	4 (1–21)
Fruits/berries, raw	25	0.4 (0–2)	2 (0–6)
Nuts, raw	5	0.3 (0.05–0.5)	0.2 (0.02–0.2)
Legumes, raw	10	1 (0.2–45)	1 (0.2–36)
Cereals	26	2 (0.3–5)	1 (0.2–3)
Dairy products	7	8 (6–45)	30 (15–38)
Human milk	1	63	211
Table salt	1	5 000	—
Sea salt	1	2 000	—
Recommended intake	—	(150 µg/day)	18
Minimum intake[a]	—	(50–75 µg/day)	7

Source: Adapted from www.slv.se.
Estimated lowest intake to prevent goitre when daily energy intake is 10 MJ (70 µg/day).

problem during human evolution, since the intake of vitamin C from plant foods is expected to have continuously exceeded requirements, making such biosynthesis redundant. The obligatory requirement of vitamin C does not necessarily suggest that early humans always consumed lots of plant foods, since organ meats from large animals can easily provide the required amounts, on condition that they are consumed raw (Table 3.5). Sometimes shellfish may also provide enough vitamin C to prevent scurvy.

Table 3.5 Content of ascorbic acid, expressed as nutrient density, in selected raw food items.

	Ascorbic acid (mg/MJ)
Game muscle	0
Fish	1 (2)
Shellfish	8 (13)
Organ meats	29 (23)
Root vegetables (cultivated)	17 (25)
Fruits (cultivated)	34 (45)
Recommended intake	≥8
Suggested lowest intake to prevent scurvy	≥4

Source: Adapted from Food composition tables, Swedish National Food Administration, 2006; www.slv.se.
Note: The values represent mean (SD) values.

Table 3.6 Content of vitamin B_{12}, expressed as nutrient density, in selected food items.

	Vitamin B_{12} (μg/MJ)
Game muscle, raw	9 (5)
Fish, raw	10 (13)
Shellfish, raw	14 (18)
Organ meats, raw	52 (61)
Vegetables, fruits, legumes, cereals	0
Dairy products	1.5 (0.9)
Recommended intake	$\geq$0.2

Source: Adapted from food composition tables, Swedish National Food Administration, 2006; www.slv.se.
Note: The values represent mean (SD) values.

Vitamin B_{12}, another indispensable (essential) nutrient, is absent in plant foods and must be supplied from meat, fish, shellfish or insects, but the required amounts are apparently small (Table 3.6). Vegans have a very high risk of vitamin B_{12} deficiency and generally need supplements[1705,1973]. Although plant foods may sometimes contain trace amounts of vitamin B_{12} analogues as a result of fermentation, most of these seem to be inactive analogues of the vitamin[716]. Even lacto-ovo-vegetarians are at substantially increased risk of deficiency despite the fact that milk products provide some vitamin B_{12}[742,934]. From the available knowledge it would seem that early humans must have had access to animal foods in order to avoid vitamin B_{12} deficiency. However, in case of irregular intake there is a high degree of retention of the vitamin in body stores, suggesting that it does not necessarily need to be supplied every week. Another relevant aspect is absorption, which may vary, not only between foods, but also between individuals. In the average healthy adult with normal stomach function, approximately 50% of vitamin B_{12} is thought to be absorbed[1973]. There seems to be a decline with increasing age in Western societies, and mild deficiency is common among elderly subjects, but this is not considered to be a consequence of normal biological ageing[263]. Non-Western populations have not been studied in this regard.

A high intake of vegetables, fruits and roots during Palaeolithic times ensured a high intake of vitamins A, B, E and K, biotin, pantothenic acid and folic acid (folate). Folic acid is found in vegetables, particularly leafy greens. Vitamin B_6 is found in both animals and vegetables. Consumption well exceeds the recommended levels for all known vitamins with one exception: vitamin D[331]. The only food habit that can compensate, to some degree, for a lack of sunlight is very high fish consumption. For most of their evolutionary history, humans spent so much time outside, and at such low latitudes, that the need for vitamin D year round was met by converting the vitamin precursors in the skin. During the winter, the rays of sunlight in Scandinavia fall to such a low angle that this mechanism was probably inadequate, even with extensive periods of time outside each day. (For more comments on vitamin D, see Section 4.12.)

Protein content

Protein intake varied considerably during human evolution. A rough estimate of average protein content, as percentage of energy (E%), in typical food groups is as follows: fruit 10 E%, leafy/cruciferous plant foods 40 E%, insects 50 E%, nuts 15 E%, roots 20 E% and wild game meat 70 E%. A diet based exclusively on (domestic) fruit would rarely meet the lower level of protein requirement (0.75 g/kg/day), while one based on other vegetables (including roots) on average would pose the risk of exceeding the presently recommended upper limit (Table 3.7). Among twentieth-century hunter-gatherers (including Arctic populations), the average protein intake was typically between 19 and 35 E%[338], compared to 14–16 E% for today's North Americans and Northern Europeans and 17–19 E% for Southern Europeans[139,872,886,1600,1810]. Even leafy and cruciferous vegetables contribute considerably to protein consumption when eaten in large amounts. Per unit of energy, spinach contains as much protein as cottage cheese and more than beans. However, only 20 g of cottage cheese is needed to get the same amount of protein as in 100 g of spinach.

National advisory bodies have for many years recommended that 10–15 E% be provided by protein and that daily intake should not be less than 0.7 g protein/kg of body weight. The current recommendation for Scandinavian adults is 10–20 E% protein[1973]. However, the debate among experts has been rather intense, and both the upper and the lower limits of recommended protein intake are being questioned by an increasing number of research groups. The lower limit recommended by these groups varies between 0.8 and 1.0 g protein per kg body weight per day (which corresponds to more than 10 E% for most adults) while their proposed upper limit varies between 20 and 35 E% or even higher[13,62,214,895]. A typical intake among elderly Scandinavians is 15 E% or 1.0 g/kg/day[1973].

Table 3.7 Protein content in selected food items.

	Protein content	
	g/100 g	E%
Meat, raw	20 (25)	59 (19)
Fish, raw	20 (12)	67 (23)
Shellfish, raw	16 (4)	78 (13)
Vegetables, raw	3 (2)	32 (14)
Root vegetables, raw	2 (1)	19 (7)
Nuts, raw	17 (8)	12 (5)
Fruits, raw	0.8 (0.4)	7 (4)
Cereal grains	10 (5)	13 (7)
Dairy products	5 (7)	24 (10)
Legumes, raw	22 (6)	31 (3)
Recommended intake	≥55 g/day	10–20

Source: Adapted from food composition tables, Swedish National Food Administration, 2006; www.slv.se.
Note: The values represent mean (SD) values.

An adaptation to very high protein diets due to long periods of dependence on large game meat during the Palaeolithic has been suggested (see Section 4.6). The proposed negative selection pressure is low blood sugar due to lack of carbohydrates in the diet, particularly when muscle insulin sensitivity is high. If future studies show that humans are more insulin resistant than other primates, the hypothesis lends support to the notion that meat intake was very high during much of hominid evolution.

Humans cannot tolerate a sudden increase in protein intake above 250 g/day (individual range 200–300 g/day) because of a limited capacity of the liver to metabolise amino acids[650]. Higher intakes may lead to nausea, diarrhoea, and finally death, in a condition which the early white American explorers called 'rabbit starvation'[338]. This name refers to their problem of surviving the winter on meat from rabbits and other small game which have very small fat depots. On a chronically high-protein intake the liver can up-regulate its enzymatic activity, but the upper limit has not been established[650,1328].

In addition to the content of protein in foods, the capacity of intestinal enzymes to digest the consumed proteins into amino acids may influence the ability to meet requirements. Edible plants contain protease inhibitors, substances that inhibit protein digestion by interfering with intestinal proteases, and particularly high concentrations are found in beans and seeds, and to some extent in roots[70,329,1856]. Heat treatment partly inactivates some of these substances, which is why cooking may sometimes have been crucial for protein balance for those early humans who relied on plant foods.

Protein quality

Dietary proteins provide amino acids for endogenous protein synthesis (and energy). Some amino acids are interchangeable while others are essential. A third group are thought to be conditionally indispensable, i.e. they must be supplied under certain physiological or pathological conditions. There has been much debate as to the role of different food types with regard to amino acid composition[1993]. A commonly held, but largely unsubstantiated, notion has been that plant proteins would be inferior to meat proteins because they lack specific amino acids. However, the bulk of evidence suggests that a mixture of root vegetables, leaves, fruits and nuts is adequate with regard to essential amino acids[1993]. Wheat and other cereal grains are low in lysine and threonine[329]. Other single plant foods may lack specific amino acids, but a varied vegetarian diet poses no obvious risk of amino acid deficiency.

Another aspect of protein quality is based on the fact that dietary proteins are not always completely broken down in the intestines. This creates a risk of whole proteins or parts thereof (peptides) being absorbed in the body causing inflammation, allergies or autoimmunity. An example is casein, the major milk protein, which apparently causes more advanced atherosclerosis, insulin resistance and lipotoxicity than other dietary proteins in animal models[76,776,993,1953]. Palaeolithic food

Table 3.8 Percentage of protein, fat and carbohydrates in selected foods in descending order based on fat content.

	Protein (E%)	Fat (E%)	Carbohydrate (E%)	Energy (MJ/kg)
Avocado	5	84	10	6.7
Walnuts	9	83	8	27.7
Salmon	41	58	0	7.6
Reindeer	59	40	0	6.0
Spinach	53	30	16	0.6
Raspberries	17	19	60	1.2
Cauliflower	48	18	32	1.1
Venison shoulder	82	17	0	4.5
Mushrooms	41	17	39	0.9
Blueberries	6	15	74	1.9
Fennel	43	13	41	1.1
Broccoli	45	13	39	1.1
Venison steak	88	11	0	4.2
Roast elk	89	11	0	5.8
Red cabbage	22	10	63	1.1
Strawberries	9	10	76	1.5
Tomatoes	19	8	67	0.9
Cod	91	8	0	3.2
Cucumber	18	8	69	0.5
Pike	92	8	0	3.4
Brussels sprouts	38	7	51	1.5
Netted melon	10	7	77	1.5
Grapes	4	7	83	3.1
Pineapple	3	7	84	2.1
Pear	3	6	85	2.3
Figs	6	5	83	2.3
Bananas	4	4	86	4.1
Eggplant	21	4	70	0.9
Cabbage	25	4	67	1.0
Onion	16	3	76	1.3
Orange	7	2	85	1.9
Apples with peel	3	2	89	2.2
Watermelon	6	0	88	1.6

provides proteins from meat, fish, shellfish and vegetables, but not from milk, grains or beans (see Table 3.8). Hence, gluten intake has increased dramatically.

Fat content

Dietary fat provides phospholipids and cholesterol for cell membranes, omega-6 and omega-3 fatty acids for various physiological functions, and concentrated fuel for energy metabolism. Depending on habitat, the total fat intake among typical prehistoric hunter-gatherers is estimated to have varied between 25 and 50 E%[338], which can be compared with 30–40 E% in most Western populations[139,872,886] and the recommended intake, which is usually 20–35 E%

Table 3.9 Total fat content in raw meat.

Fat	
g/100 g	**E%**
2.5	20
5	35
10	50
15	65
20	70
2.5	20
5	35
10	50
15	65

(http://www.who.int/nutrition/publications/nutrecomm/en/). The most important sources of fat were meat, organ meats, bone marrow, fish, nuts, insects and larvae, in various proportions (see Tables 3.8–3.11). Nuts have a high total fat content by weight, due to their low water content. The vegetables collected by traditional populations contain very little fat, with few exceptions (see Tables 3.11 and 3.12).

The total fat content, expressed in g/100 g, is relatively low in wild game, but if it is eaten in large amounts the fat intake becomes quite high[340]. This is because only 20% of muscle tissue is made up of protein (the rest is mainly water), which also provides less energy (17 kJ/g protein) than fat (37 kJ/g fat). Consequently, the fat content is very different when expressed per weight than per energy: a piece of raw meat with 10% fat by weight provides an entire 50 E% fat (Table 3.9).

Table 3.10 Total fat content in selected raw meats and sausages.

	Fat	
	g/100 g	**E%**
Elk steak, raw	1.2	11
Chicken, breast	1.2	10
Pork filet	2.6	21
Chicken, thigh	4	30
Cattle roast beef	5	34
Chicken breast with skin	7	41
Ham, 8% fat	8	49
Chicken thigh with skin	9	50
Sausage, 11% fat	11	55

Source: Adapted from food composition tables, Swedish National Food Administration, 2006; www. slv.se.

Table 3.11   Total fat content in nuts.

	Fat	
	g/100 g	E%
Coconut	34	90
Cashews	47	72
Pistachio	49	73
Sweet almond, dried	52	79
Coconut flakes, dried	62	93
Walnuts	62	85
Hazel nuts	63	88
Brazil nuts	66	90
Pecans	68	91

Frying or grilling melts a considerable amount of the fat, which decreases the fat content.

Total fat content in wild animals varies according to body size; large mammals generally have more fat than small ones. It also varies by age, sex and season, and maximal body fat is maintained only for a few months even in tropical mammals[340]. Due to continuous feeding with energy-rich cereals and slaughtering at peak body fat, the average fat percentages in modern domestic meat are several times higher than in wild game[335]. Nevertheless, there is significant overlapping, such that certain cuts of wild game provide more fat than the leanest bits of domestic meat. Trimmed, lean cuts of domestic meat can sometimes be very lean, but in most Western food stores marbled high-fat meat is much more common. Marbled meat is a product of modern animal breeding; the wild counterparts have relatively little fat inside their musculature.

The dominant sources of fat for modern Northern Europeans are dairy products, margarine, oil and fatty meat products such as sausage and paté. Only a small portion of fat comes from pure meat. The average Northern European probably

Table 3.12   Water content in hazelnut, cashew and selected foods for comparison.

	Water (g/100 g)	Energy (MJ/100 g)
Hazelnut	0.5	2.7
Cashew nut	2	2.4
Potato, boiled	77	0.4
Carrot, raw	88	0.2
Rye bread, 10% fibre	40	0.8
Hard cheese, 23% fat	43	1.4
Apple, fresh	85	0.2
Apple, dried	31	1.0

Source: Food composition tables, Swedish National Food Administration, 2006; www.slv.se.

gets roughly 15% of their fat intake from meat and poultry[139], and those that avoid chicken skin and the fatty edge of the cutlet fall well below this level. Indeed, a trimmed meat cutlet is leaner than the fattest parts of wild meat. Chicken legs with the skin removed are higher in total fat than pork tenderloin. Thus, the fat content depends to a great degree on which cuts are chosen from which type of animal, and on avoiding the most fatty parts.

Saturated fat

Ancestral human diets are expected to have varied substantially with regard to saturated fat, depending on habitat. For populations with 40–50% dependence on meat and/or fish, saturated fat is estimated to have been 5–15 E%[332]. In addition to the low total fat content in wild game, there is less saturated fat as proportion of total fat, in comparison with modern domesticated farm animals[340]. Saturated fatty acids constitute more than 50% of the fat storage depots of wild mammals, whereas the dominant fatty acids in muscle and all other organ tissues, including bone marrow, are polyunsaturated and monounsaturated fatty acids[340]. Since subcutaneous and abdominal body fat stores are depleted during most of the year in wild animals, polyunsaturated and monounsaturated fatty acids constitute the majority of the total carcass fat. The intake of saturated fat among shore-based populations was particularly low, with a high percentage of marine fat from fish and shellfish.

The percentage of saturated fat is low in most nuts. Coconut fat, however, is dominated by saturated fat. The dominant saturated fatty acids in coconut fat are lauric acid (12:0) and myristic acid (14:0), while the amount of palmitic acid (16:0), which is the main saturated fatty acid in meat and dairy products, is low. The presence of coconuts in prehistoric Africa is very uncertain[1127].

The majority of saturated fat in today's Northern European diets comes from dairy products, edible fats and delicatessen products.

Polyunsaturated fat

Omega-6 and omega-3 fatty acids must be provided but the requirements are very low, and clinical symptoms of deficiency are only seen in special circumstances, such as chronic disease or prolonged parenteral nutrition. There is no hard evidence that humans require larger amounts of long-chain omega-3 fatty acids than other mammals[756,1973]. It is also uncertain if humans, as has been suggested, have a lower capacity than rodents and herbivores to convert the predominant omega-3 fatty acid in plants, α-linolenic acid, into the long-chain omega-3 fatty acid docosahexaenoic acid[1973].

The percentage of omega-3 fatty acids from fish, shellfish and game was often considerably higher in prehistoric times than today. In contrast, the dominant polyunsaturated fatty acid in the Western world, linoleic acid (18:2 omega-6), appeared in low amounts. It is only found in the plant kingdom, but since oil was

Table 3.13 Approximate ratios of omega-6 to omega-3 fatty acids in different populations[1655].

	Omega-6/omega-3 ratio
Coastal fishing populations	<1
Hunter-gatherers	2–3
Greece in the 1900s	2
Japan today	4
Northern Europe today	15
USA today	17

not extracted from plants, the total intake during human evolution was very low. The ratio between omega-6 and omega-3 fatty acids probably lay somewhere below 2, considerable lower than is currently the case (Table 3.13). However, the addition of most nuts raises the ratio drastically. In the modern northern European diet, the ratio of omega-6 and omega-3 fatty acids is considerably higher than during the Palaeolithic, due to the high intake of oil, margarine and to a certain extent grains, while the intake of omega-3 fatty acids from fish, shellfish and game is low today.

The dominant sources of linoleic acid in Europe are margarine and various vegetable oils (see Table 3.14). The fat composition is drastically different between different oils. Compared with rapeseed oil (canola oil), sunflower oil has 3.5 times more linoleic acid, but only 1/20th as much omega-3 fatty acid, which means that the omega-6/omega-3 ratio is 70 times higher. Fish is the food that most effectively reduces the omega-6/omega-3 ratios. The more the fat in the fish, the lower the ratio in the meal (see Table 3.15). But even lean fish, such as cod, contributes to a low ratio, unless it is changed by the cooking method, which is often the case.

Human prey animals during the Palaeolithic did not generally include animals specialised on seed-eating, which meant that the meat had a low omega-6/omega-3 ratio (around 2) compared with current domestic cattle (ratio 5–10). The composition of the polyunsaturated fats in meat reflects what the animal has eaten, such

Table 3.14 Omega-6/omega-3 ratios in selected oils[1655].

	Omega-6/omega-3 ratio
Linseed oil	0.2
Rape seed oil	2
Soya oil	6
Cooking oil	7
Wheat germ oil	10
Olive oil	13
Corn oil	45
Sesame oil	109
Sunflower oil	131
Grape seed oil	173
Safflower oil, thistle oil	397

Table 3.15 Fat composition in various fish.

	Total fat (E%)	Omega-6 fat (g/100 g)	Omega-3 fat (g/100 g)	Omega-6/ omega-3 ratio
Hake	5	0.1	0.9	0.11
Haddock	7	0.1	2.3	0.04
Whiting	7	0.2	1.2	0.17
Pike	8	0.3	2.1	0.14
Cod	8	0.2	2.3	0.09
Tuna	10	0.4	2.6	0.15
Perch	14	0.7	2.8	0.25
Turbot	18	0.9	3.1	0.29
Fried coated pike	20	2.8	3.7	0.78
Cod, fried and coated	21	1.8	2.9	0.63
Flounder	21	0.8	4.4	0.18
Walleye	21	0.9	4.5	0.20
Plaice	26	1.5	6.8	0.22
Salmon trout	26	1.6	5.8	0.28
Halibut	36	1.3	11.9	0.11
Salmon, pink	36	1.0	15.6	0.06
Haddock, coated and fried	36	7.3	3.6	2.06
Plaice, coated and fried	44	9.3	8.3	1.11
Salmon lox	45	3.9	15.3	0.25
Mackerel in tomato sauce	47	1.4	10.3	0.14
Halibut, coated and fried	48	9.0	13.1	0.68
Smoke herring	50	8.4	15.7	0.54
Rainbow trout	53	4.8	25.1	0.19
Char	53	6.9	20.2	0.34
Fish sticks, fried	54	16.2	4.4	3.70
Salmon	58	5.2	20.0	0.26
Canned tuna in oil	61	84.9	11.4	7.45
Pickled herring	63	6.1	36.5	0.17
Canned sardines in oil	65	59.3	37.8	1.57
Mackerel	66	3.7	27.4	0.14
Mackerel boiled	66	4.4	32.7	0.14
Herring	71	5.0	29.8	0.17
Herring, coated and fried	71	9.2	31.9	0.29
Mackerel, canned	76	6.6	47.8	0.14
Eel	83	13.9	36.0	0.39

Source: Food composition tables, Swedish National Food Administration, 2006; www.slv.se.
Note: For comparison, the fat content is 12 g/kg in elk steak, compared to 60 g in pork chop (with 2 mm fat gristle), 87 g in chicken thigh with skin, and 280 g in cheese (28% fat content).

that animals that are raised on grain-based feeds have a high omega-6/omega-3 ratio, around 7–15 for poultry, and 5–10 for other domesticated animals[340]. Meat from free-ranging cattle (browsers feeding on high-growing vegetation and grazers feeding on grass) have the same ratio as wild game, provided they are not finished off with grain[370]. Likewise, fat composition in chicken eggs varies widely depending on the feeding of the hen. Free-range chicken, which primarily feed on grubs and grasses and are not finished off with grain, have a markedly low omega-6/omega-3 ratio[1655].

Trans fatty acids

Consumption of trans fatty acids was very low during Palaeolithic times. Trans fats are unsaturated fats with a physical rotation resembling saturated fats following the conversion of *cis* double bonds into *trans* forms. Trans fatty acids are formed during industrial processes to harden vegetable fats. The highest amounts are generally found in fats that contain partially hydrogenated vegetable or fish oils. They also develop naturally in milk and depot fat via bacteria in the first stomach of ruminators. The dominant trans fatty acid in margarines and oils is elaidic acid (*trans* 18:1n-9), while *trans*-vaccenic acid (*trans* 18:1n-7) dominates the fat in ruminants. (Both are monounsaturated fatty acids.) The fatter the cut of the meat, the larger the intake. The amount of trans fatty acids in meat animals is affected by the fatty acid compositions in the feed. *trans*-18:2 linoleic acid comes primarily from edible fats, but also from domesticated ruminants, since animal feeds provide a relatively high amount of linoleic acid.

In the West, margarine and other edible fats were the dominant sources of trans fatty acids up until 1994. Due to new regulations, however, table margarines and most household margarines in some European countries now contain relatively small amounts of trans fatty acids[137,779,1721]. Current foods on the market that contain high levels of trans fatty acids include chips, certain bakery products (biscuits, cakes, wafers, etc.), pies and pirogues, as well as snacks and candies. Pork and chicken contain a lower percentage of trans fatty acids than beef and lamb meat[74]. Game and turkey provide very small amounts.

Monounsaturated fat

Total consumption of monounsaturated fat has varied widely during evolution, depending on the human ecological niche, but has often been low because game meat, fish and shellfish do not contain very large amounts. With a low overall fat consumption, the percentage of monounsaturated fat of the total fat intake may have been at times higher than it is today. Approximately 15–35% of the total muscle fat in wild ruminants is monounsaturated, compared to around 45% in domestic meat[340]. Nuts (apart from coconut), avocado and bone marrow are very rich in monounsaturated fat, mostly more than 60 E%.

Cholesterol content

Cholesterol can be found primarily in animal cell membranes and is completely missing from plant foods. The concentration is particularly high in the musculature of meat and fish, which is why hunter-gatherers have a high intake of cholesterol

Table 3.16 Cholesterol content in selected foods.

	Cholesterol	
	mg/MJ	mg/100 g
Brain	4000	2000
Egg yolk	860	1300
Whitefish roe	680	360
Egg	680	420
Calf liver	590	300
Prawns	430	150
Elk steak, raw	185	107
Cod	158	50
Roast beef	125	70
Salmon	65	35
Cheese, 28% fat	65	100
Skim milk, 0.1% fat	14	2
Plant foods	0	0

Source: Food composition tables, Swedish National Food Administration, 2006; www.slv.se.

(but low serum cholesterol levels, see Section 4.8). Lean types of fish, such as cod and haddock, contain as much cholesterol as meat per unit of energy (Table 3.16).

Carbohydrate content

The amount of carbohydrate varied widely in the ancestral human diets. Whatever standpoint you take in the debate about carbohydrate intake and health, you seem to have a problem with the early man. When fruits or root vegetables were staple foods, carbohydrate intake was high (Table 3.17). Sometimes, honey may have been consumed in considerable amounts for a couple of months, resulting in a high intake of fructose and glucose in roughly equal amounts[43]. In most other habitats it was lower, often much lower, than the average today[338].

Today's energy-dense foods such as breakfast cereals, bread and potatoes, the dominant sources of carbohydrates in the Scandinavian diet, supply carbohydrates in a relatively concentrated form, since water content is relatively low. Glucose was originally a less dominant type of sugar than it is today and refined sugar obviously did not exist.

Carbohydrate quality

Palaeolithic foods often supply carbohydrates in a form that results in a low-to-moderate increase in blood sugar after meals, i.e. that have a low glycaemic index[1790,1791]. Today's dominant plant foods in the Western world, bread, breakfast cereals and potatoes, generally have a high glycaemic index[88,1695]. Some older

Table 3.17 Macronutrient composition in selected vegetables and fruits.

	Protein (E%)	Fat (E%)	Carbohydrate (E%)
Spinach	53	30	16
Cauliflower	48	18	32
Broccoli	45	13	39
Mushrooms	41	17	39
Brussels sprouts	38	7	51
Green beans	35	4	57
Cabbage	25	4	67
Red beets	17	3	75
Raspberries	17	19	60
Onion	16	3	76
Carrots	13	3	79
Netted melon	10	7	77
Grapefruit	9	3	82
Potato	9	1	84
Strawberries	9	10	76
Kiwifruit	8	7	80
Peach	7	2	85
Orange	7	2	85
Watermelon	6	0	88
Plums	6	10	79
Honey dew melon	6	2	86
Avocado	5	84	10
Bananas	4	4	86
Grapes	4	7	83
Pineapple	3	7	84
Apples with peel	3	2	89
Pear	3	6	85
Apple without peel	1	2	91

Source: Food composition tables, Swedish National Food Administration, 2006; www.slv.se.

varieties of potato have a low glycaemic index but these have been successively replaced by new ones, apparently due to taste preferences.

Hence, it is not the sweetness that determines the blood sugar response of carbohydrate foods. Something in the structure has decisive importance, which explains why bread and pasta can sometimes be markedly different, even when they are made from the same flour. The glycaemic index of the same kind of food can vary considerably which makes comparisons difficult[1419].

The term 'glycaemic load' indicates the amount of carbohydrates multiplied by the glycaemic index[88,1071]. Palaeolithic food carries a generally low-to-moderate glycaemic load.

Lactose (milk sugar) was not a part of the Palaeolithic diets since dairy products were absent. Lactose is digested in the small intestine to glucose and galactose by the enzyme lactase, although a significant portion of unhydrolysed lactose may hypothetically be absorbed. Free galactose is transported to the liver where it is converted to glucose, provided that the absorbed amount does not exceed hepatic capacity. The intake of galactose, which is found in minute amounts in other foods, remained low during the evolution of mammals. The percentage of simple sugars, however, was higher at the expense of starches. The starch-rich foodstuffs of the time were primarily roots and root vegetables (today, the dominant starches are grains, maize and potatoes). The percentage of starch with low digestibility (resistant starch) was probably not much higher in the Palaeolithic diet than in today's starch-rich foods. Sucrose intake was low.

Fruits, which have likely been consumed in large quantities by our primate ancestors, differ from other edible plants in that they contain appreciable amounts of fructose, a monosaccharide, which typically constitutes 20–40% of available carbohydrates in wild fruits[456,932,1226] and 10–30% in cultivated fruits[1275]. A daily fructose intake below 60 g, which is considered to be safe, corresponds to 4–5 kg of pineapples[1568,1857]. Approximately two-thirds of dietary fructose in the US population is provided by non-natural foods and additives, mainly sucrose and high fructose corn syrup[1390].

Energy density

With the exception of nuts, most food during the Palaeolithic era was voluminous, water-rich, fibre-rich, and therefore had a low-energy density (Table 3.18). This short and simple statement is possibly one of the more important ones in the book, since it may be of critical importance in terms of preventing excessive energy consumption[818,1526].

Table 3.18   Energy density in selected food groups.

	n	Energy density (MJ/kg)[a]
Vegetables	79	1.5 (1.3)
Root vegetables	13	1.7 (0.8)
Fruits	53	2.3 (0.9)
Nuts	20	23 (5.8)
Wild game	18	5.5 (2.4)
Domestic meat	120	7.7 (3.2)
Organ meats	27	6.1 (1.9)
Fish/shellfish	118	6.7 (3.4)
Cheese	31	11.8 (4.8)
Other dairy foods (except cream)	30	4.1 (4.5)
Fats and oils	58	23.5 (10.6)
Legumes	24	8.1 (4.3)
Bread and cereals	73	12.8 (2.9)
Cakes and biscuits	30	17.0 (3.4)
Sweets and sugar	43	13.2 (6.2)
Honey	1	14

Adapted from www.slv.se.
[a]The values represent mean (SD) values.

Total energy intake

It is obviously not possible to estimate the total caloric intake of prehistoric populations. The average level of physical activity was most certainly higher than in present-day humans[336], indicating that energy intake also was higher. However, the ratio between caloric intake and energy expenditure in hunter-gatherers is not known[1377]. For further discussion of energy intake, see Section 2.4 and Section 4.5.

pH

With the emphasis on the high percentage of potassium-based vegetables and the low percentage of chloride-rich foods, the original human diet was more alkalinising than the current acidifying diet[541,1493,1610]. The hypothesis about diet-dependent acid load has raised a certain amount of interest in recent years within the established scientific community after having been previously viewed with scepticism. A base-producing diet may also potentially prevent osteoporosis (see Section 4.12).

Fibre

With the exception of wild game hunters during the ice age, our ancestors during the Palaeolithic era generally had a high-fibre consumption. However, it was principally soluble fibre coming from fruits, vegetables and root vegetables. Cereals, with the exception of oats, provide primarily insoluble fibres, which have less beneficial metabolic effects[496,516,1780].

Phytochemicals

As previously mentioned, the plant kingdom contains thousands of bioactive substances and other natural chemicals, many of which are thought to be part of their defence systems against herbivores. The highest concentrations are generally found in young plants, also in the most vital parts (sprout, seeds, beans and roots). Such phytochemicals can often make up 5–10% of the plant's dry weight[1406]. Prehistoric foragers were able to limit the negative health effects by having access to a large number of various plant species, by consciously avoiding the most poisonous ones[1836], and by the use of cooking[1971].

Plant lectins are carbohydrate-binding proteins from plants. Strictly, they are defined as 'plant proteins with at least one non-catalytic domain that is bound reversibly to a specific mono or oligosaccharide'[1848]. They bind to certain sugars because they contain carbohydrate residues themselves, i.e. they are glycated (=glycosylated). The most important function of plant lectins is thought to be protection against attacks by plant-eating animals[299]. The highest concentration is found in seeds, beans, potatoes and peanuts. Unrefined grain products, on the whole, have a higher lectin content than refined seed products. Lectins in wheat, rye, rice and potatoes bind to GlcNAc-domains (GlcNAc = N-acetylglucosamine) on receptors in the 'host organism' (Table 3.19). Lectins are often not destroyed

Table 3.19 Plant lectins in selected seeds and beans.

Food	Lectin	Specificity
Wheat	Wheat germ agglutinin, WGA	$(GlcNAc)_n > GlcNAc > NANA$
Rye	Rye lectin, Secale cereale agglutinin, SCA	$GlcNAc, (GlcNAc)_n$
Barley	Hordeum vulgare agglutinin, HVA	$GlcNAc, (GlcNAc)_n$
Potato	Solanum tuberosum agglutinin, STA (STL)	$(GlcNAc)_n$
Rice	Rice lectin, Oryza sativa agglutinin, OSA	$GlcNAc, (GlcNAc)_n$
Peanuts	Peanut agglutinin*, PNA	Gal > GalNac
Jack beans	Concanavalin A, ConA	Man > Glc > GlcNAc
Soya bean	Soya bean agglutinin*, SBA	GalNac (>Gal)
Turkish beans	Phaseolus vulgaris agglutinin, PHA*	Complex specificity
Lentils	Lens culinaris agglutinin, LCA	Man > Glc > GlcNAc

>, the lectin binds stronger to the substance before the asterisk. GlcNAc, N-acetyl glucosamine; $(GlcNAc)_n$; oligomers of GlcNAc; NANA, N-acetylneuraminic acid/sialic acid; Gal, galactose; GalNac, N-acetyl galactosamine; *, one of many lectins, mannose; Glc, glucose.

during normal cooking. Cooking beans in a pressure cooker deactivates their lectin, which has been shown for Turkish beans[609] and which is expected to be true for most plant lectins.

Plant lectins are, compared to other dietary proteins, unusually resistant to enzymatic breakdown in the intestines and can penetrate the intestinal mucous membrane, finally being deposited in the internal organs. The ability to avoid destruction and be absorbed in the intestines makes plant lectins excellent carriers for pharmaceutical substances[559]. The deposition in internal organs is useful for histochemical identification of specific cell systems in the microscope[264]. A well-studied effect of a number of plant lectins is agglutination of red blood cells. The long-term, potentially negative effects of lectins on humans are addressed in the sections on atherosclerosis (Section 4.3), insulin resistance (Section 4.6), cancer (Section 4.11) and autoimmunity (Section 4.15).

During the Palaeolithic period, plant lectins were consumed on a daily basis, but probably not in the same, high concentrations of today, and not exclusively from one or a few plant species.

Protease inhibitors are substances in beans and seeds, which inhibit protein-degrading enzymes in the digestive tract such as trypsin, chymotrypsin and amylase. This very ancient defence mechanism of plants allows their seeds to pass through the entire gastrointestinal system (mouth–oesophagus–stomach–gut) undamaged, thereby surviving excretion and later to grow in the ground. The concentration of protease inhibitors in beans and cereals is so high that the digestion of dietary proteins (including other than those in the seed) can be substantially reduced[329].

Endocrine disruptors such as phytoestrogens constitute another kind of defence mechanism in the plant's struggle for survival[1976]. These hormone-like substances can interfere with the consumer's reproductive system, in which case the defence strategy may be to cause infertility rather than death. It has been suggested that isoflavones (also called flavonoids), the phytoestrogens that appear in large amounts in cereals exert an antioxidative effect, but good evidence is still lacking[754,1714].

Other hormone-like plant sterols have the effect of reducing blood lipids by hampering cholesterol absorption in the intestines[1323].

Cyanogenic glycosides are produced by more than 2500 plant species. Their production and conversion to cyanide constitutes a well-studied defence mechanism against herbivores[596]. Cyanide can be acutely toxic when consumed in high amounts, but more relevant in this context is when it is ingested regularly in low concentrations. Cyanide is then converted to thiocyanate, a potentially goitrogenic substance which can increase the need for dietary iodine and may cause goitre, even when iodine intake is high. These are well-documented consequences of certain staple foods in the Third World such as cassava, bamboo shoots, sweet potatoes, lima beans and millet. Out of the foods listed, only the edible parts of the cassava plant contain large amounts of thiocyanate, otherwise the problem is by most authors considered negligible and is not thought to be a contributing cause of goitre in Europe[397]. Even linseeds contain cyanogenic glycosides. The National Swedish Food Administration has issued a warning against consuming more than 1–2 tablespoons of linseeds on a daily basis, since 10 tablespoons daily caused mild neurological symptoms in one human, most likely through cyanide exposure (www.slv.se, in Swedish). The long-term effects of a low intake are unknown.

Pyrrolizidine alkaloids are a large group of chemicals that are produced by over 6000 plant species, some of which are used for food or herbal teas[812]. Low-level exposure to pyrrolizidine alkaloids is suspected as the underlying cause of endemic cirrhosis in certain cultural groups in Asia and Africa. The high rate of primary liver cancer in South Africa may be due to chronic low-level pyrrolizidine alkaloids. Other organs that are thought to be affected are kidneys, stomach, brain, lungs, heart and the reproductive system.

Phytic acid is found in seeds (including beans) with the aim of binding phosphorus and other minerals. The case of phytic acid may be an exception to a common rule in plant–animal interactions, that bioactive plant constituents are designed to damage the consuming 'host'. Apparently, in the case of phytate, the damage is only coincidental. When phytic acid is consumed, it binds to dietary minerals and trace metals such as iron, zinc, calcium and magnesium, to form phytate salts with these ions. As a consequence, these nutrients largely pass unabsorbed through the intestines and are excreted.

Since phytic acid is mainly found in the germ part of the seed, whole grain flour is unhealthier than refined flour in this respect. However, the seed also contains phytases that can break down the phytic acid under beneficial circumstances[259,985,1278,1570,1749]. In the best case, if the seeds are tossed in the right way, soaked and allowed to sit at proper temperature and pH for a sufficient number of hours (or days), the phytic acid can almost be eliminated. The various types of grains distinguish themselves in that, out of our four most popular cereals, it is most difficult to reduce phytic acid in oats. In today's industrially produced, rolled oats, the phytases are completely destroyed, which means that it is then impossible to reduce the phytic acid content[1569,1573]. In contrast with humans, rats have a high capacity to degrade phytates in their intestines, an apparent adaptation to regular consumption of seeds[797].

Acrylamide is formed during baking or high-temperature cooking (frying, grilling, deep-fat frying) of starchy foods, i.e. heating the surface of the food. This type of food treatment was probably uncommon during the Palaeolithic (apart from roasting carbohydrate-free foodstuffs like meat and fish). Heating meat and fish does not form acrylamide. In terms of Western food, crisps and chips have the highest amount of acrylamide, while bread, breakfast cereals and hash browns are the dominant sources of acrylamide for the average European. Acrylamide has been proposed to cause cancer, based on experiments on animals, but the connection is uncertain[1647].

Knowledge of the health effects of bioactive substances is fragmentary, and in many cases, it lacks the perspective of evolutionary biology. Research about alkyl-resorcinols and biogenic amines has concentrated on the detrimental aspects, while research on hormone-like substances and antioxidants most often has highlighted the alleged beneficial effects.

4 Modern diseases

This chapter deals with the potential prevention and treatment of common diseases in the modern world by choosing food similar to those available to ancient humans. In most cases, it is difficult, if not impossible, to gain any information about diseases among prehistoric hunter-gatherers because they seldom left any clues in the fossil record. Studies of contemporary populations with a similar lifestyle, however, strongly suggest that our modern, Western lifestyle is a very important factor in some of our most common diseases. Our own study population from Kitava, Trobriand Islands, Papua New Guinea, is discussed at length in various contexts, not because they are the optimal representatives of human's original lifestyle but because they are well characterised and because they clearly show the possibility of preventing Western disease.

A widespread misunderstanding about the lifespan of Palaeolithic humans should be addressed. It is undeniable that the average lifespan was low due to high infant and child mortality. However, at the age of 50 years, life expectancy for a Palaeolithic human was not necessarily lower than for a modern European, i.e. people who reached this age may have had a good chance of reaching 80–90 years. The average age at death in children (± a few years) and young adults (±10 years) can be estimated relatively accurately from fossil skeletons. After middle age, however, it becomes more difficult, and osteologists used to avoid making estimates any closer than simply saying '40 years or older' by using the term 'adultus'[800,1267,1581]. Whether a person reached 40 or 90 years of age could, thus, in many cases not be determined. In addition, the total number of Palaeolithic skeletons is far too low to permit any reliable comparisons of the number of elderly compared to middle-aged and young individuals.

Moreover, the skeletal material analysed is often not representative of the people that actually lived at the site. This is particularly the case if the skeleton comes from a person who was not buried, but rather was left where he died. Therefore, the probability that bones would be preserved and later recovered is very small indeed, and the special circumstances that are needed for this to occur can highly affect the available selection. For these reasons, the view that prehistoric humans always had short lives can be considered a poorly substantiated myth.

I am now changing the definition of Palaeolithic diet so that it no longer stands for the diet of prehistoric hunter-gatherers, rather it includes a modern equivalent that can be purchased in any European grocery store. A Palaeolithic diet is principally based on lean meat, fish, lots of cultivated fruits and vegetables, with a lesser amount of root vegetables, eggs and nuts.

Smoking habits, physical activity and genetics play a large role in many of the diseases to be discussed, as stated in most text books and review articles. However, I have decided to concentrate on diet and avoid commenting on these other factors. This should not be interpreted to mean that I am attributing little significance to them. On the contrary, I see it as critically important to avoid smoking and be physically active, particularly if you eat a Western diet.

As already mentioned, heredity does not exclude environment. Those who have the most to benefit from eating a Palaeolithic diet are the ones with familial tendency. The other ones, whose parents and grandparents were healthy and vital long after the age of 90 years, have a slightly greater chance of staying healthy on a Western diet.

4.1   Ischaemic heart disease (coronary heart disease)

Ischaemic heart disease is the most common type of cardiovascular disease and includes angina pectoris (chest pain due to coronary atherosclerosis) and myocardial infarction (heart attacks). The principal cause, atherosclerosis, which affects the majority of Westerners, is addressed separately in Section 4.3. The risk factors are discussed in later sections.

Incidence studies

The occurrence of ischaemic heart disease varies so widely between different countries that lifestyle obviously is a significant factor. Among populations with a Western lifestyle, the prevalence is lowest in Japan and highest in countries such as Finland, Great Britain, Sweden and the former Eastern Block countries (www.who.int).

Ischaemic heart disease is particularly rare in populations that are not under the influence of the Western lifestyle, which has been noted in a number of clinical investigations and autopsy studies in Melanesia, Malaysia, Africa, South America and the Arctic[24,99,117,126,215,255,302,320,375,407,408,429,434,454,470,620,764,798,875,940,961,1157,1263, 1347,1369,1374,1430,1482,1486,1589,1613,1632,1665,1698,1774,1788,1812,1814,1817,1870,1871,1888,1937].

A British autopsy study in Uganda, East Africa, at the beginning of the 1950s revealed only 1 in 1427 people (0.7%) above the age of 40 years with histologic signs of previous myocardial infarction[1788]. Among age-matched subjects in the USA, a high occurrence of a previous myocardial infarction was noted (Table 4.1). Consequently, a lack of elderly people does not explain the absence of ischaemic heart disease in populations without a Western lifestyle.

Table 4.1 Percentage of deceased men in USA and Uganda (1951–1956) with signs of previous myocardial infarction at autopsy[1788].

Age (years)	USA	Uganda
40–49	31 of 178 (17%)	0 of 178 (0%)
50–59	51 of 199 (26%)	1 of 199 (0.5%)
60–69	32 of 98 (33%)	0 of 98 (0%)
70–79	8 of 24 (33%)	0 of 33 (0%)
80+	2 of 9 (22%)	0 of 9 (0%)

Roughly two dozen studies from Papua New Guinea paint the same clear picture; prior to urbanisation, myocardial infarctions were unknown among the local population. These studies include two systematic reviews of 2000 and 3999 hospital case records respectively, completed during the first half of the twentieth century[255,408].

Additional support came from three systematic interviews in the original home environment[1041,1666,1817]. Sinnett noted no occurrence of retrosternal chest pains matching angina pectoris among the Murapin people in the highlands of Papua New Guinea[1666]. However, it is difficult to distinguish these pains from musculoskeletal pain in the rib cage during an interview.

Truswell found no evidence of sudden, spontaneous death when interviewing 96 adults among the San Bushmen, hunter-gatherers in Botswana, South Africa[1817]. Our own study from Kitava, Papua New Guinea, is probably the most comprehensive, systematic investigation of cardiovascular disease in a traditional environment. While their distinctive dietary habits should not be taken too seriously when considering the optimal human diet, as already stated, they do add to the evidence that coronary heart disease is fully preventable.

The Kitava study, Trobriand Islands

During an inventory in 1989, we found what appears to be one of the last populations on Earth with dietary habits matching what would have been the case for the population of *Homo sapiens* in their original habitats on the island of Kitava, one of the Trobriand Islands in Papua New Guinea's archipelago (see Figures 4.1–4.4). The Trobriander people have been thoroughly studied by social anthropologists and human ethologists such as Malinowski, Powell, Weiner and Schiefenhövel[1119–1126,1195,1234,1441–1444,1591–1593,1650,1919,1920], but medical reports have been few[855,1712].

The residents of Kitava subsisted exclusively on root vegetables (yam, sweet potato, taro, tapioca), fruits (banana, papaya, pineapple, mango, guava, water melon, pumpkin), vegetables, fish and coconuts[1051,1052,1055]. Less than 0.2% of the caloric intake came from Western food, such as edible fats, dairy products, refined sugar, cereals and alcohol, compared with roughly 75% in Sweden[136]. The intake of vitamins, minerals and soluble fibre was therefore very high, while the total fat consumption was low, about 20 E%[1055], as was the intake of salt (40–50 mmol Na/10 MJ compared with 100–250 in the Western world). Due to the high

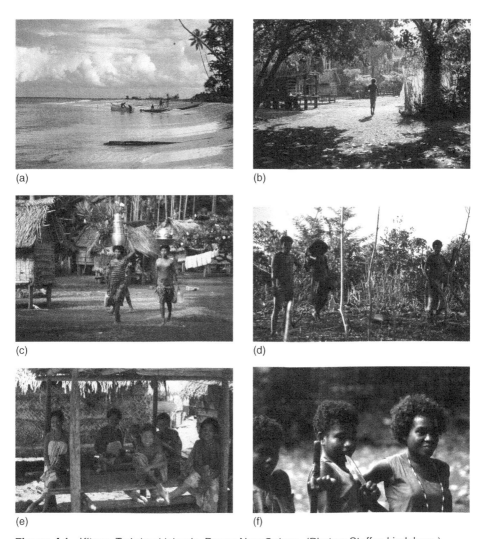

(a)

(b)

(c)

(d)

(e)

(f)

Figure 4.1   Kitava, Trobriand Islands, Papua New Guinea. (Photos: Staffan Lindeberg.)

level of coconut consumption, saturated fat made up an equally large portion of the overall caloric intake as is the case in the West. However, lauric acid was the dominant dietary saturated fatty acid as opposed to palmitic acid in Western countries. Malnutrition and famine did not seem to occur.

We noted a lack of sudden cardiac death and exertion-related retrosternal chest pain among Kitava's 2300 inhabitants (6% of which were 60–95 years old), as well as among the remaining 23 000 people on the Trobriand Islands[1041,1050].

Despite a fair number of elderly residents, none of whom showed signs of dementia or poor memory, the only cases of sudden death they could recall were accidents such as drowning or falling from a coconut tree. Homicide also occurred,

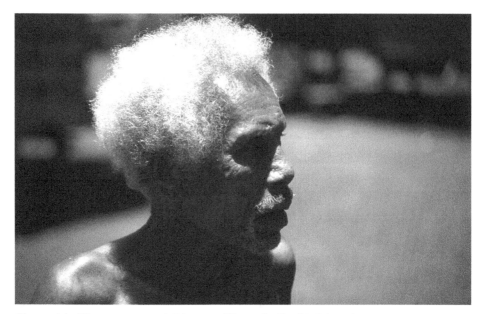

Figure 4.2   Kitavan man aged 100 years. (Photo: Staffan Lindeberg.)

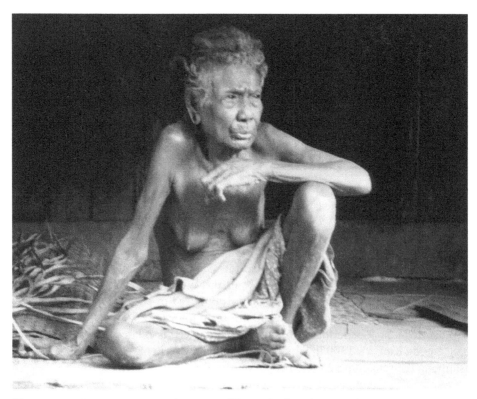

Figure 4.3   Kitavan woman aged 94 years. (Photo: Staffan Lindeberg.)

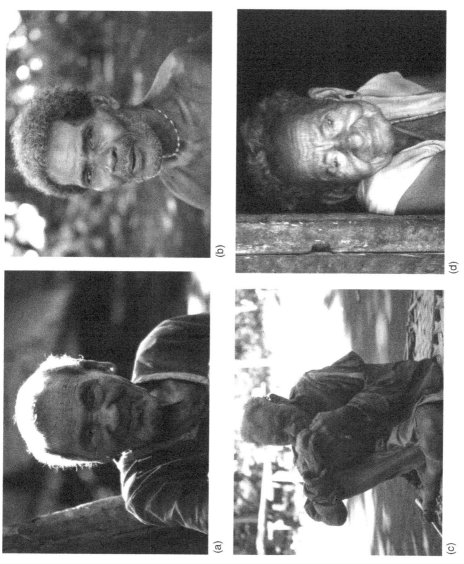

Figure 4.4 Four Kitavans aged 71–96 years. (Photos: Staffan Lindeberg.)

often during conflicts over land or mates. Infections (primarily malaria), accidents, pregnancy complications and old age were the dominant causes of death, which is in agreement with findings among other similar populations. Child mortality from malaria and other infections was relatively high, and the average lifespan was around 45 years. The remaining life expectancy at 45 years of age is more difficult to determine, but may be similar to European figures. The number of people examined with an electrocardiograph (ECG) was too small ($n = 171$) to allow for clear conclusions, but when combined with two similar studies of traditional Melanesian populations, the ECG findings provided additional support for the lack of ischaemic heart disease in the area[1369,1669].

Our age estimates were based on known historical events: (1) The arrival of Cyril Cameron, a white man from Tasmania, who established a coconut farm in 1912 and remained on the island until his death, (2) American and Australian military occupation of the area during World War II from 1942 to 1943, (3) The founding of an elementary school in 1962 and (4) Cameron's death and burial on the island in 1966. Everyone above 35 years of age could clearly remember one or more of these events, and their personal experience matched information from relatives and friends. The oldest living person during the survey was a 96-year-old woman, and during a previous visit a vital 100-year-old man was interviewed.

There is no evidence to suggest that the people who died before the age of 60 are the ones who would have otherwise suffered from cardiovascular disease. Although bacterial infections are discussed as possible (co)factors in atherosclerosis, infections which can be treated with antibiotics, the idea that present use of antibiotics in Western societies would effectively prevent ischaemic heart disease before the age of 60 is not plausible considering the remarkably high prevalence of atherosclerosis in this part of the world (see Section 4.3). Furthermore, our findings cannot be explained by positing that the truth has not been exposed. The most serious diseases that actually did occur were described carefully and in an identical manner for each of the various villages. This afforded us some measure of quality control.

The elderly residents of Kitava generally remain quite active up until the very end, when they begin to suffer fatigue for a few days and then die from what appears to be an infection or some type of rapid degeneration. Although this is seen in Western societies, it is relatively rare in elderly vital people. The quality of life among the oldest residents thus appeared to be good in the Trobriand Islands.

The main results of the Kitava study, that there is no ischaemic heart disease (and no stroke; see Section 4.2), are unanimously confirmed by medical experts with knowledge of the Trobriand Islands or other parts of Melanesia. Likewise, Jüptner noted no cases of angina pectoris, myocardial infarction or sudden death during his 5 years as a general practitioner on the islands at the beginning of the 1960s, when the population was roughly 12 000 (H. Jüptner, unpublished data). His experience is based partly on patients that visited him due to illness, and partly from systematic health examinations given in all the different villages at three separate times. The same observation was made by Schiefenhövel, physician and human ethologist from the Max Planck Institute in Munich (W. Schiefenhövel, unpublished data). He can speak the language of the Trobrianders, Kilivila, and has his own hut on Kaileuna, one of the Trobriand Islands, where he examined close to 3000 patients during his repeated visits over the course of close to 15 years. Like Jüptner, he is very familiar with the nature of cardiovascular disease and did not see any cases of the disease.

Effects of urbanisation

The emergence of ischaemic heart disease has been well documented in a number of populations after switching to a Western lifestyle[133,324,348,521,794, 897,1332,1396,1399,1450,1667,1771,1814,2008]. The first case of a myocardial infarction in New Guinea, which was verified with an autopsy, was reported in 1955. Individual cases were seen during the 1960s and 1970s[324,1698] and the number has gradually increased since then[898]. Among blacks in Africa, the first case of classic angina pectoris was recorded in 1958 in an overweight housewife with free access to Western food[578]. Later autopsy studies appeared to indicate that myocardial infarctions were more common among people with a higher income[477].

Hence, genetic factors cannot explain the lack of ischaemic heart disease in traditional cultures. Instead, heredity is an important cause of the variation in risk for ischaemic heart disease *within* a limited urbanised population, which has been shown to be the case in a number of different ethnic groups. To the extent that genetic differences between different ethnic populations exist, they are more likely to show that Europeans have a somewhat higher resistance to urbanisation than other groups (see Section 4.6).

Relevant dietary factors

Dietary habits among aboriginal populations with a documented absence of ischaemic heart disease, and/or beneficial cardiovascular risk factors, have been very different from those in the West. Their staple diet most often was based on foods that could have been part of a Palaeolithic diet. The majority of these populations had a high intake of meat or fish, while vegetables were the dominant food among some ethnic groups. Dairy products, refined fats, sugar and grains were completely missing, without exception. It is very difficult to get a well-grounded understanding of which individual foods and nutrients could be significant. In Western populations, primary prevention programmes with lifestyle modification have not been very effective, as disclosed below, and there is a need for improvement of heart-healthy dietary advice.

The following section focuses on dietary factors which are, or have been, thought to be directly related to ischaemic heart disease. Additional research related to atherosclerosis, the predominant diet-related process behind ischaemic heart disease, or risk factors such as abdominal obesity, increased blood pressure, dyslipidaemia or type 2 diabetes are discussed separately in Sections 4.3–4.8.

At present, there is uncertainty among health professionals around some of the dietary advice that has been given for the last decades in order to prevent ischaemic heart disease. Most of the current confusion relates to the intake of total fat, saturated fat, total carbohydrate, certain vitamins, eggs, milk and meat. Although there is broad consensus that vegetables and fruits are healthy, there is surprisingly little solid evidence behind any proposed food model.

Mediterranean diet

The Mediterranean diet has become the most popular diet model for the prevention of ischaemic heart disease. It was first advocated in the 1950s by Ancel Keys, the leading architect of the idea that saturated fat causes atherosclerosis[322,901]. The incidence of ischaemic heart disease in the Mediterranean countries of Europe on the whole was lower than in northern Europe up until the latter part of the twentieth century[1207]. Many experts think that this is largely due to their dietary habits. However, the extent of coronary atherosclerosis has apparently been the same as in northern Europe, at least during the late twentieth century[161]. There has also been a marked variation between different Mediterranean countries in terms of both diet and incidence of myocardial infarction. Even in Crete, one study suggests that type 2 diabetes and ischaemic heart disease are common today[1058]. The diet has varied in contents of fat, olive oil, meat, wine, milk, cheese, fruits and vegetables. Dietary habits have varied even within individual regions[859]. Greek food from the first half of the twentieth century has remained the model for what we call today the 'Mediterranean diet', as in the Lyon study discussed below[387]. The Greek diet was rich in fruit, especially wild plants, nuts and cereals, olive oil, olives, cheese, fish, meat and moderate amounts of wine[1656]. The Mediterranean diet is similar to the Palaeolithic diet in some respects.

A recent meta-analysis of observational studies, including 12 studies of 1.5 million people followed for 3–18 years, found a 9% reduced cardiovascular mortality with a high consumption of components considered to be part of a Mediterranean diet (vegetables, fruits, legumes, cereals, fish and a moderate intake of red wine during meals)[1694]. Half of the studies were from the USA, one from Australia and the rest from Europe. Another meta-analysis found a slightly greater risk reduction in people with Mediterranean-like food habits[1211]. Due to the widespread belief that Mediterranean-type foods are healthy, the risk of residual confounding is obvious.

In the Lyon Diet Heart Trial, a secondary preventive, randomised, single-blind dietary intervention trial in France, 605 men and women below the age of 70, who had undergone their first myocardial infarction, were randomly assigned either a 'Mediterranean diet' (intervention group) or a traditional low-fat, high-fibre diet according to the American Heart Association guidelines (control group)[386,388]. The intervention group received margarine made from rapeseed oil (also known as canola oil), as well as advice about increasing their intake of vegetables, fruits and whole grains. The control group received usual care and were thus less intensively educated about healthy diets, which is a methodological problem. During the follow-up period (5 years), 8 out of 303 people in the intervention group died, compared to 20 out of 302 in the control group (relative risk of death 0.30;

0.11–0.82; $P = 0.02$), of which respectively 3 and 16 died of cardiovascular disease ($P = 0.02$). The number of serious cardiovascular events was 8 and 33 respectively, (relative risk 0.27; 0.12–0.59; $P = 0.001$). The intervention group (but not the control group) showed an increase in the concentration of the omega-3 fatty acid α-linolenic acid (18:3 omega-3) and ascorbic acid in blood plasma (the fluid part of blood).

Hence, the study was very successful in terms of health benefits, although the wide confidence intervals (CI 0.11–0.82 for relative risk of death) make it uncertain how successful it were. The groups were not different at follow-up in terms of blood lipids, body weight or blood pressure, which highlights the significance of other effects of diet, regardless of these cardiovascular risk factors. Although the effect of omega-3 fat was not studied separately, this trial is sometimes cited as evidence of a benefit of omega-3 fats, which is questionable in the light of other trials on omega-3 fats (see section 'Fatty fish' below). The study's weaknesses are that the intervention group received more intensive behavioural modification and the total number of events in both groups was low.

In the THIS-DIET trial, 101 patients with myocardial infarction were randomised to follow a Mediterranean diet ($n = 51$) or a low-fat diet ($n = 50$) and were compared with 101 usual-care patients in a case–control design ($n = 101$)[1830]. The occurrence of cardiovascular disease during a median follow-up time of 46 months was 8 in each of the dietary intervention groups and 40 in the usual-care group ($P < 0.001$). Seven deaths occurred, all in the usual-care group ($P = 0.014$).

In conclusion, a Mediterranean-style diet appears to confer some protection against ischaemic heart disease, compared to an average Western diet.

Fatty fish (omega-3 fats)

The widespread notion that ischaemic heart disease is partly prevented by consumption of fatty fish 2–3 times a week (compared to no fish) because it is rich in long-chain omega-3 fatty acids has been challenged in a Cochrane meta-analysis of randomised controlled trials[756,757]. This concept originally emerged from the observed very low incidence of myocardial infarction and sudden cardiac death as well as the long bleeding time among the Eskimos of Greenland and Canada[105,1588]. Of all the characteristics of Eskimo dietary habits that could possibly explain these findings, virtually all focus has been on omega-3 fatty acids, while the absence of cereals, dairy products, refined fats, sugar and added salt has rarely been considered.

There are as yet three controlled trials where the effect of increased consumption of fatty fish on cardiovascular disease has been documented, as well as many trials on supplemental omega-3 fats[756]. In the secondary preventive Diet and Re-infarction Trial (DART), 2033 British men who had suffered a myocardial infarction were randomly assigned either a high intake of fatty fish at least twice a week or a regular diet[242]. After 2 years, a total of 94/1015 patients in the fish group had died, compared with 130/1018 in the control group ($P = 0.02$, for the difference between the groups, i.e. the probability that the difference is random is 2 in 100).

There were 78 cardiovascular deaths in the fish group and 116 in the control group ($P = 0.01$). However, in an extended follow-up study among the same persons, running until February 2000 (21 147 person-years), where 1083 men (53%) had died from any cause, the difference in favour of fatty fish no longer appeared to be the case. In contrast, the overall mortality in the fish group was higher than among controls (relative risk 1.31; 95% CI 1.01–1.70)[1285].

A second dietary trial from the same research group recruited 3114 men under 70 years of age with stable angina pectoris[241]. In the trial, which is sometimes called DART 2, the participants were randomly given one of four kinds of advice: (1) two portions of oily fish each week or three fish oil capsules daily, (2) more fruits, vegetables and oats, (3) both the above types of advice or (4) no specific dietary advice. In Group 1, fish oil capsules were supplied to men who were advised to eat fish but found it unpalatable. During the second phase of the trial, the 'fish advice' group was subrandomised to receive either fish advice or capsules. No significant effect was seen on total mortality, which was ascertained after 3–9 years. Risk of cardiac death was higher in the fish/supplement group than among those not advised to eat fish; the relative risk was 1.26 (95% CI 1.00–1.58; $P = 0.047$), and even greater for sudden cardiac death (1.54; 95% CI 1.06–2.23; $P = 0.025$). The excess risk was more evident among the 462 subjects taking fish oil capsules where the relative risk of cardiac death was 1.45 (95% CI 1.05–1.99; $P = 0.024$) as compared to 1.20 (95% CI .93–1.53; $P = 0.16$) in the real fish group. There are a number of possible explanations for the higher risk in those taking fish/fish oil, which are thoroughly discussed in the paper[241], one being risk compensation (i.e. increased risk-taking behaviour due to the feeling of belonging to the 'safe' group), a general problem with non-blinded trials.

The third controlled fish trial was small and included only 38 low-risk participants with inactive Crohn's disease and was primarily not designed to study the effect on cardiovascular disease (Maté-Jimenez et al, cited by [756]). No case of ischaemic heart disease was documented in either group during 24 months of follow-up.

Among 44 high-quality randomised controlled trials comparing at least 6 months of supplemental omega-3 fats (from capsules or oil) with placebo, there was no evidence of a lower risk of cardiovascular disease in those taking omega-3 fats[756]. Small trials were more likely to show an effect than large ones, suggesting publication bias with a number of negative small trials being unpublished. Large trials in this meta-analysis, and in others,[2016,2017] suggest that there is no clinically important preventive effect against coronary heart disease from omega-3 supplements. Five of the 44 studies provided omega-3 fats in the form of plant-based α-linolenic acid.

In contrast to these findings in intervention trials, several epidemiological observational studies have found an approximately 20% lower cardiovascular risk among Westerners who eat fatty fish at least twice a week, than among those who do not[772,1595]. However, the relationship between fatty fish and cardiovascular disease may only be evident in high-risk populations[1147].

In the light of the negative controlled trials, these findings suggest the presence of confounding factors, such that fish eaters take other preventive measures that may be more important. This would explain the substantial reduction in the association between fish intake and cardiovascular disease after adjustment for other markers of a healthy lifestyle, even in today's Japan[804].

Early studies suggested that realistic doses of fish reduce the risk of cardiac arrest from ventricular fibrillation, a major cause of sudden death[399]. However, three recent randomised placebo-controlled trials with fish oil among patients with an implantable cardioverter defibrillator, who are at very high risk of cardiac arrest, found no reduced incidence of serious arrhythmia[224]. In the first of these studies, recurrent ventricular arrythmia was more common in patients randomised to receive fish oil ($P = 0.001$)[1468], but this was not replicated in the two later studies[224].

In summary, there is presently no convincing evidence from randomised controlled trials in favour of a high intake of omega-3 fatty acids, neither from fish nor as dietary supplement, in the prevention of ischaemic heart disease.

Vegetables and fruits

Since many years, there is considerable agreement that vegetables and fruits are heart-friendly. However, it is still not known why this would be the case. Several of the minerals and vitamins that are supposed to protect against cardiovascular disease (see under 'Vitamins, minerals and trace elements'), appear in large amounts in fruits and even more in vegetables, but none of them has so far been proven to be protective against cardiovascular disease when given in double-blind placebo-controlled trials[1175].

The notion that a high consumption of fruits and vegetables has a preventive effect is to some extent supported by the Lyon Diet Heart Study (described under 'Mediterranean diet'). However, it is unknown to what extent other dietary changes explain the beneficial results in this trial. In addition, two dietary intervention studies from Moradabad, India, have been regarded as supportive[1661,1662]. Unfortunately, the first author of these two papers, published in the *British Medical Journal* and the *Lancet*, has been suspected of scientific fraud, and both papers were later questioned in editorials appearing simultaneously in the two journals[30,766,1686,1930].

There is one published controlled trial in which the advice to increase fruit intake was given randomly to men under 70 years of age with angina pectoris, the DART 2 study described under 'Fatty fish'. Control subjects were told to 'eat sensibly' without any specific advice. Despite a slightly lower percentage reporting a previous heart attack among fruit eaters, after 3–9 years of follow-up 25 more persons had died in this group than in the control group ($P = 0.07$). The total number of deaths after fruit advice was 275 (17.3%) compared to 250 (16.4%) among those who were not given such advice. The number of cardiac deaths was identical in the two groups. Advice to eat more fruit was considered by the authors to be poorly complied with, despite a 30% increase in estimated intake of vitamin C. The negative effect of fruit advice in this important trial is unexpected and it may, similar to the effect of fish advice in the same trial, be explained by risk compensation or some other effect on patients' or doctors' behaviour. Nevertheless, the study suggests that any beneficial effects of realistic amounts of fruits are small.

Epidemiological population studies indicate that roughly 15% of the variation in ischaemic heart disease in the West could be explained by differences in the intake of vegetables and fruits (or some unidentified confounder)[998,1284,1509]. Overall, 14 of the 25 published observational studies point to a primary preventive effect from fruits and vegetables[305]. Estimates of the actual size of the preventive effect are very uncertain, since this involves asking individual questions regarding dietary habits many years prior to the development of the disease.

In the American First National Health and Nutrition Examination Survey (NHANES I) Epidemiological Follow-up Study, 9608 people between the ages of 25 and 74 years, who were free of known cardiovascular disease at the start, were asked about their consumption of fruits and vegetables[132]. During an average follow-up period of 19 years, 1786 cases of new ischaemic heart disease were documented, of which 639 became fatal. The number of deaths from any cause was 2530. Subjects who initially indicated that they ate fruits and vegetables at least 3 times/day, compared with less than once a day, had a 24% lower mortality due to ischaemic heart disease (relative risk 0.76; 95% CI 0.56–1.03; P for trend = 0.07) and 15% lower overall mortality (relative risk 0.85; 95% CI 0.72–1.00; P for trend = 0.02) after correcting for established cardiovascular risk factors.

Similar results come from the Nurses' Health Study and Health Professionals' Follow-up Study on just over 126 000 people, with a relative risk for developing ischaemic heart disease of 0.80 (95% CI 0.69–0.93) in the highest quintile of fruit and vegetable consumption, i.e. 20% of the population that had the highest intake[851].

In summary, it is likely that a high intake of vegetables and fruits have a slight preventive effect against ischaemic heart disease, in particular compared to rarely consuming them. However, it is uncertain if this is due to some inherent properties of these foods or because they replace other, unhealthy foods. The possibility of confounding of other healthy lifestyle characteristics cannot be ruled out.

Vegetarianism

Vegetarians, in general, are thought to be at lower risk for developing cardiovascular disease than people who eat a mixed diet. It increasingly appears that this is more due to a healthy lifestyle in general, including high consumption of vegetables and fruits, rather than due to the absence of meat[452,1792]. A meta-analysis compiled 5 prospective observational studies, with a total of 76 000 men and women, of which almost 28 000 were vegetarians in the sense that they did not eat meat or fish[900]. A total of 2264 persons died of ischaemic heart disease. In these studies, vegetarians had, on average, a 24% lower risk of dying from ischaemic heart disease than non-vegetarians (relative risk 0.76; 95% CI 0.62–0.94; P <0.01), but the total mortality (regardless of the cause) was not lower (relative risk 0.95; 95% CI 0.82–1.11). Those persons who had been vegetarians for less than 5 years did not have a lower relative risk of dying from ischaemic heart disease (1.20; 95% CI 0.90–1.61), but the number of such cases of death was only 49, compared to 625 among those who had been vegetarians for a longer period of time (because many more such people were included in the study). In the two British studies (which had the longest average follow-up period, 18.4 and 13.7 years respectively), vegetarianism did not show any preventive effects in terms of cardiac-related death. The relative risk in one study (Health Food Shoppers Study) was 0.97 (95% CI 0.81–1.16), and in the other (Oxford Vegetarian Study) it was 0.90 (95% CI 0.68–1.20), both non-significant[63].

In a later analysis of the two English studies, the total mortality among vegetarians as well as control subjects was only 52% of the average in Great Britain (relative risk of death 0.52; 95% CI 0.49–0.56)[63]. The fact that there was not very much difference between the vegetarians and the non-vegetarians probably is due to the recruitment process and it seems to indicate the importance of a healthy lifestyle in general. In the Health Food Shoppers Study, both groups were recruited from people who were interested in health food, and in the Oxford Vegetarian Study, subjects were recruited via the Vegetarian Society and by advertising in the mass media, where non-vegetarians were recruited from the friends and family of the vegetarians. This seems to indicate that other lifestyle factors than the absence of meat are of significance.

Meat

Randomised controlled trials of the effects on ischaemic heart disease of changes in meat consumption are lacking. Hunter-gatherers have had exceptionally favourable levels of blood lipids, even with very high meat consumption (see Section 4.8). Blood pressure, glucose tolerance (ability to metabolise glucose) and body weight were also at very advantageous levels, which is discussed in later sections. However, their meat had a lower fat content and a higher percentage of omega-3 fatty acids than our domesticated meat[340,1143,1277].

An association between ischaemic heart disease and reported consumption of meat/meat products has been found in a few case–control studies[938], while other epidemiological studies have been less convincing[1211,1248]. The perception among laymen that meat and meat products is unhealthy is strongly linked to other concepts of a healthy lifestyle[1002], and the risk of confounding is particularly high in case–control studies[1687]. In the 25-year follow-up of the European Seven-Countries Study, 42% of the variation in mortality from ischaemic heart disease was statistically explained by differences in the intake of meat and meat products combined, but after adjustment for differences in other dietary factors no correlation was present, and now only butter and lard/margarine remained as explanatory variables[1207]. Similar results were noted during an extended 10-year follow-up study, where the correlation with meat disappeared altogether, while a relationship with milk remained evident when both meat and milk were included in the analysis[902]. In these studies, as well as many other observational studies, unprocessed meat was not separated from meat products such as sausage and liverwurst, and sometimes meat products were not even separated from milk products, which makes it difficult to interpret the results.

The further categorisation into red meat and white meat comes from American terminology. Red meat refers to beef, pork, lamb, roe deer, elk, etc. Chicken, turkey and other fowl are considered white meat. Ostrich meat is usually included in the red meat category because of its colour even though the ostrich is a bird. Leading experts in the USA customarily see red meat as a contributing factor for ischaemic heart disease, but the epidemiological connections are not consistent, and there is a lack of evidence to show that other nutrients besides fat, or other substances in meat, may be involved[773,1950]. Hunter-gatherers eat large amounts of lean, red meat[1143]. In many countries, domestic red meat has typically a high content of total and saturated fat.

A diet based on lean meat is high in protein. There is insufficient data to suggest that this is a health risk with regard to the heart (or kidney disease and bone fragility; see Sections 4.4 and 4.12). In a study in humans, a high intake of lean red meat in place of carbohydrate-rich foods (bread, pasta, rice, potatoes, breakfast cereals) had no adverse effects on markers of inflammation that may be relevant to ischaemic heart disease[737]. C-reactive protein tended to decrease ($P = 0.06$) during the 8-week trial. The objective in the red meat group was to achieve a 35–40 g/day (7–8% of total energy intake) higher protein intake compared with the control group.

Nuts

Five large epidemiological studies in the USA all seem to indicate that the risk of myocardial infarction is lower for people who eat nuts on a regular basis than for those who do not[947,1823]. In the three studies where nut consumption was reported in the same manner, and after adjusting for other (known) confounding dietary factors, there was a roughly 40% reduced risk by consuming nuts at least 5 times/week, compared to less than once a week[539,775,966]. One of the studies was conducted on just over 31 000 Seventh Day Adventists in California, who were interviewed about their dietary habits and tracked for 12 years. The lower risk with higher consumption was statistically significant both among overweight and lean individuals, and was not dependent on the level of other cardiovascular risk factors. In the Physicians' Health Study, the risk of sudden cardiac-related death was lower among persons who ate nuts more than 2 times/week (relative risk 0.53; 95% 95% CI 0.30–0.92) compared with those who seldom or never ate nuts (P for trend = 0.01)[31]. However, there was no apparent relation to deaths from other causes or non-fatal myocardial infarctions.

Randomised intervention studies of increased nut intake are lacking. Therefore, the presence of confounders in the observational studies cannot be ruled out. Certainly, when most of these studies were conducted, there was a general belief among

US health-conscious people that nuts are beneficial, an opinion strongly promoted by John H. Kellogg in the early twentieth century[270].

The suggested nutritional benefits of nuts include being rich in minerals, vitamins and soluble fibre. Similar to olive oil, the fat in most nuts is dominated by the monounsaturated fatty acid oleic acid (18:1n-9). The potential disadvantages include a high content of omega-6 fatty acids and phytic acid, as well as a high energy density. A handful of nuts, particularly hazel nuts, drastically increases the omega-6/omega-3 ratio. The phytate content of nuts impedes the body's ability to absorb minerals such as iron, calcium, zinc and magnesium, where a lack of the last two minerals has been suggested as a contributing factor for ischaemic heart disease[481,1639]. The low water content means that an extra handful of nuts goes down easily, which is expected to contribute to weight gain. The fact that nuts are rich in plant sterols may help to maintain beneficial levels of serum cholesterol[822], but the net effect on the heart and blood vessels is unclear (see under 'Plant sterols').

Peanuts are not nuts in the botanical sense, and should not be considered so in the context of healthy foods. They belong to the family of legumes (Leguminosae), which also includes beans, peas and lentils. Peanuts are thought to actually increase the risk of atherosclerosis via mechanisms that are partly independent of their fat (see Section 4.3).

Coconut is considerably different from other nuts in that coconut fat is dominated by saturated fatty acids (see also Section 3.2). This probably partly explains why serum cholesterol levels among some Pacific Islanders are not entirely favourable. Even if these populations apparently manage to consume large amounts of coconuts without any problems, people in the Western world are advised to be careful, particularly with coconut fat, which in contrast to coconut meat provides only calories without any vitamins, minerals or fibre.

Alcohol

A moderate intake of alcohol is sometimes highlighted, even by medical experts, as beneficial in preventing ischaemic heart disease, but the jury is still out. Alcohol in moderation increases HDL cholesterol (the 'good' cholesterol) and possibly improves insulin sensitivity (i.e. decreases insulin resistance), at least in women[850]. Several studies indeed have shown a negative relationship between wine consumption and the incidence of myocardial infarction in Western populations[412,924] and between different countries[1579], but it is uncertain if this is due to the wine itself. As indicated earlier, a low intake of milk also correlates with a high consumption of wine, which could explain the relationship. When you consider the differences in the intake of both wine and dairy products, the international relationship with wine apparently disappears, while dairy products remain as a risk factor[1431,1614].

But let us assume that the risk of myocardial infarction really is lower among those who regularly consume alcohol. Then the next question is 'Is this difference meaningful?' Probably not. If we remove abstainers and alcoholics from the analysis and only consider people with a consumption of alcohol ranging from rarely to every day, the potential benefit does not appear to be particularly interesting. A *Lancet* editorial arrived at the following conclusions[813]: 'Any coronary protection from light to moderate drinking will be very small and unlikely to outweigh the harms. While moderate to heavy drinking is probably coronary-protective, any benefit will be overwhelmed by the known harms.'

This means that those people who used to drink a glass of wine every other week, and then switch to 2 glasses/day, do not appear to reduce their risk for a myocardial infarction to any notable degree. Hence, recommending the consumption of alcohol several times per week is clearly not justified by available evidence.

Dairy products

Despite the lack of randomised controlled long-term trials (which for obvious reasons cannot be performed as double-blind studies), there is some evidence that milk products are a contributing factor for ischaemic heart disease. Much of this evidence comes from animal experiments showing that casein, the dominant milk protein, causes atherosclerosis (see Section 4.3). Furthermore, aggravation of insulin resistance and intracellular fat deposition have been noted in animal studies[76,993], and both of these disturbances are thought to increase the risk of ischaemic heart disease. In addition, milk fat is highly saturated and raises serum cholesterol although the effect is small (see Section 4.8). On the other hand, milk contains substances of potential benefit for blood pressure[523], and an independent role of milk and milk fat in ischaemic heart disease has not been established[490,1211,1904].

In the beginning of the twentieth century, it was common practice among doctors in certain parts of the USA and England to treat peptic ulcers with large amounts of milk. The most famous diet was called the Sippy diet after the physician who introduced it in 1916. In a highly publicised autopsy study of patients from 1940 to 1959, it was noted that myocardial infarctions were considerably more common among patients who had undergone the Sippy diet, than among those who had been treated at hospitals where the milk diet had not been prescribed[220]. Today, this study is seldom cited, possibly because the patients had not been randomised for one or the other treatment. Therefore, it is theoretically possible, but not particularly likely, that the two groups differed from each other in some other respect that could have affected the risk of a myocardial infarction.

In ecological studies, there is a strong, positive correlation between cardiovascular mortality and the consumption of dairy products[1612,1614]. In the late twentieth century, the European countries that reduced their milk consumption were also the ones where the incidence of mortality from myocardial infarctions had dropped the most[1249]. The strongest correlation points to components other than the fat in the milk[1190,1248,1614]. The relationship appears to be stronger for milk than for cheese[1614]. Some countries, such as France, have a low risk of developing myocardial infarction despite a high intake of dairy products. One of several proposed explanations is that the French typically eat cheese instead of drinking milk. Many cheeses have a lower content of specific milk proteins, which may be degraded enzymatically during cheesemaking[266,1472]. The absorption, metabolism and potential health effects of the resulting peptides have scarcely been studied.

The strongest international correlation between milk constituents and health appears to be with the milk protein β-casein A1, which may account for 77% of the international variation in mortality from myocardial infarctions[1190]. This structural variant of the milk protein casein can be found in the cow's milk from special breeds. In the same study, the R^2 value was 26% for total milk protein and 11% for red meat. β-Casein A1 could also explain why Iceland has a lower cardiovascular mortality than expected from the population's high intake of dairy products[1560]. Icelandic milk has a lower percentage of β-casein A1 than milk in most other parts of Europe[486,1032,1793].

Lactose, which is largely removed in cheese making (the residual is lactic acid), has also been suggested to provide an explanation for the international variation in myocardial infarctions[1614]. Asian Indians show a high incidence of myocardial infarction, as well as a high intake of dairy products and a rather high frequency of persistent lactase activity, 46% which is close to the average frequencies in the USA (51%) and Europe (61%), and higher than world average (35%)[793,1615]. It is of some relevance that lactose has been shown to promote atherosclerosis in primates[954] and insulin resistance in calves[778,1939].

Comparisons within, rather than between, countries (or ethnic groups) suggest that other lifestyle variables than milk consumption explain the variation of ischaemic heart disease in such populations[490,491]. A few cohort studies even support a lower risk among milk drinkers, although the relative risk in one meta-analysis was not significantly different than low consumers (relative risk 0.87; 95% CI 0.77–0.90)[490]. At further odds with the understanding that milk fat is unhealthy are studies showing a lower risk of ischaemic heart disease and more beneficial risk factor levels among those who prefer high-fat milk[168,1670,1684,1904]. However, this may relate to the possible risks of other milk components than fat, rather than to the question of whether milk as such is harmful or beneficial.

In the DASH trial (Dietary Approaches to Stop Hypertension), a reduction in blood pressure was achieved using a diet that included low-fat milk products but the specific effect of milk was not investigated, and the suggested beneficial nutrients are easily provided by vegetables, fruits and lean meat[1554]. In the prospective epidemiological CARDIA study (Coronary Artery Risk Development in Young Adults), the risk for developing the metabolic syndromes (abdominal obesity, glucose intolerance, hypertension and dyslipidaemia) among overweight, young Americans was lower with a higher intake of dairy products[1408]. It is highly probable that milk, in particular low-fat milk, has certain nutritional advantages over other energy-supplying drinks, which can have a beneficial effect on cardiovascular risk factors. However, much evidence points to milk as a contributing factor in ischaemic heart disease, and that it should be avoided. Today, many authorities do not agree on this, partly because they rely heavily on the above cohort studies.

Refined fats

The effect of different types of margarines and oils, and lard, on myocardial infarction and angina pectoris is insufficiently documented. All margarines and oils contribute to excess calories and probably to atherosclerosis. It used to previously be thought that the polyunsaturated omega-6 fat linoleic acid (18:2 omega-6) could prevent cardiovascular disease[1349,1657], but the majority of studies now point to the opposite effect[159,417,588,736,1111]. From an evolutionary perspective, the current intake of linoleic acid is very high.

Monounsaturated fat

Monounsaturated fat from olive oil, for example, is often presented as beneficial[946], but randomised studies of clinically significant events are still pending. Any potential benefit may have been exaggerated. Advocates of a high intake of olive oil base their opinion primarily on epidemiological studies, and on the fact that monounsaturated fat, in exchange for saturated fat, has a greater beneficial effect on insulin sensitivity and serum triglycerides than if carbohydrate consumption is increased[946,1479] (see Section 4.8). The support from the cooking oil industry, by sponsoring symposiums and supplements of scientific nutrition journals, may have potentially facilitated the widespread dissemination of this hypothesis.

Total fat and saturated fat

Despite that dietary fat has been shown to promote atherosclerosis, insulin resistance and lipotoxicity in animal experiments (see Sections 4.3 and 4.6), randomised studies on humans provide rather weak support for the notion that the total fat intake or the amount of dietary saturated fat markedly increases the risk for angina pectoris, myocardial infarction or sudden cardiac death[755,1211]. In the majority of human trials, the intervention diet corresponded on the whole with the recommendations of the American Heart Association as of the second half of the twentieth century[944]. The emphasis was placed on reducing the intake of total fat ($\leq$30 E%), saturated fat (8–19 E%) and dietary cholesterol (<300 mg/day) and on increasing the intake of polyunsaturated fat (up to 10 E%). (These guidelines have since been modified somewhat, and now focus more on whole foods, energy balance, soluble fibre, trans fatty acids and dietary salt, but also propose an even lower intake of saturated fats down to less than 10 E%[945].)

The results of a Cochrane meta-analysis of 27 randomised controlled trials, which satisfied generally accepted scientific requirements, showed that the above-mentioned changes in fat intake did not affect overall mortality (relative risk of death 0.98; 95% CI 0.86–1.12)[755]. The 9% drop in cardiovascular mortality (relative risk 0.91; 95% CI 0.77–1.07) was non-significant, while the risk of any cardiovascular event (cardiovascular death, non-fatal myocardial infarction, stroke, angina pectoris, heart failure, peripheral arterial disease and coronary bypass or angioplasty) was significantly lowered by 16% (relative risk 0.84; 95% CI 0.72–0.99). However, studies with a follow-up period greater than 2 years provided stronger support for protection against cardiovascular events (relative risk 0.76; 95% CI 0.65–0.90), which agrees with the notion that this type of dietary change limits the development of atherosclerosis by improving blood lipids[1141].

In the more recent Women's Health Initiative Dietary Modification Trial, intensive nutritional counselling on the merits of a low-fat, high-fibre diet had no beneficial effect on cardiovascular disease and actually increased the risk among those with known cardiovascular disease at entry (see 'Old and new concepts of healthy diets' under Section 2.4)[768].

The support from epidemiological studies is not consistent, and not as strong as one could expect from the high level of consensus that was previously the case among health authorities[962,1476].

A possible explanation of the inconsistent research findings is that dietary fat alone is insufficient to cause cardiovascular disease, but that it acts in liaison with other dietary factors. Until this possibility has been properly addressed in dietary intervention trials, high-fat diets should probably be avoided in order to prevent ischaemic heart disease.

Trans fats

Epidemiological studies indicate that trans fatty acids, primarily elaidic acid (*trans*-18:1n-9) in partially hydrogenated margarines and oils, can contribute to ischaemic heart disease[1251,1357]. In the studies where the intake of *trans*-vaccenic acid was analysed separately, this did not appear to be linked with increased cardiovascular risks. *Trans*-vaccenic acid is the dominant trans fatty acid in depot fat of ruminants. In an intervention study with two kinds of margarine (9.4% or 0.4% trans fat), consumption of margarine rich in trans fat in exchange for saturated fat led to impaired endothelial function in humans, which provides further evidence of a difference between these two types of fat[392]. The majority of the research in this area has otherwise concentrated on the adverse effect on blood lipids[73]. Elaidic acid and *trans*-vaccenic acid raise LDL cholesterol (the 'bad' cholesterol) and decrease HDL cholesterol[282,878,1250,1300].

In a case–control study from Seattle, a high percentage of *trans*-isomers from linoleic acid (18:2 omega-6) in red blood cells (as measured upon admission) was linked to a sharply increased risk for cardiac arrest[1011]. Consuming pizza, barbecued chicken and biscuits explained 33% of the variation in *trans*-18:2 levels. The intake of elaidic acid and *trans*-vaccenic acid did not show any relation to the risk of cardiac arrest in this study.

Dietary cholesterol

The percentage of cholesterol in food seems to have little effect on the risk for cardiovascular disease[517,1194]. A reduced cholesterol intake has been a part of many of the studies in the Cochrane review mentioned under 'Total fat and saturated fat' above[755]. The effect of cholesterol intake on blood lipids is modest in most people, mainly because the major part of circulating serum cholesterol has been produced by the liver, rather than absorbed from the diet (see Section 4.8). For this reason, advising against a high intake of eggs or meat or, for that matter, fish or seafood is not justified.

Plant sterols

Plant sterols (phytosterols) such as sitosterol and campesterol have been proposed to prevent cardiovascular disease by way of lowering serum cholesterol (see Section 4.8). Certain exclusive margarines have therefore been enriched with plant sterols. However, their long-term safety has not been tested, and there is some concern about their possible *pro*-atherosclerotic effect[82,1075]. In a nested case–control study in Germany, analysing plasma samples collected 10 years earlier, people suffering from myocardial infarction or sudden death had elevated levels of plasma sitosterol[82]. In this study, increased levels of plasma sitosterol showed to be a cardiovascular risk factor of the same magnitude as hypertension, diabetes or family history of premature ischaemic heart disease. In other studies, patients with abnormally elevated absorption of dietary plant sterols have had advanced atherosclerosis in early life despite normal cholesterol levels[154]. A recent experiment found β-sitosterol, a plant sterol, to be cytotoxic in human aorta endothelial cells[1540].

Energy intake

A food model based on lean meat, fish and lots of fruits, vegetables and root vegetables has a low energy density (few calories per gram) and is, in our clinical experience, very difficult to consume in excess of caloric needs. This apparent satiating property reduces the risk of overweight, which could theoretically prevent ischaemic heart disease[975,1182,1500]. However, it is unclear whether being overweight, independently of waist circumference and insulin resistance, contributes to ischaemic heart disease[35,975].

Long-term rigorous calorie restriction has resulted in markedly beneficial cardiovascular risk factor levels in non-human primates (randomised controlled trials)[189,274] and in humans (observational studies)[529]. In the human studies, processed foods containing *trans* fatty acids and high glycaemic loads (e.g. refined carbohydrates, desserts, snacks and soft drinks) were strictly avoided, which makes the independent role of energy intake questionable. In addition, low calorie consumers in Malmö, Sweden, had higher cardiovascular mortality than those in the third (women) and fourth (men) quartiles[1015]. The increased mortality after weight loss, in particular muscle loss, discussed on pages 121–22 under 'Potential consequences' (of overweight and obesity), is highly relevant to this issue.

Glycaemic index and carbohydrate intake

The dominance of bread, breakfast cereals and potatoes in the typical Western diet results in large amounts of carbohydrates being supplied in a concentrated form, and often with a high glycaemic index (GI). The product of the GI and the absolute amount of carbohydrate is called the glycaemic load[88,1558]. A higher glycaemic load means that blood sugar increases more after a meal.

It has been suggested that recurrent high blood glucose levels (hyperglycaemia) after meals contribute to ischaemic heart disease[207,639,1007]. The proposed mechanisms include high serum insulin (hyperinsulinaemia)[1401], impaired fibrinolysis[465,817], low HDL cholesterol[530], high triglycerides[1876], increased appetite[201] and intracellular glucose toxicity in the heart and arteries[226,639].

A continuous positive relationship between post-prandial blood sugar and ischaemic heart disease has been found in observational studies. Thus, in the Nurses' Health Study, a high glycaemic load was positively associated with developing ischaemic heart disease after correcting for age, smoking, total energy intake and other cardiovascular risk factors[1071]. The relative risk from the lowest to the highest quintile of glycaemic load was 1.00, 1.01, 1.23, 1.51 and 1.98 (95% CI, 1.41–2.77 for the highest quintile, P for trend < 0.0001).

However, clear-cut evidence for 'the-lower-the-better' (for the heart) from controlled trials is still lacking. Furthermore, randomised controlled studies of the effect of low-carbohydrate diets on the incidence of cardiovascular disease are lacking. Pharmacological studies in patients with type 2 diabetes suggest that a decrease in blood sugar is less efficient for the prevention of ischaemic heart disease than expected from the observed correlation between blood sugar and the incidence of such disease in the population[1174,1834]. In 2008, three large randomised controlled trials found that intensive lowering of blood sugar lacks benefits (for the patients) and increases adverse effects[442,582,1394].

Diets that prevent an excessive increase in blood sugar can be low-GI, low-carbohydrate, high-protein or high-fat diets in various combinations, compared to a defined control diet, and they can be either energy-restricted or not. Consequently, there is much uncertainty as to the role of each of these variables with regard to ischaemic heart disease and its related disorders.

In a large, well-controlled trial of 129 overweight or obese young adults, a high-carbohydrate, low-GI diet resulted in more beneficial cardiovascular risk factor levels than a high-protein diet despite similar loss of body fat[1192]. In this study, subjects were randomly assigned to one of four reduced-fat, high-fibre diets for 12 weeks. Diets 1 and 2 were high carbohydrate (55% of total energy intake), with high and low GIs, respectively; Diets 3 and 4 were high protein (25% of total energy intake), with high and low GIs, respectively. The glycaemic load was highest in Diet 1 and lowest in Diet 4. While weight loss was similar in all groups, the proportion of subjects in each group who lost 5% or more of body weight varied significantly by diet (Diet 1, 31%; Diet 2, 56%; Diet 3, 66%; and Diet 4, 33%; $P = 0.01$). Women on Diets 2 and 3 lost approximately 80% more fat mass, –4.5 ± 0.5 (mean ± standard error) kg and –4.6 ± 0.5 kg, than those on Diet 1 (–2.5 ± 0.5 kg; $P = 0.007$). Low-density lipoprotein cholesterol levels declined significantly in the Diet 2 group (–0.17 ± 0.10 mmol/L) but increased in the Diet 3 group (+0.26 ± 0.10 mmol/L; $P = 0.02$). Goals for energy distribution were not achieved exactly: both carbohydrate groups ate less fat, and the Diet 2 group ate more fibre. Hence, both high-protein and low-GI regimens increased body fat loss, but cardiovascular risk reduction was optimised by a high-carbohydrate, low-GI diet.

The Kitavans of Papua New Guinea have a very high intake of carbohydrate, 65–70 E%, mainly from starchy root vegetables and from fruits. The conspicuous absence of ischaemic heart disease in this population strongly contradicts the idea that carbohydrates are dangerous, at least in that setting. Among the Kitavans, as well as among other high consumers of starch, serum triglyceride levels are relatively high, a circumstance which is discussed in Section 4.8.

A sensible dietary approach in order to prevent ischaemic heart disease is to avoid carbohydrate-rich foods with a high GI, especially for people with diabetes or abdominal obesity. When carbohydrate restriction is desired, it seems prudent to increase the intake of protein rather than fat, and to reduce caloric intake. Further discussions on these matters with regard to type 2 diabetes and overweight are found in Sections 4.4 and 4.5.

Sugar

Consumption of sugar, i.e. added sucrose and monosaccharides, mainly from sweets, candy, soft drinks, cookies and ice cream is high in the West, approximately 10–15% of total caloric intake (www.usda.gov, www.slv.se). Much of this sugar is in the form of sucrose, a disaccharide containing glucose and fructose units. An increasing proportion of sugar in soft drinks in USA is glucose and fructose from maize (high fructose corn syrup).

If sugar increases the risk of ischaemic heart disease, it might be because it provides energy without essential nutrients, although their value in this context is as yet unproven. Another possibility could be that sugary foods trigger overeating and thereby cause obesity. The glycaemic load from sucrose is relatively high.

Fructose constitutes one half of sucrose. A high intake of fructose contributes to insulin resistance and type 2 diabetes in certain rat models, but this effect has not been established in humans (see Sections 4.4 and 4.6). Unlike rodents, our pre-human ancestors were supposedly specialised fruit eaters for 60 million years since the time of early primates until early Palaeolithic modern humans. In addition, fructose has not been investigated as part of a diet, which the studied animals would eat in their original habitat, and it is conceivable that some other dietary factor may have influenced the results.

Salt

An increased risk for developing ischaemic heart disease from a high salt intake has been observed among overweight men in both Finland and USA[693,1827]. Both of these studies analysed urinary sodium excretions for 24 hours, which provide a good measure of the sodium intake at the group level. In the Finnish study it was noted that among 1173 men and 1263 women aged 25–64 years, there was a more than 50% increased risk for developing ischaemic heart disease when urinary sodium excretions increased by 100 mmol/24 hours (relative risk 1.51; 95% CI 1.14–2.00), and just over a 25% increased risk for all-cause death (relative risk 1.26; 95% CI 1.06–1.50)[1827]. When the sexes were analysed separately, a significant effect was only seen in men, and the effect was most evident in overweight men.

Another prospective cohort study, the American NHANES I Epidemiological Follow-up Study, provided similar results with a study covering just over 14 400 people aged 25–74 years who were tracked for 19 years[693]. The numbers are relatively reliable since a total of 1727 subjects developed ischaemic heart disease, 614 cases of which were fatal. Among overweight people, a 100 mmol sodium excretion was linked with a 44% increased risk of heart-related death (relative risk 1.44; 95% CI 1.14–1.81; $P = 0.002$), and a 39% increased total mortality (relative risk 1.39; 95% CI 1.23–1.58; $P = 0.001$). There was no increased risk among subjects with a normal weight (BMI < 25).

In contrast, some epidemiological studies have found no association, or even an inverse one, between salt intake and risk of ischaemic heart disease[311]. Consequently, there is some disagreement as to the influence of dietary sodium in ischaemic heart disease[33,753,1030]. On the one hand, salt raises blood pressure (see Section 4.7) and may increase the risk of left ventricular hypertrophy (see Section 4.9). On the other hand, salt restriction activates the renin–angiotensin system which could hypothetically be unfavourable[33]. However, traditional populations do very well on life-long, intense activation of the renin–angiotensin system, the most extreme example being the Yanomamo hunter-gatherers of South America[546]. Nevertheless, people treated with antihypertensive drugs, particularly angiotensin-converting enzyme (ACE) inhibitors, need to be cautious and not change their salt intake too drastically from one day to another (see Section 5.3).

Whole grains

There are no randomised intervention studies to support recommending a high intake of whole-grain bread or cereals, and a recent trial did not find any beneficial effect on cardiovascular risk factors from increasing whole-grain foods among 316 overweight subjects (who consumed less than 30 g whole grains per day before the study) (Brownlee IA et al. Cereal Foods World 2008; 53(4 Suppl):Abstract 22). Instead, this recommendation is based on observational studies, where people who prefer whole grains have a lower cardiovascular risk[1201,1683,1816]. This can either mean that whole-grain cereals are healthier than the foods they are replacing (such as refined cereals), or that people who choose whole grains have a healthier lifestyle in other respects. Both statements are probably true. Whole-grain cereals are more nutritious and filling than the refined varieties. Compared with staple foods available during human evolution, however, they do not have any known benefits. If Palaeolithic food is supplemented with cereals, the intake and/or bioavailability of several relevant nutrients drops. Furthermore, cereals contain lectins and other bioactive substances that can hypothetically increase the risk of atherosclerosis.

These issues are discussed in more detail in the section dealing with atherosclerosis (Section 4.3).

Dietary fibre

There is insufficient high-quality research on the importance of dietary fibre for ischaemic heart disease. If people who prefer whole grains have less heart disease, it may be because of other elements of their healthy lifestyle. The only published controlled trial of dietary fibre on the risk of developing ischaemic heart disease, the DART study mentioned above, showed a tendency towards *increased* mortality from cardiovascular diseases in people eating more dietary cereal fibre[242]. The study took roughly 2000 British men, who had had a previous myocardial infarction, and randomly assigned them either a high intake of dietary fibre (≥ 18 g/day) or an ordinary diet. After 2 years, a total of 123/1017 patients in the fibre group had died, compared with 101/1016 ($P = 0.16$) from the other group. The number of subjects who developed cardiovascular disease were, respectively, 109 and 85 ($P = 0.10$). After adjustment for possible confounding factors such as health state and medication, the increased risk of developing ischaemic heart disease was statistically significant (hazard ratio 1.35; 95% CI 1.02–1.80), although it subsided after more than 10 years (hazard ratio 1.11; 95% CI 0.96–1.29)[1285]. Since cereals made up the main source of fibre, it should not be ruled out that the tendency towards increased mortality was a detrimental effect of the increased grain consumption.

The widely accepted hypothesis that dietary fibre, including cereal fibre, prevents ischaemic heart disease is based on epidemiological studies[1409,1735]. However, one of the largest, and most often cited, prospective observational studies points to the appearance of confounders that could possibly explain a large part of the relationship[1068]. The study recorded the dietary habits of close to 40 000 healthy women, primarily nurses, by means of frequency formulas. During the 6-year follow-up period, 570 new cases of disease were noted, including myocardial infarction (177), stroke, percutaneous transluminal coronary angioplasty, coronary bypass operations or cardiovascular death. Women in the quintile with the highest fibre intake (median 26.3 g/day) had, compared with the lowest quintile (median 12.5 fibre/day), a relative risk for developing any type of cardiovascular disease of 0.65 (95% CI 0.51–0.84), and 0.46 (0.30–0.72) for undergoing a myocardial infarction. After correcting for differences in cardiovascular risk factors, however, the relative risk dropped to 0.79 (95% CI 0.58–1.09, not significant) and 0.68 (95% CI 0.36–1.22, not significant) respectively.

It should be noted that there are two kinds of dietary fibre. The first is insoluble fibre, which is mainly found in cereals, and which does not appear to affect cardiovascular risk factors very much[225,516,1929,1959]. The other kind is soluble fibre, which dominates in fruits, root vegetables and nuts, and has been shown to improve blood lipids and glucose metabolism, particularly when ingested in high amounts[1780]. Insoluble dietary fibre has two main benefits, it is satiating due to its filling capacity in the stomach[769], and it prevents constipation[471]. Soluble fibre has the same effects, but it is thought to improve blood lipids and carbohydrate metabolism more than insoluble fibre[225,516,1780], hence it probably has a greater ability to prevent cardiovascular disease and diabetes. A case–control study in Italy found fruit fibre to be protective against myocardial infarction, while no such effect was found for cereal fibre[1281]. In contrast, a pooled analysis of cohort studies found both kinds of fibre to be inversely related to ischaemic heart disease mortality[1409].

Tea

In clinical human experiments, black tea has been found to improve endothelial function[448] in ways that can theoretically prevent ischaemic heart disease. In contrast, black tea increased aortic wall stiffness in a supposedly unfavourable manner, while green tea had no such effect[1874]. There seems to be no effect of black or green tea, or tea polyphenols, on markers of inflammation, coagulation, fibrinolysis or endothelial function[390,1414]. Although tea polyphenols had a potent antioxidant activity on LDL oxidation in the laboratory test tube (in vitro), no effect was found on LDL oxidation in humans after consumption of green or black tea or intake of a green tea polyphenol isolate[1449]. Tea does not reduce blood pressure or serum cholesterol in well-controlled human trials[1507].

Epidemiological studies are equivocal, usually showing an inverse association, or none, between tea drinking and incidence of ischaemic heart disease[1254,1414,1507,1624]. The studies that did find a relationship were usually European studies, while US studies generally failed to do so. This may indicate the presence of confounders, since tea drinking is associated with cultural, ethnic and social customs in a different manner across various countries. In a US study showing a lower 3.8-year mortality among tea drinkers after myocardial infarction[1254], it is possible that the habit of drinking tea may have been a consequence of increased lifestyle awareness. In a study in Wales, tea intake did not correlate with ischaemic heart disease incidence in a 14-year follow-up of 334 men, 45–59 years of age, and there was actually a positive association with total mortality (relative risk 1.4; 95% CI 1.0–2.0; $P = 0.014$)[722]. High social class and healthy lifestyle were negatively associated with tea drinking in the Welsh study, as opposed to a positive association in a Dutch study[723].

Although some studies show interesting results, including reduced atherosclerosis in hypercholesterolaemic rabbits[883], drinking black or green tea cannot currently be recommended as a means to prevent ischaemic heart disease.

Coffee

Available evidence does not support an important effect of coffee relevant to cardiovascular disease[651,1414,1693]. In epidemiological case–control studies, heavy coffee drinkers had increased risk of ischaemic heart disease, while no significant association emerged for low daily coffee intake ($\leq$2 cups/day). A meta-analysis of ten long-term prospective studies did not show any association between the consumption of coffee and ischaemic heart disease, with a relative risk of 1.16 (95% CI 0.95–1.41; $P = 0.14$) for the highest category, and 1.05 (95% CI 0.90–1.22; $P = 0.57$) and 1.04 (95% CI 0.90–1.19; $P = 0.60$) for the second and third highest categories, respectively[1693]. A later prospective study found a non-significantly ($P = 0.07$) lower risk of myocardial infarction with increasing coffee consumption[1534].

Vitamins, minerals and trace elements

There are two major concepts related to ischaemic heart disease and vitamins: the antioxidant hypothesis and the homocysteine hypothesis, but neither seems to hold up against recent evidence from randomised controlled trials. It was thought for many years that ischaemic heart disease could be prevented by means of dietary antioxidants such as vitamins A, C and E, and selenium. However, no effect has been seen in several large-scale randomised controlled trials[174,1175,1623]. These include the Heart Protection Study (HPS), in which roughly 20 500 high-risk cardiovascular patients were treated for more than 5 years with a combination of vitamins C, E and A (250 mg vitamin C, 650 mg vitamin E and 20 mg β-carotene per day)[5]. These findings may mean that the positive effects that were noted in observational studies are due to other lifestyle factors[80], or that the effects of the vitamins in pill form are different from vitamins in food. These findings justify a certain amount of scepticism regarding the antioxidant hypothesis for now[1175,1719].

A Cochrane meta-analysis found that supplementation with vitamins A and E may actually increase mortality, while the impact of vitamin C and selenium was thought to need further study[174]. A later randomised controlled trial of selenium supplementation found an increased risk of diabetes in the selenium supplement group[1733]. Two recent large trials, again, found no benefit from antioxidant supplementation and one of them found an increased risk of diabetes in the selenium group and prostate cancer in the vitamin E group[575,1060].

The hypothesis that lowering blood homocysteine with *folic acid* and *vitamins B_6 and B_{12}* prevents ischaemic heart disease was strongly refuted by the findings of large-scale randomised trials[192,467,1079]. The hypothesis has been based on observational studies showing that lower homocysteine levels are associated with lower rates of cardiovascular disease. Folic acid and vitamins B_6 and B_{12} do lower homocysteine levels, but these two large randomised controlled trials now failed to show any protection against ischaemic heart disease[192,1079]. In one of the trials, more patients in the active-treatment group than in the placebo group were hospitalised for unstable angina (relative risk 1.24; 95% CI 1.04–1.49). Since the doses used were higher than what is found in a well-balanced diet, it cannot be excluded that such a diet is beneficial through lowering homocysteine[1887]. A Palaeolithic diet is rich in all three of these vitamins. Vitamin B_6 and folate are usually considered to have the largest effect on homocysteine. However, vegans and ovo-lacto vegetarians had higher levels of homocysteine (and lower levels of vitamin B_{12}) than meat eaters in three different studies[172,1113,1144].

Other nutrients/dietary factors that have been suggested to prevent ischaemic heart disease include *magnesium*[1191,1639,1699] and *potassium*[687,1100]. A diet based on lean meat, fish, fruits, root vegetables and nuts effectively supplies both of these minerals.

There has been a long debate about increased body stores of *iron* as a risk factor for ischaemic heart disease, but after much research most studies do not suggest an increased risk[367,1101,1462,1767]. A meta-analysis of prospective studies actually found a decreased risk with high iron intake: the relative risk of ischaemic heart disease among individuals in top thirds of total dietary iron was 0.8 (95% CI 0.7–1.1; not significant)[367]. For serum iron, a tendency for decreased risk was noted in the top third (relative risk 0.8; 95% CI 0.7–1.0). Furthermore, one Italian study found an inverse association between iron intake and risk of myocardial infarction[1767]. These findings make sense, since the ancient human diet would otherwise seem hazardous, due to its excess of highly absorbable iron. Not even carriers of the gene for hereditary haemochromatosis, a disorder of enhanced iron absorption (see Section 5.1), seem to have an increased risk of ischaemic heart disease[483,1852].

Soya protein

Soya has gained much attention with regard to Western disease, including ischaemic heart disease. In 2006, the Nutrition Committee of the American Heart Association came to the conclusion that 'earlier research indicating that soya protein has clinically important favourable effects as compared with other proteins has not been confirmed' [1553]. The overall effect on serum cholesterol is very small, even with very high amounts of soya protein, and possible adverse effects need to be considered, as stated in two independent meta-analyses from 2006[409,1553]. The interpretation of intervention studies is problematic since the control protein has usually been casein (see 'Dairy products' above).

Conclusion

Available evidence does not contradict the notion that an ancestral-like diet based on fruits, vegetables, root vegetables, nuts, lean meat, fish and shellfish is safe and effective for the prevention of ischaemic heart disease. A Mediterranean-like dietary pattern based on vegetables, fruits, legumes, low-GI cereals and fish seems to be only one step in the right direction, compared to a typical Western dietary pattern. However, in order to minimise the risk, it is obviously not enough.

Tobacco smoking

Stopping smoking at age 50 years reduces by 50% the risk of premature death, and cessation at age 30 almost eliminates it[433]. Much of this life extension is due to a lower risk of ischaemic heart disease. Cigarette smoking is associated with an increased risk for developing ischaemic heart disease in a number of Western populations[902,1646,1944]. The proposed mechanisms include atherosclerosis[1185]; vasoconstriction (contraction of the blood vessels)[1740]; increased haemostasis (blood clotting)[992], hypertension[1753] and insulin resistance[480]. Nevertheless, the incidence of ischaemic heart disease has been low in Japan and China despite widespread smoking. In the Seven Countries Study, cardiovascular mortality did not appear to be related to smoking habits within the Mediterranean populations, in contrast to the populations in northern Europe and USA[902].

In Kitava, 76% of the men and 80% of the women were smokers, but we still found no sign of ischaemic heart disease[1050]. Smoking was introduced on the island approximately 100 years ago. The blood lipid levels of smokers differed just as much from those of non-smokers as they do in the West[1051]. Similarly, the Bushmen of South Africa appeared to be free of myocardial infarctions despite the fact that they were heavy smokers[1817].

Tobacco smoking in combination with unhealthy food promotes the development of atherosclerosis in animal models, but it is not thought to be a sufficient cause by itself[1524]. Correspondingly, the development of cardiovascular disease is only weakly correlated to smoking among those Westerners with the lowest blood pressure and serum cholesterol[1943].

These findings can potentially be interpreted to mean that smoking works in combination with an unhealthy diet to cause the development of cardiovascular disease.

Physical activity

Regular physical activity is a very important way for Westerners to increase lifespan and postpone cardiovascular disease. My interpretation of the available evidence is that exercise is more effective than most standard models of healthy diets.

The average level of physical activity in general was higher prior to the switch to the Western lifestyle, and even the psychosocial environment has changed. Energy expenditure among adult men on Kitava was estimated to be approximately 1.7 times the basal metabolic rate (BMR). The corresponding value for Western men and women with low physical activity at work, and who are inactive during their leisure time, was 1.4 times the BMR[401]. Among those with a moderate amount of activity on the job and during leisure time, it is 1.7 for men and 1.6 for women. This means that many Westerners have a level of physical activity that is well within the range of the Kitava population. Hence, physical activity does not seem to explain most of the differences in disease pattern between Kitava and the Western world.

4.2   Stroke

Discussions of the significance of dietary habits for cardiovascular disease have primarily focused on ischaemic heart disease, while stroke has largely been ignored. Studies of non-Western populations can provide important insights in this regard.

Table 4.2 Important risk factors for stroke and their impact at the population level in Sweden.

Risk factor	Relative risk	Population attributable risk	Number of cases/100 000 per year caused by the risk factor
Hypertension	3.5	30	50–80
Smoking	Men: 1.5	Men: 10	20–30
	Women: 2.6	Women: 15	
Diabetes	5	10–20	20–40
Atrial fibrillation	5	15–20	30–40
TIA/minor stroke	5	2	4
TIA/minor stroke *and* complicated carotid stenosis	10	1	2–3

Note: The figures are similar for most other Western countries[600], although the relatively low smoking rates in Sweden (19% of women and 16% of men) attenuates this burden. TIA, transient ischaemic attack.

Stroke most often depends on a cerebral infarction caused by blood clots in one of the brain's blood vessels. Bleeding is a less frequent cause. The diet-related risk factors that are most closely related to stroke are hypertension and type 2 diabetes[3,600] (see Table 4.2). Both of these risk factors seem to be absent among traditional populations[1048,1051].

Incidence studies

The Kitava study is probably the only published attempt to examine the incidence of stroke among a traditional population in its home environment unaffected by Western eating habits. In our systematic questioning (see Section 4.1), we did not find any cases of alert persons with paralysis of one side of the body (hemiplegia), inability to speak (aphasia) or sudden loss of balance. The answers covered at least two generations in the past, probably more, due to detailed knowledge of living and dead fellow residents. Clinical examinations did not reveal any manifestations of stroke.

Our results match the experiences of other physicians on the Trobriand Islands (H. Jüptner and W. Schiefenhövel, personal communication) and in other parts of Papua New Guinea (M. Alpers and I. Kevau, personal communication.) All of them consider it a well-established and generally accepted fact that stroke has been non-existent among aboriginal populations in the area, and that it cannot be explained by a lack of elderly residents. These types of unpublished observations by experienced, clinically active doctors and researchers sometimes tend to be undervalued. Professor Michael Alpers had more than 30 years of experience as a researcher in Papua New Guinea, with 25 years as the head of the Papua New Guinea Institute of Medical Research in Goroka (he is now at the Centre for International Health at Perth, Australia). He and Isi Kevau, professor of cardiology and active at Port Moresby General Hospital, have confirmed that no case of stroke among the native population in the area was ever reported prior to

Table 4.3 Percentage of stroke among patients with neurological disease in Kampala, Uganda, in three consecutive series.

Year	n	%	Reference
1942	0	0	1263
1954	11/100	11	786
1968	17/50	34	166

1975. The medical literature also highlights the absence of stroke in Papua New Guinea[99,215,255,302,408,763,764,1268,1374,1482,1665,1669,1712,1870].

The medical records from Kenya and Uganda, which became British protectorates in 1920, are equally convincing. Non-infectious stroke apparently did not appear in these countries before 1940[1042,1814]. British doctors in the 1920s, who worked in East Africa after receiving their training in Great Britain, have documented this very convincingly. At the medical clinic in Kampala, Uganda, there was no case of non-infectious stroke among 269 consecutive patients with neurological diseases[1263]. Furthermore, in an overview of 3000 careful autopsies in Uganda during the 1930s and 1940s, a total of four cases of cerebral haemorrhaging were uncovered, but no case of ischaemic stroke[375]. In addition, Hugh Trowell, in his meticulous accounts of non-infectious diseases of East Africa, did not record any case of ischaemic stroke among the aboriginal population there in almost 30 years as a doctor and researcher in Uganda[1812].

Table 4.3 shows the almost explosive growth of stroke, a previously unknown illness, among the native population of Uganda. By 1955, stroke already made up 11% of the neurological cases[786], and by 1968, it became the most prevalent neurological diagnosis[166]. At the same time, hypertension, another previously unknown phenomenon, began to spread, a curious development that was lively debated by British doctors in Uganda and Kenya at the time[1814]. Parallel with the changes in the landscape of diseases, these countries also underwent rapid social change from original traditional societies to Western-style colonial societies.

The East African pattern is now in the process of being repeated in Papua New Guinea[1042]. The first known case of stroke at Port Moresby General Hospital was seen in 1975 (I. Kevau, personal communication), a few years after the first documented case in Lae[1157]. Since then, cases became increasingly more common, and in 1998 there were almost two cases per week at the Port Moresby General Hospital. When I was visiting, I noted that local physicians had good knowledge of the symptoms of stroke. The clinical picture of a 47-year-old man with hemiplegia and total aphasia (Figure 4.5) was recorded completely and adequately by the hospital's assistant physician.

Recent estimates show that stroke is now more common in low- than high-income countries, with an average threefold higher incidence in the former group of countries[843]. Most of this difference has not been explained, but a partial explanation is probably variations in management of risk factors as well as cases of developing stroke. Among high-income countries, stroke does not appear to have as much

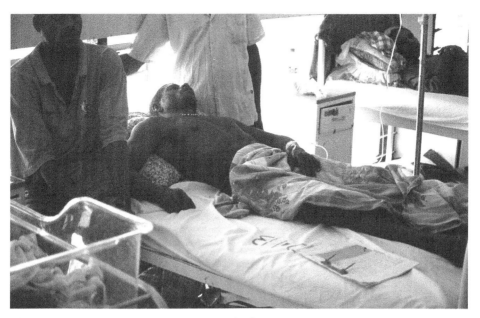

Figure 4.5 A 47-year-old man in Port Moresby, Papua New Guinea, with stroke, causing paralysis of the right extremities and complete expressive aphasia (inability to express speech). (Photo: Staffan Lindeberg.)

variation internationally as ischaemic heart disease. Rather, it is almost equally common in the majority of developed countries[511,1205,1794]. The incidence appears to be at least as high in Japan, Italy and Greece as in other Western countries (Figure 4.6)[511]. The lifestyles that are thought to prevent myocardial infarction, such as Mediterranean and Japanese dietary habits, thus seem to have a limited value in preventing stroke. Migration studies of Japanese in USA, in Hawaii or at home in Japan show that the incidence of stroke decreases the further away from Japan they move, while the reverse trend is seen for myocardial infarction [1483].

In urbanised populations, blood pressure is a very strong predictor for stroke, both at the national population level and in international comparisons (Table 4.2)[2,3,1717]. Blood pressure medication among high-risk persons with hypertension reduces the risk of stroke by at least 35%[1948]. The occurrence of atherosclerosis in the large cervical arteries accounts for a roughly 50% increased risk for stroke[745], and blood lipid regulation using statins decreases the risk of stroke among high-risk patients[46,702].

Increasing evidence suggests that hyperglycaemia and impaired glucose tolerance are risk factors for stroke, even in the absence of diabetes[600]. In one Austrian study, 286 acute stroke patients were screened for glucose tolerance within two weeks after the stroke event[1162]. Severely ill patients were not screened ($n = 48$). Of the remaining 238 patients, 20.2% had previously known diabetes, 16.4% were classified as having newly diagnosed diabetes, 23.1% as having impaired glucose tolerance, 0.8% as having impaired fasting glucose and only 19.7% showed normal

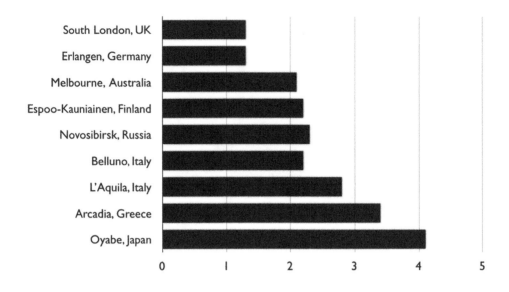

Stroke incidence per 1000 person-years

Figure 4.6   Stroke incidence in some Western countries with good quality data. (Adapted from Reference 511.)

glucose levels. Since the majority of people without stroke have normal glucose levels, and since these are strongly influenced by food habits, the study adds to the evidence that stroke prevention can be optimised by increased understanding of the role of diet.

Likewise, epidemiological studies have found an increased risk of stroke in people with abdominal obesity or other components of the metabolic syndrome[188,1897,1955]. Similar findings were reported already in the early twentieth century. According to Folke Henschen, professor of pathology between 1920 and 1946, it was a known fact that even before he began his career, stroke was overrepresented in people with a certain body type: '*habitus apoplecticus*, the short, stout, short-necked, fat, type of person with a tendency for apoplexy, i.e. "a candidate for stroke" '[714].

Of the total number of strokes in Sweden, it is estimated that approximately 30% are due to hypertension, 10–20% due to diabetes and 10–15% due to smoking (Table 4.2). The increased risk for smokers is higher among women than among men. Diabetes has been defined according to older criteria – using the new, lower threshold values (fasting blood sugar less than 6.1 mmol/L), probably more than 20% of cases can be attributed to diabetes.

A noteworthy observation is that stroke appears to be more common than myocardial infarction in populations that have recently transitioned to a Western lifestyle, which is indeed the situation for Africa[1256,1888,1889], and also seems to apply to Papua New Guinea. In the USA, atherosclerosis in the cerebral blood vessels in the 1960s was considerably more pronounced among African Americans than among whites[1696], but it is doubtful that this difference still prevails[360,964]. One can only speculate the extent to which these findings reflect an ongoing process of natural selection.

Relevant dietary factors

The effect of diet on stroke has not been evaluated in randomised controlled trials. One would expect a Palaeolithic diet to be beneficial because it is low in salt and rich in vegetables and fruits[600,624,689]. It also helps to combat major underlying disorders such as hypertension, overweight, type 2 diabetes, insulin resistance, atherosclerosis and dyslipidaemia[600]. The impact of diet on these conditions is discussed under their respective headings. A Cochrane review concluded that randomised controlled trials of weight reduction for stroke prevention are urgently needed[358].

Salt restriction may prevent stroke independently of blood pressure. A direct connection between sodium intake and stroke was noted in comparisons between different regions in Europe[1411], as well as China and Japan[1833]. In the previously mentioned NHANES I Epidemiological Follow-Up Study, a 100 mmol increase in urinary sodium excretion was linked with a 32% increased incidence of stroke (relative risk 1.32; 95% CI 1.07–1.64; $P = 0.01$) and an 89% increase in fatal stroke (relative risk 1.89; 95% CI 1.31–2.74; $P = 0.001$); however, this was only among overweight subjects[693].

In Finland, where stroke mortality has decreased by 80% among middle-aged men and women in the past 30 years, average salt intake has dropped from 14 to 8 g/day in the same period, along with other lifestyle improvements and a 10-mm Hg fall in blood pressure[876]. Smoking rates decreased in men but increased in women.

Epidemiological studies in the West also support the role of *fruits and vegetables* in stroke prevention[689]. Eight studies, consisting of 9 independent populations, which included 257 551 individuals and 4917 stroke events, with a mean follow-up of 13 years, found an average risk reduction of 26% (95% CI 21–31%) among people consuming >5 servings/day, compared to <3 servings/day. In the middle group, consuming 3–5 servings/day, risk reduction was 11% (95% CI 3–17%). Subgroup analyses showed that fruits and vegetables had a significant protective effect on both ischaemic and haemorrhagic stroke.

One of the possible explanations is that fruits and vegetables are rich in *potassium*. In a large cohort study of 43 738 US men, 40–75 years old, who completed a semi-quantitative food frequency questionnaire in 1986 were followed for 8 years, during which time 328 cases of stroke were documented, the relative risk of stroke for men in the top fifth of potassium intake (median intake 4.3 g/day) versus those in the bottom (median 2.4 g/day) was 0.62 (95% CI 0.43–0.88; P for trend = 0.007)[77]. These inverse associations were all stronger in hypertensive than normotensive men and were not materially altered by adjustment for blood pressure levels. A smaller study of 859 men and women found similar results[904].

Potassium supplementation dramatically lowers stroke mortality in stroke-prone spontaneously hypertensive (salt-fed) rats, an effect that is independent of blood pressure[1800,1801]. If this animal model is relevant to humans, an adequate intake of potassium levels may be critical to prevent stroke, although the benefit for blood pressure has not been established in humans[418]. The association is supported by a study in humans where the incidence of stroke was increased among people with a tendency for low serum potassium (<4.1 mmol/L)[614].

It has long been debated whether treatments that lower homocysteine concentrations can reduce the risk of stroke. One relevant agent is *folic acid*. A recent meta-analysis found 8 randomised trials of folic acid supplementation in the prevention of stroke[1899]. Folic acid supplementation significantly reduced the risk of stroke by 18% (relative risk 0.82; 95% CI 0.68–1.00; $P = 0.045$). A greater beneficial effect was seen in four trials with a treatment duration of more than 3 years (relative risk 0.71; 95% CI 0.57–0.87; $P = 0.001$). Since the risk of cancer (or pre-cancer) has shown a tendency (usually not significant) to increase in various trials of folate supplementation[192,283,314,908,1079], the most prudent way to keep homocysteine under control is by means of a diet rich in fruits and vegetables. The effect of vitamins B_6 and B_{12}, which also reduce homocysteine, is more uncertain[1489].

In the light of the apparent role of glucose intolerance for stroke, the epidemiological observation of increasing risk of stroke with increasing *glycaemic load* among overweight or obese US women may also be relevant[1341]. In Japan, stroke has long been a major health problem. In addition to reduced salt intake, the official Japanese nutritional recommendations have included increased consumption of protein and fat (which were both at very low levels) in order to reduce the occurrence of stroke in society. The recommendations for an increased intake of protein and fat have been based on negative correlations with the development of stroke, primarily haemorrhagic stroke, in some cohort studies[592,805,1235,1582,1645], but not in others[698]. The variation in protein intake in Japan has probably largely been attributed to differences in the consumption of *fish*, a major protein source, which has shown a negative correlation with stroke mortality in Japan[2004]. In the later part of the twentieth century, the incidence of stroke in Japan declined sharply[916]. This drop occurred in parallel with an increased intake of fat (from a very low intake of 20 g/day in 1955 to 58 g/day in 1988) and protein (from 70 g/day in 1955 to 79 g/day in 1988), as well as a reduced salt intake[1230,1761].

In summary, it is highly plausible that an energy-restricted, low-salt diet with a relatively low glycaemic load, such as a Palaeolithic diet, is helpful in the prevention of stroke.

4.3 Atherosclerosis

Atherosclerosis is the most important underlying cause of cardiovascular disease, in particular angina pectoris and myocardial infarction, but also many cases of stroke, heart failure and dementia. Most middle-aged and elderly Westerners are affected by atherosclerosis, even in the absence of known cardiovascular disease (see below). There is good evidence that atherosclerosis can be countered by lifestyle changes emphasising dietary adjustments. The importance of diet is particularly clear in animal experiments. Much attention has been paid to dietary fat and dyslipidaemia, but many studies indicate that other nutrients may be equally or more important.

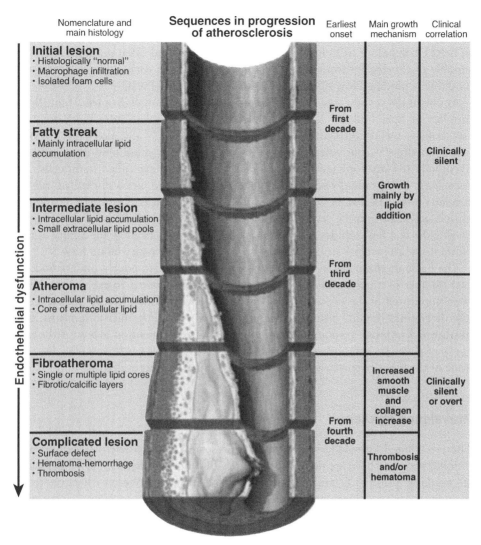

Nomenclature and main histology	Sequences in progression of atherosclerosis	Earliest onset	Main growth mechanism	Clinical correlation
Initial lesion • Histologically "normal" • Macrophage infiltration • Isolated foam cells				
Fatty streak • Mainly intracellular lipid accumulation		From first decade		Clinically silent
Intermediate lesion • Intracellular lipid accumulation • Small extracellular lipid pools			Growth mainly by lipid addition	
Atheroma • Intracellular lipid accumulation • Core of extracellular lipid		From third decade		
Fibroatheroma • Single or multiple lipid cores • Fibrotic/calcific layers			Increased smooth muscle and collagen increase	Clinically silent or overt
Complicated lesion • Surface defect • Hematoma-hemorrhage • Thrombosis		From fourth decade	Thrombosis and/or hematoma	

Endothehelial dysfunction

Figure 4.7 The time course of atherosclerosis in a representative model. Note that the glycocalyx is not depicted. (Adapted from Wikimedia Commons.)

The very first step in atherosclerosis is not known. When the process starts to become visible microscopically, there is thickening of the walls of blood vessels, in the intima layer, which is closest to the blood stream[595,663,1028,1096,1756,1938] (see Figure 4.7). White blood cells enter the arterial wall at roughly the same time, perhaps earlier, and are converted to macrophages, a type of cell with a great capacity to absorb and break down particles of foreign material. This can be seen as an indication that atherosclerosis starts as an inflammatory reaction to foreign (or foreign-like) substances, either because there is too much of them or because they too easily cross the endothelial barrier and enter the wall. The first barrier is the often forgotten glycocalyx, a gel-like mesh located between the flowing blood and the endothelium[222,1313,1492,1850,1916]. The second line of defence is the endothelium, through which foreign-like substances (proteins, lipoproteins, proteoglycans and so forth) originating from inside or outside the body, and often modified, may be capable of causing inflammation. One of the suspects in early atherosclerosis are oxidatively modified low-density lipoproteins in the vessel wall.

At one of the earliest stages, the macrophages contain small droplets of fat (lipid droplets or lipid bodies)[1715]. In normal cells, these droplets store lipids for cell metabolism, membrane synthesis and steroid synthesis[1152] and also exert various other functions[602], but when there is too much they can cause lipid overload[1838]. Eventually the macrophages become filled with fat and are called foam cells. As these foam cells gradually accumulate, plaques are formed, i.e. well-defined, raised patches on the vessel wall, which eventually calcify. An excessive growth of smooth muscle cells can even be seen in the blood vessel wall at a relatively early stage. During the first few decades of life, this process is compensated by the ability of the blood vessel to increase its outer diameter to ensure the proper blood flow[594].

The basic mechanisms in the atherosclerotic process are poorly understood. A vast number of biochemical factors, often inextricably linked to each other, have been implicated in the process. These include blood pressure, lipids, glucose, various hormones (leptin, insulin and many others), invading microorganisms and misdirected immune response (autoimmunity), only to mention a few. Although many of them are established predisposing risk factors for cardiovascular disease, none of them has been shown to be the prime cause of atherosclerosis.

Prevalence studies

There is limited knowledge regarding the presence of atherosclerosis among traditional people. There are no autopsy studies of hunter-gatherers. However, studies available prior to urbanisation and the transition to a Western lifestyle seem to indicate that coronary atherosclerosis was relatively rare in New Guinea and Africa[24,99,117,255,324,375,408,728,875,898,940,1022,1157,1374,1486,1667,1698,1788,1812,1871].

In autopsy studies from Rabaul, one of New Guinea's towns, significant constriction of the coronary artery was seen in only 3 out of 724 individuals, while atherosclerosis of the aorta was considerably more common (97 of 724)[99].

An international autopsy study in the 1960s comparing middle-aged men in four countries revealed a marked difference depending on lifestyle[1774]. Among whites in the USA, only 9% were completely or almost completely free of atherosclerosis (<2% vascular area in the left descending coronary artery afflicted), compared with 76% of blacks in South Africa. Today, African Americans in the USA have more pronounced atherosclerosis than whites, which shows that genetic differences are not the primary explanation[360,964].

Autopsy studies from Sweden in the 1930s showed that residents of the northern, poorer, territories had markedly less pronounced atherosclerosis and a lower rate of obesity than in Stockholm and Malmö, Southern Sweden[714,1094]. Notably, cow's milk, barley, oat and potato were staple foods at the time (http://www.ksla.se/atlas1900/). Wheat was absent and cow's milk was mainly from Swedish Mountain cattle[873]. Milk from this breed does not appear to have been low in β-casein A1, in contrast to closely related Finnish breeds[1032]. By the middle of the century, Henschen and other pathologists noticed that these differences in atherosclerotic disease disappeared, which Henschen attributed primarily to changing dietary habits[714]. At the end of the twentieth century, cardiovascular disease instead had become more common in the same northern regions than in the south of Sweden, something that led to large-scale public health projects in the province of Västerbotten[1918].

Today, atherosclerosis can be considered a normal part of ageing in all parts of the modern world, where majority of the people are affected at an early age[1181,1715]. Even by 16–19 years of age, 15% of North Americans display early stages of coronary atherosclerosis, and more than 50% show deposits of foam cells in the walls of the blood vessels[1715]. The majority of Westerners over the age of 60 have fully developed atherosclerosis[1311,1774,1831,1858–1860], including Southern Europeans[161]. Even Japanese and Chinese people are affected at an early age, although their atherosclerosis is less pronounced than that of Westerners[1,751,1017]. In 1930, the pathologist Ito believed that atherosclerotic changes appeared somewhat later in life among the Japanese than among Europeans (cited by Henschen)[714].

A traditional X-ray with an injected contrasting agent (angiography) can easily fail to visualise atherosclerosis, even when it is at a fairly advanced stage[1831]. When the radiopaque substance fills the blood vessel, occlusions can be highlighted, but the degree to which the vascular wall has thickened outwards is not visible. An autopsy was previously the only reliable method for measuring thickening of the walls due to atherosclerosis. However, in recent years, an intravascular ultrasound method has been developed, where a small transducer is inserted into the coronary artery via a thin catheter[1311]. Examinations of apparently healthy people have confirmed what autopsies of traffic accident victims have previously shown, namely that atherosclerosis is an insidious disease that affects the majority of us[1311,1831], almost regardless of blood lipid levels[752,1398,1718]. Hence, atherosclerosis is a 'normal' phenomenon among middle-aged and elderly Westerners with 'normal' levels of blood pressure or serum lipids. But who wants to be normal[1043]?

During the first half of the twentieth century, there was widespread curiosity among researchers regarding the significance of dietary habits behind the large geographic and temporal differences in the spread of atherosclerosis throughout the world. However, for some unknown reason, researchers avoided analysing the dietary habits among the populations in question in a systematic way that would allow an assessment of which foods might have been involved.

Appearance in animals

An extremely important finding is that *other free-ranging mammals do not seem to be affected by fully developed coronary atherosclerosis*. Fatty streaks are sometimes seen in vulnerable species, particularly in the aorta, but advanced atherosclerosis in (captive) animals seems to require that they be raised on feed other than what they would find in their actual ecological niche[71,1176,1184,1515,1730,1934]. High age, stress or smoking are apparently not sufficient causes by themselves (though important promoting factors), and a reversal of the disease requires that the animal returns to its original food[874,1118,1232].

Elephants have been widely debated in this regard. Widespread atherosclerosis, even in a mild form, has been noted in the coronary artery of the animal's heart, and it is pronounced in other blood vessels among East African elephants over 25–30 years of age[1177]. This is often interpreted as natural ageing, but studies in the 1960s by Sylvia Sikes from London University show that the issue is actually more complicated. Sikes performed autopsies on elephants from two different environments, where one of them represented the elephant's original, undisturbed ecological niche[1652]. This 'natural' environment consisted of extensive, forested, mountainous areas and Alpine moorlands, with plenty of streams and a rich and varied plant mix including different types of trees. The other environment, which she characterised as 'disturbed', consisted of savannah, which was partly overgrown with bushes. This niche, where elephants originally used to only reside temporarily, was now overpopulated by elephant herds that were squeezed in from the surrounding developments. Since there were not enough natural resources for them, these elephants fed on hay, which made up their principal and unbalanced feed. Advanced atherosclerosis was only seen in elephants from the 'disturbed' environment. Mild forms of atherosclerosis, however, were seen in elephants from both environments, primarily among young, suckling elephants or females who were pregnant or breastfeeding. This form of early atherosclerosis can be easily reversed, and it is also seen in humans[1372,1715] (M.F. Oliver, unpublished observations).

It is noteworthy that domesticated dogs do not develop coronary atherosclerosis as easily, but they can have hyaline sclerosis in the smaller blood vessels running through the cardiac musculature[847]. This type of thickening of the blood vessels probably plays a part in the development of small infarctions and heart failure in domestic dogs. It is also interesting that serum cholesterol does not appear to rise as easily in dogs as in other animals[622], and that HDL cholesterol makes up most of the serum cholesterol, while LDL cholesterol makes up a smaller percentage (a trait that they share with rats and mice)[1115,1116]. Certain dog breeds, such as Doberman Pinscher and Labrador Retriever, appear to be more susceptible to atherosclerosis and hypercholesterolaemia[1072].

Dogs were domesticated early in human cultural history, probably between 10 000 and 20 000 years ago[1351,1583] (a considerable number of generations before the current species of dog), and since they were often supposedly fed human food, they could have adapted genetically over time. One would wonder if dog breeds with the least tendency for atherosclerosis, obesity and insulin resistance could be the ones who were first consuming agrarian diets, and thus have had most time to adapt.

Regression studies

Palaeolithic food has not been studied in terms of reversing the process of atherosclerosis. In animal experiments, the disease can apparently be regressed by returning to the type of food that the animal eats in its original environment[874,1118,1232].

In the Lifestyle Heart Trial, 28 highly motivated atherosclerotic human subjects were apparently able to reverse the process of coronary atherosclerosis by means of a vegetarian diet that was extremely low in fat and salt[1359,1360]. The diet was based on vegetables, fruits, legumes, unprocessed cereals (primarily grains other than wheat) and egg white. The reported drop in fat intake was from 30 E% to less than 10 E%. Atherosclerosis regression was documented by means of coronary angiography. During the 5-year follow-up period, the control group continued to develop atherosclerosis, despite the fact that the total estimated fat intake decreased from 30 to 25 E% (the average for most Western populations is around 35 E% and the recommended intake is usually 25–35 E%).

One possible interpretation of the Lifestyle Heart Trial is that a lacto-vegetarian diet can prevent atherosclerosis, assuming that the fat intake remains extremely low. Most patients probably have a harder time complying with this type of diet than with a Palaeolithic diet. It is also highly debatable whether a fat intake below 15 E% is advisable for a person's overall health. Another more hypothetical conclusion, based on Richard Fienne's hypothesis below regarding a connection between cereals and atherosclerosis, is that a diet based on grains necessitates an extremely low intake of fat and cholesterol. To what extent avoiding wheat played a part in the study cannot be determined.

In another dietary intervention study, the St. Thomas' Atherosclerosis Regression Study, STARS, the development of atherosclerosis could be slowed in 54 men with ischaemic heart disease and high serum cholesterol (7.2 ± 0.8 mmol/L)[1909]. The intervention consisted of a 3.5-year period aiming on a fat intake of 27 E%, where saturated fat was 8–10 E%, polyunsaturated fat 8 E%, dietary cholesterol 100 mg/1000 kcal, a high intake of soluble fibre and weight loss as necessary. In 15% of the study group, atherosclerosis continued to advance, as compared with 46% of the control group. The inner diameter of the blood vessel in both groups increased by 3 nm in one group and decreased by 103 nm ($P < 0.05$) in the control group.

The Heidelberg study examined 36 men (around 51 years old) with atherosclerosis of the coronary artery documented with an angiography[1598]. An intervention under 1 year attempted to bring the total fat intake to <20 E%, dietary cholesterol <200 mg/day, as well as do more than 3 hours of physical activity/week. Regression of atherosclerosis occurred among 7 of the 18 trial subjects, compared with 1 out of 18 control subjects ($P < 0.05$). A statistically significant reduction of stress-induced myocardial ischaemia (lack of oxygen in the heart muscles) was obtained, regardless of whether full regression was achieved.

Overall, there is strong support for studying the effect of a Palaeolithic diet. The dietary models that have been studied so far are either difficult to comply with or insufficient to prevent atherosclerosis.

Relevant dietary factors

The fundamental characteristics of atherosclerosis remain poorly understood. Therefore, it should not come as a surprise that the picture is vague in terms of how diet can affect the initiation and enhancement of atherosclerosis, particularly in humans. Furthermore, in the majority of animal experiments, scientists have not compared different diets, but have rather used one atherogenic (atherosclerosis-causing) diet as a means to produce atherosclerosis in order to study its basic mechanisms. When diet has been the primary research target, dietary fat has usually been at the centre of attention. For many years, the rabbit was a preferred animal model in atherosclerosis research, despite that it differs markedly from humans in its response to various dietary factors[122,952]. In order to accelerate the development of atherosclerosis, which normally would take decades, researchers have often used feeds unrealistically high in one or several dietary components. In addition, evolutionary aspects of diet have rarely been considered, which means that the control diet in animal experiments has not been one that the animal would eat in its natural habitat. With regard to rodents, genetically modified varieties have generally been used (otherwise there would be no or little atherosclerosis in this species; see below), which makes comparisons with humans even more difficult. After many decades of research, available evidence does not yet point to any particular individual dietary factor being a primary cause of atherosclerosis in Western societies.

Fat

In a number of animal experiments, the process of atherosclerosis has been accelerated by a high-fat diet[952,1542,1748]. Although saturated fat usually increases blood lipids slightly more than unsaturated fat (see Section 4.8), both these types of fat are able to enhance atherosclerosis. Inconsistent results have been noted in some studies but, in general, no dramatic differences have been found when comparing various refined fats with each other, including olive oil and its dominant type of fat, monounsaturated fat[20,960,1541,1543].

In some experiments on primates, rats and rabbits, peanut oil has been more effective at producing atherosclerosis than other fats, a difference which seems to be due to the peanut lectin (see below). In some other animal studies, fats rich in omega-6 fatty acids have been particularly atherogenic, possibly more so at early stages of atherosclerosis, and hypothetically because they are more easily oxidised than monounsaturated or saturated fatty acids[953,1299]. A cross-sectional survey in Alaskan Eskimos found increased prevalence of atherosclerotic plaque with higher consumption of saturated fatty acids, especially palmitic acid, as estimated from food frequency questionnaires[466]. In the same study, a high intake of omega-3 fat did not protect against plaque formation although it was associated with decreased thickness of the intima-media layer of the carotid artery.

In one cohort study among postmenopausal US women, the progression of coronary atherosclerosis was actually greater in those with the lowest intake of saturated fat[1253]. During 3.1 years of follow-up, there was a 0.22-mm decline in the quartile (quarter) of women with the lowest intake of saturated fat, compared with a 0.10-mm decline in the second quartile ($P = 0.002$), a 0.07-mm decline in the third quartile ($P = 0.002$), and no decline in the fourth quartile ($p < 0.001$).

Monounsaturated and total fat intakes were not associated with progression. The mean overall fat intake in the total population was rather low, 25 E%.

Additional evidence of the atherogenic effects of any kind of fat can be found in human prospective observational studies using coronary angiography[183], as well as in studies of Mediterranean populations with a high intake of monounsaturated fat and among whom the prevalence of atherosclerosis is comparable with that of other Europeans or North Americans[161,943].

Dairy products

Casein, the major protein in milk, aggravates atherosclerosis in animal experiments[950]. A literature search yielded 25 studies comparing casein with soya protein in terms of progression of atherosclerosis or endothelial dysfunction, and all of these found casein to be more atherogenic[16,56,57,130,156,267,268,364,365,422,423,776, 948-950,955,956,958,959,1076,1505,1565,1566,1883,1884]. It is interesting, however, that the authors of all publications, except one, reached the conclusion that soya protein prevented atherosclerosis rather than casein causing it. Since experiments on hamsters showed that meat protein (from bison and beef, respectively) resulted in less pronounced atherosclerosis than soya protein, it seems that this conclusion is misleading[1953]. However, experiments on rabbits showed that casein and meat protein had similar effects in terms of atherosclerosis, and they were a worse alternative than vegetable protein[955]. Since rabbits are exclusive plant eaters in the wild, while hamsters feed on vegetables as well as lizards, frogs, mice, small birds and snakes, rabbits are expected to be less genetically adapted to meat proteins[1102]. Compared to most other species used in atherosclerosis research, rabbits are particularly responsive to dietary cholesterol[1547].

In experiments in primates, cynomolgus monkeys have developed coronary atherosclerosis after repeated injections of bovine serum albumin[1727], which indicates that other milk proteins, besides casein, may be significant. In humans, the appearance of immunoglobulin A antibodies, such as β-lactoglobulin, casein and α-lactalbumin is common in patients with advanced atherosclerosis[1260]. The findings are consistent with the hypothesis that atherosclerosis is an inflammatory disease with early activation of the immune system[664]. They also suggest that the interaction between various nutrients is of significance[952]. The case against casein is further strengthened by its apparent role in insulin resistance and lipotoxicity (see Section 4.6).

The largest constituent of milk by weight (second to water) is lactose. A study in baboons showed that lactose produced more pronounced atherosclerosis than fructose, sucrose, starch or glucose[954]. All diets contained equally high amounts of casein (25%) and coconut oil (14%). The authors hypothesised that dietary lactose modifies aortic wall metabolism, possibly through the formation of glycosaminoglycans. One proposed type of such modification is galactosylation of structural proteins in the arterial wall[1616]. Lactose is digested in the small intestine to glucose and galactose, although a significant portion (of unknown magnitude) of unhydrolysed lactose may hypothetically be absorbed. Free galactose is transported to the liver where it is converted to glucose, provided that the absorbed amounts do not exceed hepatic capacity. Galactose has a greater potential than glucose for binding to proteins[237], and the resulting proteoglycans could hypothetically enhance atherosclerosis, would they enter the arterial wall[1354]. Galactosylated matrix proteins in arterial walls could contribute to atherosclerosis by attachment of lipoprotein particles from the bloodstream[632]. Another possible effect of lactose on atherosclerosis could be through insulin resistance (see Section 4.6).

Another bioactive substance which is abundant in milk is β-cellulin, a member of the epidermal growth factor (EGF) family and a possible growth promoter in the bovine foetus[129]. Since β-cellulin activates EGF receptors in the glycocalyx which may lead to shedding of this barrier, it is quite possibly another way through which milk can cause atherosclerosis[440].

Milk fat has received a lot of attention over the years, but its role in atherosclerotic disease may have been overemphasised[168,581,1670,1904]. Although some fatty acids in milk increase serum cholesterol, others could potentially have opposite effects[1208]. Some bioactive components in milk have been proposed to be beneficial and even prevent atherosclerosis[1418].

Nilo-hamitic African herding populations, such as the Masai, have a high intake of fermented milk from Zebu cows (*Bos indicus*), often more than 3 L/day. A limited number of autopsies ($n = 50$) were performed in one study, which showed pronounced, generalised coronary atherosclerosis but no plaques[1140]. McLachlan attempted to explain this fact by pointing out that Zebu milk is very low in β-casein A1[1190]. Segall instead attributes the lack of atherosclerotic plaque to the low lactose content after fermenting the milk[1614]. The low serum cholesterol level among the Masai is discussed in the section on dyslipidaemia (see Section 4.8).

Calorie restriction

An observational study in 50-year-old men, who had been on a calorie-restricted diet for an average of 6 years, suggests that the atherosclerotic process can be attenuated[529]. In that study, the thickness of the intima-media layer of the carotid artery was 37% lower after rigorous calorie restriction, 0.5 ± 0.1 mm compared to 0.8 ± 0.1 mm in comparison subjects of the same age. However, in studies on non-human primates, calorie restriction has not been shown to retard atherosclerosis[189,274], pointing to the importance of other dietary factors as well.

Nutritional deficiencies

Similar to the situation for ischaemic heart disease, available studies do not suggest that deficiency of vitamins, minerals or trace elements is a widespread cause of atherosclerosis[184]. This is once again in contrast to epidemiological studies and laboratory research that led to the belief that such nutrients prevent atherosclerosis, either by acting as antioxidants (vitamins E and C, β-carotene and selenium), or by decreasing homocysteine (vitamins B6, B12 and folate). Other nutrients of proposed benefit include magnesium[808], zinc[713], potassium[1990], taurine[1259] and lutein[453]. All these nutrients are effectively provided with a Palaeolithic diet.

Cereals

Richard Fiennes, a veterinary pathologist, noted that mammals and birds (mice, rats, passerines, ostriches, etc.) which subsist on grass seeds are typically resistant to atherosclerosis when they are fed grain-based, atherogenic food, while non-seed eaters (primates, pigs, guinea pigs, parrots, etc.) are more susceptible[519]. Therefore, he postulated more than 40 years ago that cereals could contribute to atherosclerosis among *Homo sapiens* and other non-adapted species. Coronary atherosclerosis among free-ranging elephants has already been discussed. In laboratory animal experiments, atherosclerosis has developed in non-seed eaters which were raised on grain-based, low-fat diets[71,844,1515,1730,1934]. Unfortunately, the feed in such animal experiments was almost exclusively based on cereals, and no study controlled for cereal intake, a fact that makes comparisons difficult.

One plausible, but unproven, atherogenic factor is the plant lectins, which can bind to glycosylated proteins at human cell surfaces. A large number of studies indirectly support the role of plant lectins as being capable of causing disease, for instance by way of inflammatory and hormonal disturbances[543]. Lectins in cereals and beans increase the permeability of the intestinal barrier[1033,1460] and gliadin, the lectin-like gluten protein in wheat, apparently has the same effect[438,978]. Thereby, they (or other large molecules simultaneously present) can enter the blood stream when supplied from food[1461,1898]. The wheat lectin (wheat germ agglutinin, WGA) binds to macrophages and smooth muscle cells of the vessel wall[376,860], both of which are players in the atherosclerotic process. WGA has a growth-inducing effect by activating the EGF receptor[1900], which is considered a potential contributing factor in the development of atherosclerosis[1845]. In addition, WGA has a strong activating effect on platelets and cell adhesion molecules[1342], which may also play a part in atherosclerosis[359]. The peanut lectin (PNA) obviously contributes to atherosclerosis in primates, rabbits and rats, since removal of PNA makes peanut oil less atherogenic[957]. The fact that plant lectins have demonstrated an insulin-like effect (see Section 4.6) may also be considered a contributing factor in atherosclerosis. Another relevant line of thought concerns the glycocalyx, the protective barrier covering the inside of blood vessels. By activating the EGF receptor[1900], wheat lectin may cause shedding of the glycocalyx and increased flux of harmful substances (bacteria, oxidized lipids, etc.) into the arterial wall, hypothetically leading to atherosclerosis[1850,1855].

Seed lectins are often not destroyed by normal cooking but some of them by pressure cooking[609], and they are highly resistant to digestive enzymes in the gastrointestinal tract[543]. Common breakfast cereals in the US diet have been found to cause haemagglutination (clumping together of red blood cells) when ingested in realistic amounts, an effect most certainly attributed to WGA and other chitin-binding lectins[1264]. On 10 December 2007, 6271 publications were identified in PubMed by the search term 'wheat germ agglutinin', dating back to 1965. Only 50 of these citations and abstracts included the word 'nutrition' which is surprisingly few in the light of the bulk of evidence that ingested WGA from food is biologically active. A comparable search on 'saturated fat' yielded 3395 papers of which 2121 included the word 'nutrition'. Although WGA is present in the endosperm, the starchy part of the wheat grain, the content is much higher in the germ (embryo)[1644]. If, in the future, there will be strong and consistent evidence of a dose-dependent anti-atherosclerotic effect of whole grain wheat, compared to more refined wheat (where the germ has been removed), the role of WGA in atherosclerosis seems questionable.

Another group of wheat lectins are the gliadins, although they are usually designated proteins or prolamins with lectin-like properties. If wheat lectins are to be suspected of causing atherosclerosis, it would perhaps make more sense to consider the gliadins, which are present in the endosperm, than WGA, which is more abundant in the germ. The endosperm is the starchy part of a seed that acts as a food store for the developing embryo. Modern, smooth steel roller wheels finely crush the endosperm while flattening the waxy germ in one piece so that it can later be removed from the flour.

Gliadins, which belong to the larger family of gluten proteins, are a well-established cause of coeliac disease and are suspected of causing other autoimmune diseases as well (see Section 4.15). This is relevant for atherosclerosis, which is seen by many experts as having an autoimmune basis[663]. The leptin receptor, which is activated by the satiety hormone leptin, is glycosylated[660] and is thus expected to bind to lectins, including lectin-like molecules like gliadin. As a matter of fact, wheat lectin has been shown to bind to the leptin receptor[867], and our research group suspect gliadin-derived peptides to bind as well. If such binding will be confirmed, the next question is if the leptin receptor is activated or blocked. In the latter case, wheat lectins could hypothetically be a cause of reduced leptin action (leptin resistance), which, in turn, has been proposed to aggravate lipotoxicity[1840] and atherosclerosis[144]. Another pertinent finding is cytotoxicity and accumulation of intracellular lipid droplets in cell cultures exposed to gliadins[432]. This could be highly relevant to the lipid-laden foam cells of early atherosclerosis.

Cereals lack several of the minerals, vitamins and trace elements mentioned above, although, at this stage, a low intake of none of them seems to explain the omnipresence of atherosclerosis in Western societies. Cereals contain no vitamin C or vitamin B_{12}. Compared with a diet based on meat, fish, vegetables and fruits, cereals also contribute towards a lack of zinc, selenium, carotenoids, folic acid, vitamin B_6 (low bioavailability), magnesium (through chelate binding with phytic acid), potassium, biotin, vitamin D and taurine. The proportion of omega-6 fatty acids is high, and the content of omega-3 fatty acids is low. Several of these nutrients are further depleted in refined cereals, compared to whole grain cereals[1683,1816].

If cereals have undesired health effects, animal species that are specialised seed eaters can be expected to differ from non-seed eaters in terms of digestion and/or metabolism. Several of the characteristics of rats and mice should be analysed in this respect. The fact that the intestinal phytase activity of rats is 30 times higher than that of humans[797] can be seen as an indication that cereals rich in phytic acid can impair the bioavailability of dietary minerals[289]. Among the other examples of the special traits of rats and/or mice (some of which, however, they do not share with non-seed eaters) include, for those who are particularly interested, the fact that HDL is the dominant lipoprotein instead of LDL in humans[633,1115]; that cholesterol is converted to a large degree to bile through LXR-mediated stimulation of *CYP7A1* transcription[292]; that Wy-14643 and ETYA are relatively weak PPAR-α-agonists[987]; that the genetic expression for resistin is high[1266]; that the formation of pancreatic islet amyloid is absent[163]; that the release of GLP-1 after consuming protein or fat is high[98]; and that the regulation of LXRα in macrophages is quite different[971]. A special feature in glucose metabolism has been noted in seed-eating birds compared to meat-eating birds. If the pancreas is removed while retaining the α-cells, seed-eating birds will develop a temporary form of insulin-dependent diabetes, in contrast to the type of diabetes that affects non-seed eating birds[1085].

On the plus side, cereals are often high in fibre and low in fat, with a low percentage of saturated fat. The high fibre content has been proposed to slow down the atherosclerotic process, possibly through reduced absorption of lipids in the gut, but the evidence is equivocal[458].

4.4   Type 2 diabetes

Persistently high blood sugar (hyperglycaemia), due to failing production and action of insulin, is the main characteristic of type 2 diabetes. After consumption of a carbohydrate-rich meal, blood sugar increases considerably and does not decrease as rapidly as in the non-diabetic state. An intermediate state is called glucose intolerance, where blood sugar is only slightly elevated after carbohydrate-rich meals. Glucose intolerance precedes frank diabetes, usually by several years, and is therefore sometimes called pre-diabetes, although in many cases diabetes never develops. Both conditions are also characterised by insulin resistance, a disturbance which is discussed in Section 4.6.

People with type 2 diabetes run a several-fold increased risk of cardiovascular disease such as stroke, myocardial infarction, angina pectoris, heart failure and impaired arterial circulation in the legs (peripheral arterial disease), compared to those with normal glucose tolerance[231,343,774,1549]. Even in the state of glucose intolerance, a sharply increased risk is apparent[1463]. Furthermore, in people with normal glucose tolerance, one study found a continuous positive association between blood glucose and risk of ischaemic heart disease[583]. These findings explain why the definition of type 2 diabetes, based on fasting blood sugar, has been changed to a fasting blood sugar above 6 mmol/L, which is 1 mmol/L lower than before[1549]. Since the risk increases gradually, any particular level of hyperglycaemia (such as the present limit of diabetes) can be disputed, in analogy to the situation for hypertension, high cholesterol and overweight. Similar to these risk factors, it is worse to have an average blood sugar level than a low level.

Accordingly, most people with cardiovascular disease are glucose intolerant or have diabetes. In fact, various observational studies have found only 35–54% of ischaemic heart disease patients to have normal glucose tolerance[125,666,678,771,801,833,1322]. In addition, increasing evidence suggests that glucose intolerance and type 2 diabetes are important risk factors for stroke, as shown in one study where only 20% of stroke patients had normal glucose tolerance[1162]. This often passes unnoticed, because routine examination with the oral glucose tolerance test (which analyses the increase in blood sugar after glucose intake) is uncommon in such patients, and because many cases are not detected by casual blood sugar assessment.

Diabetes and glucose intolerance negatively affect the long-term prognosis after myocardial infarction[124,522], and there is a gradual increase in mortality with increasing blood sugar even among those with normal glucose tolerance[1434]. Therefore, prevention should aim at improving glucose metabolism in addition to dealing with other risk factors. Unfortunately, the ability to prevent cardiovascular disease by controlling blood sugar with medication is limited, while the effect on other, less common complications, such as blindness and renal failure, appears to be greater[1174]. In fact, serious damage to the kidneys, eyes or peripheral nervous system is the main reason for intervening with glucose-regulating medication.

Thus, in the United Kingdom Prospective Diabetes Study (UKPDS), encompassing 3867 middle-aged patients with type 2 diabetes, the risk of myocardial infarction was lowered by only 16% ($P = 0.052$) in those assigned a more intensive control of blood sugar with glucose-regulating drugs[1834]. If we translate the findings from this study, we would expect, among 100 people with type 2 diabetes who are treated for 10 years, that only 2 of 17 myocardial infarctions were prevented ($P = 0.052$). For other cardiovascular calamities the situation is even worse: no effect would be expected on stroke (0 of 5 cases prevented), heart failure (0 of 3) or angina pectoris (0 of 7)[1834].

Prevalence studies

The prevalence of diabetes among hunter-gatherers has not been studied using current methods, but indirect studies of glucose tolerance, blood sugar, serum insulin, waist circumference and other related variables provide evidence of an extremely low prevalence of type 2 diabetes[832,1048,1213,1702,2008]. On Kitava, Trobriand Islands, Papua New Guinea (see Section 4.1), diabetes does not seem to occur, and the average fasting blood sugar is approximately 2 standard deviations (SD) below the average among the Swedish population (Figures 4.8 and 4.9)[1048]. This means that approximately 98% of Swedes have a higher fasting blood sugar than any of the Kitavans, and the divergence is similar or larger if other Western populations are used for comparison. In addition, roughly the same difference (–2 SD) was noted between migrants and non-migrants from Cameroon, West Africa[350].

From a global ethnic perspective, there is a very large variation in the prevalence of diabetes[910] with a positive correlation to the average BMI across populations[327].

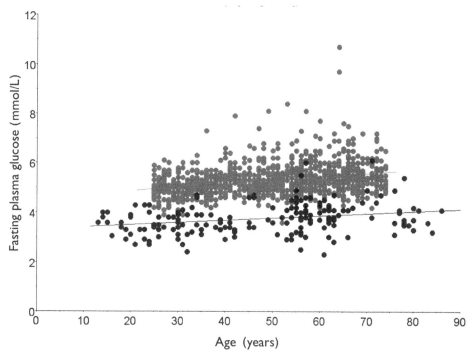

Figure 4.8 Fasting plasma glucose samples in Kitava, Trobriand Islands, Papua New Guinea (black) and Sweden (grey). No sex difference was found; therefore, data for men and women were combined. (Adapted from Reference 1048.)

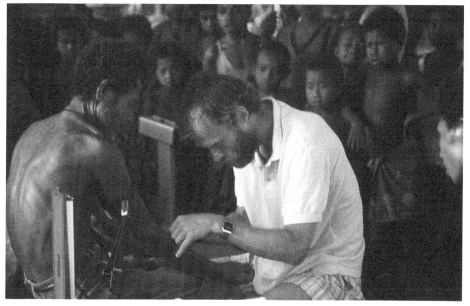

Figure 4.9 The author taking blood samples in Kitava in 1990. (Photo courtesy of Eva Lindsten.)

After urbanisation, blood sugar levels among the entire population increase to higher levels and the prevalence of diabetes increases dramatically[350]. The first known case of diabetes in Uganda, East Africa, was noted in the 1940s in an obese woman who was employed by a British colonial officer[1813]. Among the Pima Indians of the Gila River in Arizona, USA, the first confirmed case of diabetes was in 1908. Thirty years later, 21 cases were reported, and by 1965 the number had risen to 500[150]. A similar increase in death rates of diabetes among the urban population of New York between 1866 and 1922, likely including type 2, has been reported[493]. There have been various attempts to relate such increases to changes in lifestyle without finding any consistent pattern[493,715,841,1813,2009].

Today, we are seeing an explosion of diabetes in the developing world following the introduction of a Western lifestyle[1941]. The situation in the South Pacific is somewhat bizarre with an extremely high occurrence of diabetes among young people in countries such as Fiji, Samoa and Tonga, yet with the Trobriand Islands as one of the few protected enclaves in a sea of 'Coca colonisation'. Even in North America and Europe the prevalence of diabetes is increasing as obesity becomes more common[1941]. Thus, in Canada the diabetes prevalence increased from 5.2 to 8.8% between 1995 and 2005, a staggering 69% increase[1062].

Obviously, genetic changes do not explain such alterations. Likewise, the apparent absence of excessive weight and diabetes in aboriginal populations is not due to some inherited protection. If anything, several studies provide evidence that populations of non-European origin have lower resistance to the modern lifestyle, which is discussed in Section 4.6. Instead, heredity is an important cause for the variation in risk of diabetes *within* a limited, Westernised population, which has been shown for a number of different ethnic groups[245].

Mediterranean countries have, somewhat unexpectedly, a high prevalence of type 2 diabetes (and overweight). In a study in rural Crete around the turn of the century, 7% of an adult population of 4282 inhabitants were found to have type 2 diabetes (5.2% after age standardisation to the world population)[1058]. After age 65, the prevalence was 30%. A survey from mainland Greece found similar levels[1376]. In a study from Catalonia, Spain, the prevalence of diabetes (known and unknown) in the 30–89-year-old population was 10.3% (95% CI 9.1–11.6) in a random sample of 3839 subjects[271]. The prevalence of impaired glucose tolerance was 12% in men and women. The age-adjusted prevalence to the world population for the 30–64-year-old age group was 6.1% (7.1% in men and 5.2% in women). These prevalence rates are similar to those observed in other Mediterranean countries and not lower than in northern European populations.

Preventive/causative dietary factors

There is general agreement that improvement of glucose tolerance lowers the risk of diabetes. However, given the uncertainty about the basic mechanisms behind glucose intolerance, there is no good evidence showing any particular dietary factor as an independent cause of type 2 diabetes[8,892,1142,1312,1480,1958]. A recent Cochrane review found no high-quality randomised controlled trials on the efficacy of dietary intervention for the prevention of type 2 diabetes[1303]. Virtually all experts agree on one point: being overweight is a contributing factor, but perhaps not essential, to glucose intolerance and type 2 diabetes. Available evidence supports the benefits of a combination of physical activity and healthy foods by standard dietary advice, although the independent effect of each has yet to be proven[591,928,1828,1979]. Standard dietary advice includes whole grain cereals, low-fat dairy products, vegetables, fruits, legumes, oily fish and refined fats that are rich in monounsaturated fatty acids and α-linolenic acid (omega-3) while low in saturated and trans-unsaturated fatty acids. Most authorities advocate high-fibre diets with low GI, especially when carbohydrate intake is close to the proposed upper limit (60 E%). Much of the dietary advice aims at other cardiovascular risk factors than high blood sugar, such as abdominal obesity, dyslipidaemia (high cholesterol, low HDL, high triglycerides) and high blood pressure, since these other risk factors may be more important to manage than high blood sugar[1274,1682].

As a consequence of the apparent negative impact of excess body fat, avoiding overweight by eating a nutrient-rich, satiating diet with a limited amount of calories is expected to prevent type 2 diabetes. An example of such a diet is a Palaeolithic diet, although it cannot be excluded that other low-calorie diets are equally effective to obtain a certain amount of weight loss (see Section 4.5).

Weight management

There is a broad consensus that weight management (weight loss among the overweight and avoidance of weight gain among the lean) lowers the risk of type 2 diabetes. In randomised controlled lifestyle trials, weight loss and a reduced waistline have apparently been critical for the beneficial effect on glucose tolerance. The largest of these studies, the US Diabetes Prevention Project ($n = 3324$), found weight loss to be the dominant predictor of reduced diabetes incidence among glucose intolerant subjects who were randomised to intensive lifestyle modification (low-calorie, low-fat diet plus moderately intensive physical activity 150 min/week)[652,928]. After adjustment for weight loss, neither physical activity nor dietary change was predictive of diabetes development in that study. Similar results were found in a study from Finland ($n = 522$), where weight loss (or increased exercise) was crucial for success, irrespective of assignment to control group or lifestyle intervention[1828]. Since physical activity was part of the lifestyle intervention in both trials, the independent effect of the applied dietary models (low-fat, high-fibre diets) is uncertain.

However, weight change does not explain all, or even most, of the improvement in glucose tolerance in such trials, and in a meta-analysis on the efficacy of lifestyle education to prevent type 2 diabetes in high-risk individuals, 4 out of 8 trials did not find any effect on 2-hour plasma glucose despite significant weight loss[1979]. Furthermore, in epidemiological studies, most of the variation in glucose tolerance among the general population is not explained by adiposity[1186]. Therefore, an improvement in glucose tolerance that is independent of weight change would not be entirely unexpected.

Palaeolithic-style diet

There is a paucity of clinical trials with ancestral-like diets in subjects at risk for diabetes. In a randomised controlled trial among 29 patients with ischaemic heart disease and glucose intolerance or diabetes, we compared a Palaeolithic diet ($n = 14$) based on lean meat, fish, fruits, vegetables, root vegetables, eggs and nuts, with a Consensus (Mediterranean-like) diet ($n = 15$) based on whole grains, low-fat dairy products, vegetables, fruits, fish, and oils and margarines generally assumed to be healthy[1049]. After 12 weeks, in the Palaeolithic group there was a 26% decrease ($P = 0.0001$) in the area under the glucose curve during 2 hours after intake of glucose solution (glucose tolerance test), while the 7% decrease among Consensus subjects was no longer statistically significant ($P = 0.08$) (Figure 4.10). The difference between the two groups was highly significant ($P < 0.0001$). This corresponded with a 36% decrease in 2-hour plasma glucose in the Palaeolithic group (from 8.9 to 5.6 mmol/L; $P = 0.0003$), while the 7% decrease in the Consensus group was not significant (from 8.8 to 7.9 mmol/L; $P = 0.10$).

At baseline, 10 of 14 Palaeolithic and 9 of 15 Consensus subjects had diabetic plasma glucose values. After 12 weeks, all 14 subjects in the Palaeolithic group had normal values, compared with 7 of 15 subjects in the Consensus group ($P = 0.0007$ for group difference). After 12 weeks, 5 Consensus subjects still had diabetic values.

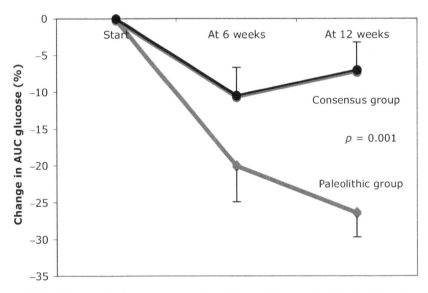

Figure 4.10   Changes in glucose response to a 75 g oral glucose load during 12 weeks of Palaeolithic or Consensus diet. Values are means ± standard errors. (Adapted from Reference 1049.)

The markedly better result in the Palaeolithic group was not due to greater weight loss. Although loss of waist circumference was greater in that group, 5.8 cm compared with 2.9 cm in the Consensus group ($P = 0.03$ for difference), and despite large variation in weight loss (between –10.7 and +1.3 kg), there was no relationship between changes in glucose tolerance and changes in waist circumference ($r = 0.01$; $P = 1.0$) or weight ($r = -0.06$; $P = 0.9$). Subjects in the Palaeolithic group lost on average 5.0 kg compared to 3.8 kg in the Consensus group ($P = 0.3$ for difference).

A recent non-controlled trial with Palaeolithic diet in healthy volunteers found improved glucose tolerance, decreased insulin secretion, increased insulin sensitivity, decreased blood pressure and improved lipid profiles without significant weight loss[2018]. These findings suggest that weight loss may not be the most important goal to eliminate the fundamental cause of type 2 diabetes. Possibly, a Palaeolithic diet improves glucose tolerance beyond weight loss by some unknown mechanism, and that an energy-restricted diet based on cereals and dairy products is not the best choice.

Calorie restriction

An observational study in 36 middle-aged people, 18 of which had been on long-term rigorous calorie restriction, suggests that this is a powerful way to keep your blood sugar low[529]. At age 50 years, after an average of 6 years of calorie restriction, fasting plasma glucose was 2 standard deviations lower in the calorie restricted group, 4.5 ± 0.4 mmol/L compared to 5.3 ± 0.4 mmol/L in the control group. In a normal Western population of the same age, less than 3% would be expected to have a blood sugar lower than 4.5 mmol/L. The average BMI was 20 in the calorie restricted group, compared to 26 in the control group. Thus, half of the calorie-restricted group were below 'normal' weight (BMI 20).

Low-fat diet

According to the 2004 guidelines of the Diabetes and Nutrition Study Group (DNSG) of the European Association for the Study of Diabetes (EASD), total fat intake should be restricted in order to prevent type 2 diabetes[1142]. Two reasons are given, the risk of increased body weight in people on high-fat diets and a possible adverse influence on insulin sensitivity by total fat intake. However, the only reference provided to substantiate the latter notion is a study on fat quality, not quantity[1866]. According to the American Diabetes Association position statements, reduced-fat diets, when maintained over the long term, contribute to modest waist loss and improvement in dyslipidaemia, while studies on diabetes incidence are inconclusive[8,538]. The effect of total fat on weight is discussed in Section 4.5. One large randomised controlled trial, the Women's Health Initiative Dietary Modification Trial, did not find a reduced incidence of diabetes after 8.1 years of a low-fat diet[1797]. In summary, if weight management fails on a traditional fat-reduced diet, no favourable effect on blood glucose should be expected. On the other hand, animal experiments have shown that high-fat diets can cause glucose intolerance in dogs[863] and various strains of rats and mice[235], but the full impact of other dietary factors has not been elucidated.

Glycaemic load

One of the longest held debates in clinical medicine concerns the role of dietary carbohydrate in glucose intolerance. The name of the disorder tends to guide your thought: if you are intolerant to glucose, why not avoid it, or at least choose low-glycaemic index foods? Starch, the dominant type of carbohydrate in Western diets, is built up of long chains of glucose. When you eat starch, your blood sugar goes up. The logic seems to be simple. However, the main cause of an individual's inability to limit blood sugar rise after eating carbohydrates remains obscure, and it is questionable if dietary glucose/starch per se plays a causative role[446,892,1312,1480]. Insulin resistance, which is a proposed but as yet unproven cause of glucose intolerance, has not been shown to be affected by varying the amount of dietary carbohydrate, as discussed in Section 4.6. Furthermore, you must eat something, and the replacements are not always safe, particularly the high-fat alternatives[892]. Nevertheless, for many Westerners it may be beneficial to avoid the hyperinsulinaemia (high blood insulin) and glycation (attachment of carbohydrate residues) of proteins that are discussed in the same section. Furthermore, once the process has developed as far as type 2 diabetes, it is certainly sensible to avoid foods that raise blood sugar too much, as discussed below.

Experiments in rats have shown that very high-fat diets cause glucose intolerance and insulin resistance even when carbohydrate intake is extremely low[1664]. In contrast, other experiments in rats, in whom parts of the pancreas (including some of the insulin-producing β-cells) have been surgically removed, suggest that amylopectin, the major form of starch with a high GI, can aggravate glucose intolerance when incorporated into a very high-carbohydrate (69 E%) diet based on starch, casein, sucrose, soya bean oil, wheat bran and gelatin[1401]. Control rats were given a diet which differed only in being rich in amylose (low-GI starch) in exchange for amylopectin. It is conceivable, but speculative, that there might be an interaction between amylopectin and some of the other dietary components and that the amylopectin content of the control diet was too low to elicit this interaction. Thus, a possible interpretation from these animal experiments is that a high GI is one of several contributing causes of glucose intolerance, and that it may be harmful in concert with other factors but not in isolation. One of the factors that may have contributed is casein (which constituted 20% of the feed per weight), as discussed below.

Fructose

Another matter of debate concerns (very) high-fructose diets, which have been shown to cause glucose intolerance in rats[487], while studies in mice have shown varying results, in some cases even improvement of glucose tolerance[1358]. Other rodent experiments suggest that this negative effect of fructose is mainly seen in taurine-deficient animals[1272]. In addition, studies in humans suggest that dietary fructose in quantities corresponding to a high intake of fruit are not harmful[1857]. Much of the concern about dietary fructose in Western societies relates to soft drinks and other non-natural foods, which provide 2/3 of dietary fructose in the USA, mainly in the form of sucrose and high fructose corn syrup[841,1390].

Unlike rodents, the primate ancestors of humans likely consumed considerable quantities of fruits during 50 million years or more, particularly until the emergence of *Australopithecines* 4 million years ago. After this date, it is questionable if there would have been any disadvantage of a high capacity to handle fructose, which may therefore still characterise the human species. Therefore, findings in rodents, which are not descendants of specialised fruit eaters, should be interpreted with caution. A daily fructose intake below 60 g, corresponding to 4–5 kg of pineapples, appears safe[841,1857].

In our study with Palaeolithic diet, average fruit intake in the Palaeolithic group was 493 g, corresponding to 4–5 apples, and twice as high as in the Consensus group. This is almost sevenfold higher than the median intake among Swedish men (75 g/day)[138], although rather low from an evolutionary perspective. Despite large variation in fruit intake (range 160–1435 g/day in the Palaeolithic group and 53–679 g/day in the Consensus group), fruit intake was not associated with change in area under the curves of glucose ($r = -0.06$; $P = 0.8$) or insulin ($r = -0.19$; $P = 0.4$) during the glucose tolerance test. Thus, our study lends no support to the notion that fruit intake should be restricted in people with glucose intolerance.

Dairy products

Studies of dairy products in connection with the development of type 2 diabetes are contradictory. Among US health professionals, a lower risk of type 2 diabetes has been observed among those who regularly consume dairy products, in particular those who choose low-fat varieties[296,1069]. In contrast to these prospective studies, a cross-sectional survey of 4024 British women aged 60–79 years, randomly selected from primary care centres in 23 towns, found diabetes to be less common ($P = 0.06$) among those who avoided milk (0.9%) than among milk-drinkers (5.6%), despite no difference in waist-to-hip ratio ($P = 0.45$)[1001].

Animal studies have found lactose to cause high blood sugar and insulin resistance in calves[777,778,1375]. Galactose, one half of the disaccharide lactose, has a more unstable ring structure than glucose and is therefore more prone to glycosylate proteins[237]. Glycosylation of proteins has been discussed mainly with regard to diabetes complications, but it is also highly relevant in the context of progressive β-cell failure[1343]. In rats, casein, which is the dominant protein in milk, apparently causes insulin resistance[993,1808], and in liver cells it contributes to fat overload[76,1804]. Since fat overload in pancreatic β-cells is thought to contribute to type 2 diabetes by way of lipotoxicity[395,1428], further studies of casein are clearly warranted in this aspect. It is obvious that such studies have been delayed by the fact that casein traditionally has been regarded as a neutral reference protein.

In humans, milk stimulates insulin release from the pancreas, an effect mainly mediated by whey protein[1307], but the long-term effects of the ensuing hyperinsulinaemia have not been studied. Some experts suggest the effect to be beneficial, even in healthy people, but no one would recommend healthy people to take sulfonylurea or other insulin-releasing drugs in order to prevent diabetes. In an evolutionary perspective, stimulation of pancreatic release of insulin with milk and medication are both artificial. Some authorities assume that unnaturally high levels of serum insulin are harmful and may be responsible for most of the abnormalities that are associated with glucose intolerance[1480].

The idea that milk aggravates glucose intolerance is not new. Allen and Cheer noted a strong inverse correlation between prevalence of adult lactase persistence and type 2 diabetes, such that ethnic groups who are largely able to drink milk as adults also have a relatively low prevalence of type 2 diabetes[39]. A plausible explanation is that milk causes type 2 diabetes or related disorders, which reduce biological fitness (see Section 4.6). Obviously, there are other causes as well, since many Westernised people apparently acquire glucose intolerance without having consumed dairy products.

Cereals

Epidemiological studies suggest that high-fibre diets reduce the risk of type 2 diabetes, while data on Mediterranean diets, fat quality, minerals, vitamins, micronutrients and phytochemicals are inconsistent[8,1142]. An increase in dietary fibre typically means more grains. However, most evidence favours soluble fibre from fruits and vegetables, while insoluble fibre, the dominant type of fibre in grains, seems less beneficial[500,1142,1514].

A possible disadvantage of whole grains (and beans) is their content of plant lectins. The best studied cereal lectin is WGA, while gliadin, which also has lectin properties, has scarcely been investigated (see Section 4.3 for speculations on gliadin and atherosclerosis). As outlined in Section 4.6, wheat lectin binds strongly to the insulin receptor and activates it more intensively than insulin, and with longer duration, which suggests that it may cause insulin resistance. However, the relevance of these findings for glucose tolerance is unclear.

Observations among birds indicate that cereals can affect glucose metabolism in a potentially negative way. Those species of birds that are natural seed eaters regulate their blood sugar differently compared with other birds, and can manage quite well after the insulin-producing β-cells have been removed from their pancreas[1085]. Shortly after removal, temporary insulin-dependent diabetes develops and insulin treatment is mandatory, but after a period of recovery, insulin therapy is no longer needed to maintain normal blood sugar levels. In contrast, non seed-eating birds behave like humans and are continually dependent on supplementary insulin after removal of the β-cells. Now, why should seed-eating animals have this particular feature unless it is a defence against something in the seed (or something that is connected with seed-eating) that can eventually destroy their β-cells?

Diet in established type 2 diabetes

No specific diet is known to prevent the serious complications of type 2 diabetes. The most important thing (in terms of survival and life quality) is usually to prevent cardiovascular disease, and therefore the conclusions drawn in Sections 4.1–4.3 are highly relevant for people with diabetes. In order to keep blood sugar low, available evidence suggests that being physically active can be more important than complying with traditional low-fat, high-fibre diets[1236,1302]. Prevailing concepts are based on the well-known associations between cardiovascular complications and high blood sugar, abdominal obesity, dyslipidaemia and high blood pressure[8,1142]. The current disagreement on other aspects of nutrition is largely based on shortcomings of each of the prevailing dietary models with regard to one or more of these four variables.

For reasons given above and below, a diet based on lean meat, fish, vegetables, fruits and nuts, such as a Palaeolithic diet, can be expected to stabilise weight, blood sugar, blood pressure and blood lipids, and to prevent cardiovascular disease, in people with type 2 diabetes.

In the early 1980s, the Australian scientist Kerin O'Dea, one of the first researchers to realise the potential of ancient human diets, persuaded a group of Aborigines with type 2 diabetes to revert to their hunter-gatherer lifestyle. During the trial, the consumption of meat, fish and shellfish increased considerably, as did physical activity, whereas Western food was absent. The effects she noted were dramatic, in particular with regard to blood sugar, fasting insulin, weight and serum triglycerides (Table 4.4)[1331].

Recently, we performed a 3-month trial in 13 men and women with long-standing type 2 diabetes[848a]. Using cross-over design, where each individual tested both the

Table 4.4 Effect of returning to a hunter-gatherer lifestyle for 7 weeks among ten Australian Aborigines with type 2 diabetes[1331].

	Before	After	p
Weight	82 ± 3	74 ± 3	<0.001
BMI	27.2 ± 1.1	24.5 ± 0.8	<0.001
Fasting blood glucose	12 ± 1.2	6.6 ± 0.5	<0.001
2-hour blood glucose	18.5 ± 1.3	11.9 ± 0.9	<0.001
Fasting insulin	23 ± 3	12 ± 1	<0.001
2-hour insulin	49 ± 9	59 ± 11	n.s.
Triglycerides	4.0 ± 0.5	1.2 ± 0.1	<0.001
Cholesterol	5.7 ± 0.2	5.0 ± 0.3	n.s.
Systolic blood pressure	121 ± 5	114 ± 4	<0.08
Diastolic blood pressure	80 ± 2	72 ± 2	<0.02

n.s., not significant.

Palaeolithic diet and a diet generally prescribed for patients with type 2 diabetes, we found the Palaeolithic diet to be superior for the control of blood sugar, blood pressure, triglycerides, HDL cholesterol and abdominal obesity.

In type 2 diabetes, the total amount of calories should be kept low in order to manage body weight. In our experience, this is achieved more or less automatically with a Palaeolithic diet, since it works against overeating (see Section 4.5).

Glycaemic load

A traditional starch-based, whole-grain, low-fat diet often fails to lower blood sugar[363,455,565,686,892,913,1383,1628,1960,1981,2019,2020,2021] and serum triglycerides[1876]. On the other hand, a low-carbohydrate, high-fat diet may increase LDL choles-terol[1876] and, in animals, aggravate atherosclerosis[952], insulin resistance[276] and lipotoxicity[1386,1927]. A widely accepted compromise in recent years is a diet moderately high in monounsaturated fat and carbohydrate, while low in saturated and trans-unsaturated fat[8,244,445,1530] but, again, the support is indirect and open for debate[469,580].

Several factors determine the GI of food, i.e. how much blood sugar increases after a meal, and how quickly it returns to normal. These factors include the type of sugar (glucose, fructose, galactose), the type of starch (amylose, amylopectin), food processing and the addition of other components during the meal (protein content, etc.)[538]. In addition, fermented foods or food products with added organic acids seem to result in lower glucose and insulin responses, possibly by delaying the passage of food from the stomach to the small intestine[1038,1362]. Finally, the blood sugar response is also affected by the character of the previous meal (second-meal effect)[221,1363,1961].

A beneficial effect, usually modest, of food with a low GI on glycated haemoglobin (HbA1c) and other markers for the control of diabetes has been noted in some studies[8,208,826,1510,1783,1960]. A Cochrane review of randomised controlled trials found a mean decrease of 0.5% units of HbA1c with low, compared to high-GI diets (95% CI −0.9 to −0.1; $P = 0.02$)[1783]. All studies favoured the low-GI diet, but only one was statistically significant in its own power. The effect on blood lipids is apparently marginal[538]. Of greater interest is perhaps the pronounced reduction of the activity of the plasminogen activator inhibitor-1 (PAI-1) in plasma, an indicator of impaired fibrinolysis which is associated with insulin resistance[817]. It should be noted that the levels of PAI-1 were extremely beneficial in the Kitava population[1045]. The influence of GI and type of carbohydrate (starch, sucrose, fructose, glucose, etc.) on diabetes progression is much debated.

Fat intake

A reasonable goal is to keep total fat intake at around 25–35 E%, which also aims at countering weight gain. However, in case of successful weight loss and improved blood glucose and other risk factors, a higher fat intake may be acceptable. It may be more important to avoid energy-dense foods, in particular high-fat processed foods, than to actually calculate the percentage of energy coming from fat[2022,2023,2024]. In the case of a diet high in meat, it may be relevant to emphasise lean portion sizes (<10 g fat/100 g). The intake of saturated fat and trans fatty acids should preferably be limited in order to reduce serum cholesterol. This is achieved by excluding dairy products, fatty delicatessen products, fatty cuts of meat, margarine and oil.

Protein content

An increased intake of protein in exchange for starch and glucose leads to lower blood sugar after a meal, as shown in several studies with high-protein diets[8,565]. In addition, available evidence suggests that protein is more satiating than carbohydrates or fat and thereby may foster weight loss[84] (see Section 4.5). However, the extent to which a high-protein intake (>20 E%) is beneficial (or detrimental) for the long-term progression of diabetes and its complications has not been extensively studied.

In the case of calorie restriction, the absolute protein intake in g/day is often not increased despite a higher intake relative to other macronutrients. In our study in patients with glucose intolerance and ischaemic heart disease, where we compared a Palaeolithic diet with a Mediterranean-style diet, absolute protein intake was identical in the two groups, 1.0 g/kg body weight/day, while relative protein intake was 27 ± 7 E% in the Palaeolithic group and 20 ± 3 E% in the Mediterranean-style diet group.

It has been proposed that elevated blood sugar at the levels common to type 2 diabetes can contribute to increased turnover of the body's own proteins, which can potentially increase the need for protein in the diet, particularly in the case of a low energy intake[538]. A consumption level below 0.6 mg protein/kg body weight/day has even been suggested to carry a risk of malnutrition[1202]. In the case of restricted energy for the purpose of weight loss, the suggested recommendation for protein requirement should probably be in the range of 0.9 – 1.0 g/kg/day[538].

The proposed benefits of high-protein consumption should be weighed against the potential risk of kidney damage[838,1133]. In the event of manifest kidney failure, many experts have advocated protein restriction, particularly in people without diabetes or with type 1 diabetes[534,662]. However, for the majority of people with type 2 diabetes there is not much evidence of a beneficial effect on the kidneys of a low protein intake[838,1133,1153,1202,1273,2025]. A recent meta-analysis did not find that low protein dies improved kidney function in patients with either type 1 or type 2 diabetic nephropathy. In animals, two experiments actually showed that calorie restriction with a high percentage of protein prevented the development of kidney failure[933,1765].

Among northern Europeans with type 2 diabetes, serious kidney damage is considerably less common than myocardial infarction, cardiac failure and stroke[232,1529]. In fact, these cardiovascular complications generally kill the patients before they develop advanced kidney failure that requires dialysis or kidney transplant. Even among those who develop kidney failure, cardiovascular disease is the dominant cause of death[425,1021,1722]. For each person with diabetes who passes away from kidney failure, there are at least 50 who die of cardiovascular disease. In the general population, patients with uraemia requiring dialysis have a cardiovascular mortality rate that is 10–20 times higher than the normal population after adjusting for age, sex and the appearance of diabetes[527]. Cardiovascular prevention, therefore, has the highest priority among these patients. This also applies in the case of microalbuminuria, a condition that primarily signals an increased risk for cardiovascular disease and, secondarily, progressive renal failure[1704]. The people who develop diabetes before the age of 50, as well as those of non-European ethnicity, however, have a more obvious risk for serious kidney failure that cannot be overlooked[1499].

Protein quality

From an evolutionary perspective, it is reasonable to wonder whether protein from meat and fish is different from protein in milk, grains and beans in terms of preventing and treating type 2 diabetes. This has scarcely been studied, and none of the published studies on protein restriction have made this distinction. Furthermore, casein (milk protein) is often lumped together with meat protein. These 'animal' proteins are then compared with vegetable protein (usually soya protein). In one such study on Zucker rats, a rat strain with inherited tendency for obesity and insulin resistance, a higher level of kidney failure was noted using casein compared to soya protein[1110]. Several other animal experiments have found similar results[377,1556,1802,1815,1947]. In contrast, one study in humans found no effect on blood sugar or serum insulin of substituting 50 g casein with 50 g soya protein for 3 weeks[718]. The possible link between kidney failure, insulin resistance, lipotoxicity and Western disease, including the possible untoward effects of dietary casein, is discussed in Section 4.6.

Patients with type 2 diabetes who wish to try a Palaeolithic diet should preferably do so in consultation with their physician or diabetes nurse and schedule evaluations on a regular basis. If body weight starts to drop and the blood pressure, blood sugar and blood lipids improve, the net effect will probably be beneficial even with a high-protein intake, especially if urinary albumin excretion does not increase. If the goal is to restrict protein, it may be wise to reduce milk protein.

Dietary salt

A low salt intake is particularly desirable in the case of diabetes, not just to fight hypertension. Studies on rats with artificially generated type 1 diabetes (streptozotocin diabetic rats) have shown that salt restriction can effectively prevent reduced kidney function in this animal model[40]. One diet that was extremely low in salt did not impair kidney function at all, whereas adding salt in realistic amounts (0.4% NaCl) did have a negative effect. The concentration of angiotensin II, a protein involved in high blood pressure, in the plasma was normalised, as well as the size of the kidneys, and later experiments showed that urinary leakage of albumin could be prevented. In other rat studies, salt restriction prevented pathologic changes in connective tissue of the renal parenchyma (and cardiac musculature), which may be the actual mechanism involved in declining kidney function[1994]. It has been suggested that inadequate reduction of dietary salt may explain why some people do not obtain any benefit from ACE-inhibiting drugs in delaying progression of renal disease[1922].

Food choice

From all we know, fruits, vegetables, nuts, fish and lean meat can be eaten without restrictions. The beneficial effects of a Palaeolithic diet in our study mentioned above are probably applicable to most people with type 2 diabetes. Fruit has a high water content and therefore facilitates caloric restriction. It is also low in fat and salt, while high in soluble fibre, vitamins and minerals. Furthermore, most fruits have a low GI (melons are relatively high GI)[88,617]. Even ripe bananas are acceptable with a mean GI of 50 (glucose = 100)[88,498,717]. However, fruits are considerably less protein-rich (per unit of energy) than vegetables, which therefore results in a higher glycaemic load. When fruits replace cereal grains, as will be the case for most Westerners with diabetes, the total glycaemic load decreases. Nevertheless, blood sugar should be carefully monitored, particularly when fruit consumption exceeds 500 g/day and in case of high intakes of grapes or ripe bananas. Serum triglyceride levels can rise in sensitive patients since fruit contains relatively high levels of fructose[1843]. The fructose content in fruit is apparently too low to pose a significant problem for most people with type 2 diabetes. The amount of fructose in 500 g of fruit is approximately 25 g[88], while available evidence suggests that a fructose intake below 60 g is safe[1568,1857].

Although the role of cereals and dairy products in type 2 diabetes is uncertain, restriction of these foods can be tried without obvious risks (calcium intake and bone health is discussed in Section 4.12).

4.5   Overweight and obesity

Middle-age spread is a normal phenomenon – assuming that you live in the West. Few people are able to maintain their juvenile waistline after age 50. The usual explanation – too little exercise and too much food – does not fully take into account the situation among traditional populations. Such people are usually not as physically active as you may think, and they usually eat large quantities of food.

Prevalence studies

Overweight (see Table 4.5) has been extremely rare among hunter-gatherers and other traditional cultures[118,126,816,821,1046,1051,1065,1108,1132,1139, 1369,1631,1634,1668,1736,1814,1817,1937]. This simple fact has been quickly apparent to all foreign visitors. The average BMI at 40 years of age has typically been around

Table 4.5 Lower limits for being overweight and obese in three different body heights.

Body height stature (cm)	Limit for being overweight (kg) (BMI 25)	Limit of obesity (kg) (BMI 30)
160	64	77
170	73	87
180	81	98

Note: Overweight is defined as a BMI (body mass index) > 25 kg/m² and obesity is a BMI > 30 kg/m².

20 kg/m² for men and 19 kg/m² for women. After the age of 40, the BMI for both sexes drops because muscle mass and water content decrease with age and because fat is not increasingly accumulated[562,1545].

The Kitava study measured height, weight, waist circumference, subcutaneous fat thickness at the back of the upper arm (triceps skinfold) and upper arm circumference on 272 persons ages 4–86 years[1051]. Overweight and obesity were absent and average BMI was low across all age groups (Table 4.6, Figures 4.11 and 4.12). A 50-year-old Swedish man would weigh 19 kg less if he had the same BMI as on Kitava, and the corresponding difference for women would be 22 kg. The average waist circumference was much lower in Kitava (Figures 4.13 and 4.14 show values adjusted for height), where no one was larger around their waist than around their hips.

Among Kitavans aged 40–60 years, 87% of men and 93% of women had a BMI below the 10th percentile for Swedish men and women, i.e. 22 kg/m² for men and 21 kg/m² for women. (The definition of the 10th percentile for any measurement is the level below which 10% find themselves.) The corresponding numbers for triceps skinfolds was 50% of men and 80% of women on Kitava. The circumference of the upper arm was only negligibly smaller on Kitava, which indicates that there was no malnutrition. It is obvious from our investigations that lack of food is an unknown concept, and that the surplus of fruits and vegetables regularly rots or is eaten by dogs.

The population of Kitava occupies a unique position in the world in terms of the negligible effect that the Western lifestyle has had on the island. A comparison can be made to a study of the so-called 'original' Pima Indians in Mexico, whose average BMI was as high as 25 kg/m²[2535], which indicates a significantly greater

Table 4.6 Definition of weight classes and their occurrence in the 40–60-year age group in Sweden and on Kitava.

Weight class	BMI (kg/m²)	Sweden (%)	Kitava (%)
Underweight	<20	3	72
Normal weight	20–25	45	28
Overweight	25–30	38	0
Obese	30–35	10	0
Morbidly obese	≥35	2	0

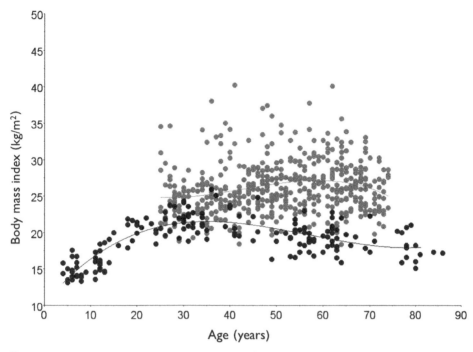

Figure 4.11   Body mass index among males in Kitava, Trobriand Islands, Papua New Guinea (black) and Sweden (grey). (Adapted from Reference 1051.)

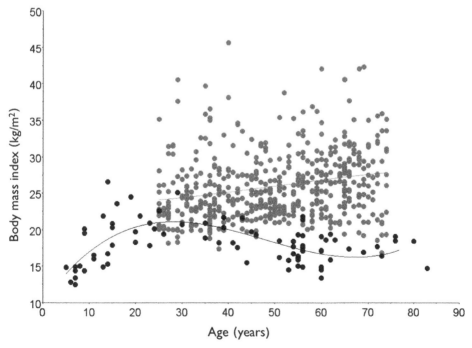

Figure 4.12   Body mass index among females in Kitava (black) and Sweden (grey). (Adapted from Reference 1051.)

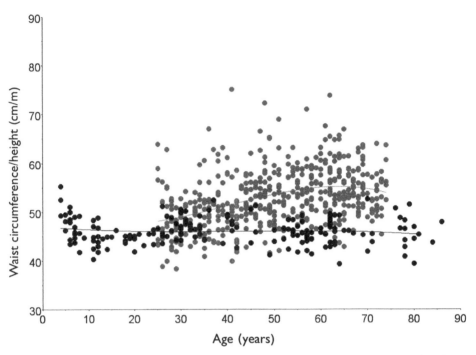

Figure 4.13 Waist circumference-to-body height ratio among males in Kitava (black) and Sweden (grey). (Adapted from Reference 1051.)

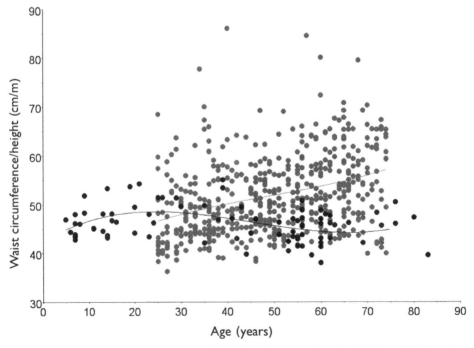

Figure 4.14 Waist circumference-to-body height ratio among females in Kitava (black) and Sweden (grey). (Adapted from Reference 1051).

effect of a Western lifestyle than on the Trobriand Islands, where the BMI in the corresponding age groups was 20 among men and 18 among women. Likewise, in the well-known Tokelau Island Migrant Study, men in their 40s had a BMI of 26 before migration[1451] versus 22 on Kitava.

At the time of our survey in Kitava, we observed two cases of abdominal obesity, both in urbanised male migrants who had grown up in Kitava and now came for a visit. We managed to examine one of them, a businessman aged 44 who differed in four variables from all other adults regardless of sex: he had the highest BMI (28.0), the highest waist-to-hip ratio (1.06), the highest diastolic blood pressure (92) and the highest PAI-1 in blood plasma, an indicator of impaired fibrinolysis (increased tendency towards clotting). The most obvious difference in his lifestyle, as compared with non-migrant Kitavans, was the adoption of Western dietary habits.

During the twentieth century, an epidemic of obesity and weight gain has occurred in former traditional populations that transitioned to a Western lifestyle[22,44,315,457,472,521,1137,1271,1334,1450,1559,1769,1770,1795,1814,1890,2008]. Which lifestyle changes played the largest role cannot be fully determined but, in my opinion, the importance of food choice has often been underestimated. The level of physical activity has generally been higher in the traditional setting, but often not higher than among Western manual workers.

In the modern world, the prevalence of overweight and obesity is increasing at a frightening rate (http://www.who.int/topics/obesity/en/) (Table 4.7). Globally, approximately 1.6 billion adults (age > 15 years) were overweight in 2005, and at least 400 million were obese.

Potential consequences

The relationship between body weight and health is more complex than generally depicted. While an increased waistline undoubtedly poses a threat, even in 'normal'-weight people, crude body weight, as measured in kilograms or BMI, is a poorer predictor of serious health problems among Western populations (notable exceptions are morbidly obese or young people). Furthermore, it is often difficult to differentiate a beneficial weight loss from a harmful one.

Early death

Among a group of North American men aged 50–70 years, with a BMI of 24 and who have never been smoking, roughly 93% will be alive after 10 years, and for an equivalent group of women the number is 95%[14]. The corresponding percentages are not very different for a group of people who are on the verge of obesity (BMI 30): 91% for men and 94% for women. With increasing age, overweight becomes progressively less important as risk factor until it disappears after age 75[524,1724]. In two prospective studies from the US National Health and Nutrition Examination Survey, NHANES II and NHANES III, 10-year survival

Table 4.7 The age-standardised estimated prevalence
(%) of obesity (BMI > 30 kg/m^2) among adults (age >
15 years) in selected countries in 2005 (www.who.int).

	Women	Men
USA	42	37
Egypt	46	22
Mexico	34	24
Jordan	36	20
Greece	25	28
Australia	24	25
UK	24	23
Canada	23	24
Peru	31	13
South Africa	35	7
Germany	20	21
Finland	18	19
Iran	27	10
Fiji	33	9
Spain	16	16
Poland	18	13
Russian federation	24	10
Italy	13	13
Brazil	18	9
Sweden	11	12
Netherlands	12	10
Zimbabwe	15	0.6
France	7	8
Thailand	8	3
Angola	7	1.9
Papua New Guinea	4	3
Pakistan	4	1.0
China	1.9	1.6
Japan	1.5	1.8
India	1.4	1.1

rate among men and women aged 60 or more was identical in the three groups
with BMI 30–35, 25–30 and 18.5–25 at baseline[524]. After age 70, not even BMI
≥35 was associated with reduced survival. Slightly contrasting results were found
in the recent Prospective Studies Collaboration (PSC), where the investigators of
61 prospective studies have shared individual data for a million adults[1933]. After
excluding the first 5 years of follow-up, 66 552 deaths of known cause occurred
during a mean of 8 further years of follow-up. At all ages, all-cause mortality
was lowest at BMI about 22.5–25 kg/m^2. Above this minimum, mortality was on
average about 30% higher for every 5 kg/m^2 higher BMI. Although the proportional
increase was somewhat greater at younger ages (35–59 years), each 5 kg/m^2 higher
BMI was still associated with almost 30% higher mortality at 70–79 years of age.

In younger people, the relative risk of early death is more clearly increased in
obesity[145]. In US non-smoking whites aged 30–55, the risk of early death increases

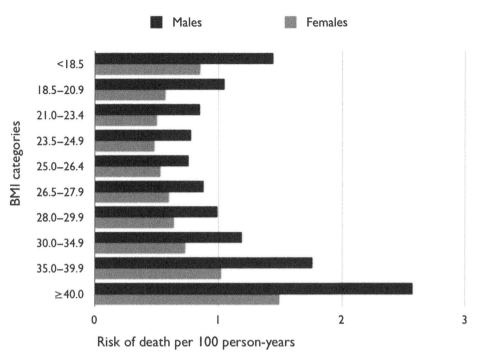

Figure 4.15 Risk of early death among 50–71-year-old never-smoking US men and women according to BMI at study start (10-years of follow-up, $n = 527\,265$). (Adapted from Reference 14.)

by approximately 5% for each additional unit of BMI, starting around BMI 25[1724]. Another study from Germany suggests that the increase of death from having a BMI above 40 increases threefold in men (mean relative risk 3.1; 95% CI 2.5–3.7) and more than twofold in women (mean relative risk 2.3; 95% CI 2.0–2.6) during 14 years of follow-up[146]. Young people evidently have a very high probability of being alive 10 years later, and therefore a relative risk of 2–3 may not seem very frightening.

An increased mortality is often found among people with a low body weight, an issue which has been much discussed[577,1057] (Figure 4.15). In young and middle-aged people, the relationship between BMI and early death tends to be U-shaped, while in older people the right leg of the U is often flat or points downwards in a continuous negative relationship[1057,1448,1724,1933].

While the significance of crude body weight is complex, the adverse impact of abdominal obesity on mortality is more straightforward, although the risk is usually not very different with different levels of waist circumference (Figure 4.16). Many studies have consistently found a continuous positive association between waist (or waist-to-hip ratio) and all-cause mortality [165,345,861,880,881,1057,1423,1448,1617,1872,1923].

In studies of weight loss, a paradox similar to the one concerning BMI, as described above, is apparent. In several large-scale prospective studies in Denmark, Sweden, Norway, Finland and the USA, the risk of early death gradually

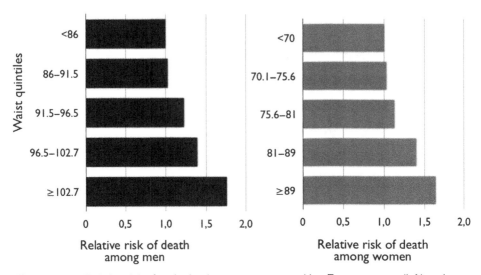

Figure 4.16 Relative risk of early death among never-smoking European men (left) and women (right) according to waist circumference at study start (age 52 ± 10 years, 10 years of follow-up, n = 359 387). (Adapted from Reference 1423.)

increases with increasing weight loss among overweight or moderately obese people[441,930,1224,1308,1700]. In one of these studies, almost 3000 healthy Finnish men and women above average weight were asked in 1975 if they intended to lose weight[1700]. Those who answered 'yes' and, in the following 25 years, had succeeded to lose weight had a higher risk of death (relative risk 1.86; 95% CI 1.22–2.87) than those who said 'no' and were weight stable.

However, a British study found that intentional weight loss for personal reasons was beneficial while intentional weight loss on a doctor's recommendation was not[1903]. Possibly, we have here a confounding factor such that the latter group had a higher risk to start with, a risk which they did not manage to eliminate (although they lost weight). Nevertheless, it cannot be excluded that intentional weight loss sometimes is harmful, depending on the method.

Furthermore, two American studies that also quantified loss of fat tissue suggest that such loss may actually prevent premature death, while loss of muscle tissue (sarcopenia) seems to shorten it[41]. This distinction is particularly important in old age, when sarcopenia is considered to be a common cause of frailty and preventable death[103].

In the Swedish Obese Subjects Study, 2010 individuals who decided to undergo surgery for their extreme obesity were compared with 2037 subjects who declined such treatment[1673]. During 10 years of follow-up, there were 101 deaths in the surgery group and 129 deaths in the control group. The relative risk of death in the surgery group was 0.76 (95% CI 0.59–0.99; p = 0.04). The most common causes of death were myocardial infarction (surgery group, 13 subjects; control group, 25 subjects) and cancer (surgery group, 29; control group, 47) and these two causes of death explained all of the difference between the two groups. The main methodological problem was the lack of randomisation procedure which basically makes this study an epidemiological study.

Ischaemic heart disease

The main risk with increased waistline or high BMI is ischaemic heart disease, as shown in many studies[1427,1933]. In one study of 1346 healthy Finnish men aged 42–60 years, waist circumference was more predictive than BMI of future acute coronary events (myocardial infarction or prolonged chest pain)[975]. In fact, no matter if BMI was below or above 25 kg/m^2, there was a threefold higher coronary risk with a waist-to-hip ratio above 0.9, compared to those with waist-to-hip ratio <0.9 and BMI <25. In a large international case–control study with 27 098 participants in 52 countries (12 461 cases and 14 637 controls), waist-to-hip ratio showed a graded and highly significant association with myocardial infarction risk worldwide[1995]. For waist-to-hip ratio, the odds ratios for every successive quintile were significantly greater than that of the previous one (2nd quintile: relative risk 1.15, 95% CI 1.05–1.26; 3rd quintile: 1.39; 1.28–1.52; 4th quintile: 1.90, 1.74–2.07; and 5th quintiles: 2.52, 2.31–2.74).

Several studies suggest that among people with established ischaemic heart disease, the prognosis is better, not worse, in overweight or mildly obese subjects. A meta-analysis of 40 studies with more than 250 000 patients found that those with a BMI <20 had the highest risk for total mortality (relative risk 1.37; 95% CI 1.32–1.43), and for cardiovascular mortality (relative risk 1.45; 95% CI 1.16–1.81)[1527]. Overweight patients (BMI 25–30) had the lowest risk for total mortality (relative risk 0.87; 95% CI 0.81–0.94) and cardiovascular mortality (relative risk 0.88; 95% CI 0.75–1.02) compared with those with a normal BMI. Obese patients (BMI 30–35) had no increased risk for total mortality (relative risk 0.93; 95% CI 0.85–1.03) or cardiovascular mortality (relative risk 0.97; 95% CI 0.82–1.15). Patients with severe obesity (≥ 35) did not have increased total mortality (relative risk 1.10; 95% CI 0.87–1.41), but they had the highest risk for cardiovascular mortality (relative risk 1.88, 95% CI 1.05–3.34). The better outcomes for cardiovascular and total mortality seen in the overweight and mildly obese groups could not be explained by adjustment for confounding factors. These findings support the notion that weight loss should be carefully monitored in overweight patients with ischaemic heart disease. If there is loss of fat tissue instead of muscle (as measured by bio-impedance analysis or other equipment) and concomitant improvement of cardiovascular risk factors (preferably including glucose tolerance), weight loss is probably safe. Loss of waist circumference is probably beneficial in most cases. A South Korean study found that a high waist-to-hip ratio was associated with increased mortality after myocardial infarction while the opposite relationship was seen for BMI[1006].

Traditional populations where no one is overweight have a negligible risk of myocardial infarction. In contrast, among populations with a high prevalence of these diseases, overweight is very common. Nevertheless, the relationship between weight and myocardial infarction is not particularly strong on a global scale, which means that the most obese populations are not necessarily the ones with the highest rates of myocardial infarction. Once again it is appropriate to talk about sick and healthy populations (see Section 2.2). If you have the same kind of lifestyle as the overweight people around you, you carry a considerable risk of Western disease even if you are not overweight yourself.

Stroke

Several studies have shown that obese people have an approximately twofold risk of stroke[599]. The American Heart Association/American Stroke Association Stroke Council has estimated that 12–20% of annual stroke cases in the USA are caused by obesity[599]. A Japanese study of 9526 men and women found a two- to threefold increased risk of stroke in the highest BMI category (BMI $\geq$30)[1346]. A Cochrane review came to the conclusion that obesity seems to be associated with an increased risk of stroke and that randomised controlled trials of weight reduction are urgently needed[358].

Cancer

Overweight and obesity are risk factors for several types of cancer, including cancer of the colon and rectum (large intestine), breast, endometrium (inner lining of the uterus), kidney and oesophagus[275], although not in all studies[147]. In a large study of 1.2 million UK women, each 10-unit increase in BMI was associated with a threefold higher risk of endometrial cancer (relative risk 2.89; 95% CI 2.62–3.18), as well as higher risk of oesophagus cancer (2.38; 1.59–3.56), kidney cancer (1.53; 1.27–1.84), leukaemia (1.50; 1.23–1.83), multiple myeloma (1.31; 1.04–1.65), pancreatic cancer (1.24; 1.03–1.48), non-Hodgkin's lymphoma (1.17; 1.03–1.34), ovarian cancer (1.14; 1.03–1.27), all cancers combined (1.12; 1.09–1.14), breast cancer in postmenopausal women (1.40; 1.31–1.49) and cancer of colon and rectum in premenopausal women (1.61; 1.05–2.48)[1488]. In Europe, it has been estimated that excess body weight causes around 4% of all cancers[157]. Some cancers, such as prostate cancer, are more closely related to increased waistline than to crude body weight (see Section 4.6).

Diabetes type 2

A large number of studies have consistently shown a substantial increase in the risk for type 2 diabetes in obese people, in particular in cases of abdominal obesity[262,279,1912]. When populations transition from a traditional to an urban lifestyle, the prevalence of obesity and diabetes increase in parallel[327,910]. Among people with glucose intolerance, weight loss has been shown to prevent diabetes and, in some cases, improve glucose tolerance. For further discussion, see Section 4.4.

Ethnic populations of non-European heritage seem to suffer a particularly large amount of damage from being overweight[443,1567], which has prompted some of the experts at the WHO to suggest a BMI of 23 (instead of 25) as a threshold for being overweight among Asian populations. A lower threshold for dangerous waist circumference may also be pertinent in such ethnic groups[684].

Gallstones

Overweight and obesity are well-established risk factors for gallstones, which are very common in modern populations with the highest known rate, 60–70%, among Pima Indians[218,704,1627]. Autopsy studies in the twentieth century found an exceptionally low prevalence of gallstones in traditional lean populations[703,1424]. In Uganda, East Africa, an autopsy study of more than 2000 subjects in the 1940s found only one single gallstone, an exceedingly low prevalence compared to Western populations[1812]. The incidence of gallstones increased dramatically among Canadian Eskimos after transition to a Western lifestyle[1589] and the same consequence of urbanisation has been noted elsewhere[703,1424]. Slightly contrasting findings from mummies have shown a few scattered prehistoric cases in Egypt, China, Italy and South America[307].

No particular food is known to cause gallstones[704]. Insulin resistance and reduced intestinal transit time are among the suggested contributing factors[704,1626]. Foods like cucumber, pears, onions, eggs and fatty foods cause contraction of the bile ducts but do not directly produce the stones. Rapid weight loss can induce attacks and is best avoided in obese people with gallstones.

Fatty liver

Overweight is often accompanied by liver steatosis, or non-alcoholic fatty liver disease (NAFLD), a disorder which is caused by accumulation of fat inside the principal operating liver cells, the hepatocytes. However, fatty liver is often seen in people of normal weight, and strong evidence indicates a connection with insulin resistance, as discussed in Section 4.6.

Breathing difficulties

Breathing disorders are common in obesity and are sometimes due to heart failure (see Section 4.9). In old age, obesity is probably the most common cause of shortness of breath[158,733]. Obstructive sleep apnoea is a potentially serious disorder by causing daytime sleepiness, and obesity is often an underlying cause[621]. Some studies suggest a connection between overweight and asthma, and one systematic review found that weight loss leads to improvement of asthma in many cases[494].

Other consequences

Osteoarthritis, degeneration of the cartilage in certain joints, a common disease in middle-aged and elderly people, is slightly more common among overweight or obese persons[378,513].

Sex hormone disturbances, sometimes causing infertility, are often seen in obesity, in particular abdominal obesity in women[1393]. This is usually connected with insulin resistance as discussed in Section 4.6. Several studies suggest that fertility increases after weight loss in obese women[1393].

Birth defects such as spina bifida and cardiac defects are considerably more common in children born to obese mothers[1907]. There appears to be a 7% increase in the risk of foetal anomaly for each 1 unit incremental increase in BMI above $25 \, kg/m^2$. Other complications of maternal obesity are miscarriage, preeclampsia, stillbirth, caesarean delivery, early neonatal death and abnormally large babies[273,585].

Kidney disease and renal failure are more common in people with abdominal obesity, while general obesity does not increase the risk[489].

Inflammation is increasingly being regarded as a hallmark of obesity, due to the findings of increased levels of inflammatory markers such as C-reactive protein and the identification of macrophage cells infiltrating the white adipose tissue in obese people[256]. We found increased levels of subcutaneous fat and C-reactive protein in pigs which were fed a cereal-based swine feed, as compared with another group raised on vegetables, fruits, root vegetables and meat[848].

Other problems include low self-esteem and depression, sometimes caused by physical impairment, unemployment or social isolation. In one Swedish study, the perceived health of morbidly obese people was similar to that of spinal cord injured persons or cancer survivors[1742].

Relevant dietary factors

Substantial evidence indicates that dietary habits are a major explanation for the absence of overweight in non-Western populations[1967]. Most experts would agree that a diet based on lean meat, vegetables, fruits, root vegetables and nuts is helpful in the prevention and treatment of overweight and obesity. Unfortunately, dietary intervention trials have rarely contrasted such ancestral-like foodstuffs with modern staple foods. Instead, nutritional research has been mainly concerned with comparing different processed foods or different amounts of fat versus carbohydrate. Currently, many experts have concluded from available studies that an evidence-based advice is simply to eat less, which is a rather equivocal recommendation.

Controlled trials of weight loss from a Palaeolithic diet are scarce. We found a larger decrease of waist circumference, but a similar degree of weight loss, during 12 weeks on a Palaeolithic diet compared with a prudent Western diet, as seen in Figures 4.17 and 4.18 and Section 4.4. In the study on Australian Aborigines who returned to a hunter-gatherer lifestyle for 7 weeks (mentioned in Section 4.4), a sharp reduction in weight was seen (Table 4.4)[1331]. However, they had

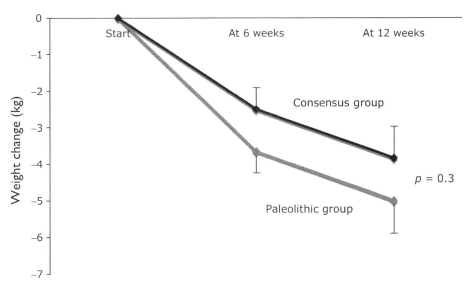

Figure 4.17   Weight change during 12 weeks in patients randomised to eat a Palaeolithic diet or a Consensus (Mediterranean-like) diet. Values are means ± standard errors. Body weight before dietary change was 91.7 ± 11.2 kg in the Palaeolithic group and 96.1 ± 12.4 kg in the Consensus group. (Adapted from Reference 1049.)

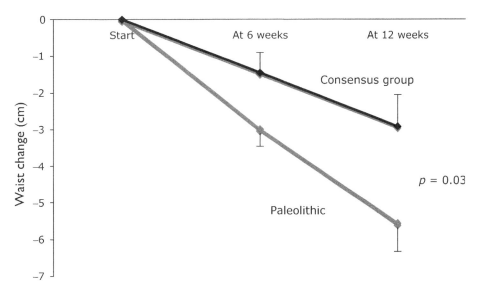

Figure 4.18   Waist loss on a Palaeolithic or Consensus (Mediterranean-like) diet. Values are means ± standard errors. Waist circumference before dietary change was 105.8 ± 7.6 cm in the Palaeolithic group and 106.6 ± 8.0 cm in the Consensus group. (Adapted from Reference 1049.)

sometimes trouble finding enough food to eat. In a non-controlled 3 week trial with palaeolithic diet, healthy volunteers consumed 36% less calories and lost 2.3 kg of weight[2026].

Calorie restriction

Meta-analyses and large weight loss trials with various dietary interventions (based on Western food patterns) suggest that for weight management, energy restriction is more important than other known dietary factors[86,371,446,572, 818,1321,1415,1422,1552,1628]. They also suggest that adherence to the new diet is more important than the diet itself. The average weight loss in long-term studies of low-calorie diets is virtually always smaller than expected, a finding which was explained by lack of adherence in one meta-analysis[726].

A satiating diet, i.e. one that satisfies the appetite with a lower amount of calories, is a crucial factor in preventing and treating obesity in the population. A Palaeolithic diet in this sense appears to be particularly satiating, although this has not been systematically investigated. In our study of a Palaeolithic diet, the reported energy intake was 25% lower in the Palaeolithic group than in the Consensus despite no difference in satiation as reported by the participants[1049]. We have hypothesised that grains may interfere with satiety and promote excess consumption of calories by way of grain-derived endocrine-disrupting substances interfering with the satiety hormone leptin[849]. Traditional explanations of such findings would be that the diet is voluminous (water-rich, fibre-rich), rich in protein or low in fat[1433,1585]. It should also be noted that under-reporting is thought to be common in assessments of food intake under free-living conditions, and that energy-dense junk food appears to be more commonly underreported than other items.

As already noted in Section 2.4, the first law of thermodynamics is often misinterpreted in the context of restricted food intake. The law states that energy can be transformed and that it can neither be created nor destroyed. However, it also states that transformation from one form of energy into another results in more or less heat being produced. This is termed diet-induced thermogenesis, a phenomenon which is well known in the inner circle of scientists. It certainly does not imply that when physical activity is kept constant, the amount of weight loss is exclusively determined by the reduction in energy intake. Animal experiments have shown that (forced) calorie restriction lowers body temperature[980], and the resulting weight loss may therefore be less than expected from dietary energy. Contrariwise, two foods with the same amount of calories may not necessarily have the same effect on energy balance, because they may differ in terms of diet-induced thermogenesis. Even a difference in body temperature which is too small to be practically measurable can be crucial for long-term weight maintenance.

The generally accepted notion that energy-dense foods (foods with a high energy content per unit of weight, such as many processed foods) increase the risk of weight gain and obesity[1526] makes more sense in the context of a typical Western diet than for someone who eats an ancestral-like diet. However, it should be noted that soft drinks, which are considered energy-dense, and apples, which are not, have the same concentration of sugar (10%).

Macronutrient composition

Many researchers have explored various proportions of fat, carbohydrate and protein without arriving at any consensus, and most studies support the notion that calorie restriction is more important than the proportion of macronutrients for the prevention of overweight and obesity[818,1415,2024]. A 2002 Cochrane review of high-quality studies, and a systematic review by the same authors, did not find a reduced fat intake to be more effective for weight loss than other types of energy restriction, rather quite the opposite[1421,1422]. The Cochrane review was withdrawn in 2008 with the stated reason of being 'very much out of date'[1743]. (It was also stated that there were no plans to update it.) One meta-analysis of low-fat, ad-lib diets (i.e. without intentional energy restriction), published in 2000, found a beneficial effect on weight in non-obese subjects (studies in obese subjects did not fulfil inclusion criteria)[85]. More recent studies have generally found that carbohydrate-restricted, high-fat diets produce more pronounced weight loss in the first 6 months but possibly not after 1 year, and they suggest that energy intake and adherence to the respective dietary program are more important than macronutrient composition for long-term weight maintenance[86,371,446,572,1321,1628]. In these studies, the individual variation of weight loss has been considerably larger than the small or non-existent differences between the dietary models. One randomised controlled trial in obese young adults found that a low-glycaemic load, starch-restricted diet resulted in more pronounced weight loss than a low-fat diet, but only among subjects with high post-meal insulin secretion[464]. This is in line with the idea that insulin-resistant overweight people may benefit from restriction of certain starchy foods.

For those who consider restricting carbohydrate intake, an increase in dietary protein may be preferable to an increase in fat[84]. Compared to protein or carbohydrate, fat contains more than double the amount of energy on a weight basis. Protein appears to provide the highest sense of appetite satisfaction per unit of energy while fat provides the least. Diet-induced thermogenesis is also considered to be highest from protein, which would hypothetically facilitate weight loss[349,842,1681].

A recent, large, 2-year trial found a similar degree of weight loss (3–4 kg) with different proportions of carbohydrates, proteins and fats[1552]. Although macronutrient composition did not differ as much as intended between the diets, the study adds to the evidence that other factors are more important for weight loss. The results have been taken as evidence that future interventions should not focus on comparing food models, and one editorial even suggests that we do not need another diet trial (but, instead, community action)[879]. Another common conclusion has been that overweight people 'only' need to eat less (of the same food), but the study was not designed to explore this issue. Some experts conclude that dietary counseling needs to be intense, since participants who attended many counseling sessions lost more weight, but here could obviously be a confounding factor: enthusiasm, which caused both high attendance rate and larger weight loss. It should also be noted that all groups were advised to consume the same type of foods. Therefore, an expansion of the above conclusions might be as follows: (1) Macronutrients are of minor importance for weight management; (2) if we eat a Western diet we need to stop eating before we are satisfied; (3) in order to lose weight on a traditional healthy Western diet, we need to be highly motivated and attend many counselling sessions. In any event, I think the time is ripe to consider food choices rather than macronutrients.

Glycaemic index

High blood sugar and the ensuing hyperinsulinaemia have been proposed to contribute to overweight, even when total carbohydrate intake is not altered[211,1091]. A Cochrane review found that overweight or obese people lost slightly more weight during 5–12 weeks of low-GI diets, as compared to high-GI diets[1784]. However, three trials that were not included in the review (two of them were published afterwards) did not show any such benefit during 12–18 months[83,1465,1649]. One recent trial in 32 subjects found greater weight loss but no effect on changes in fat mass or waist circumference of low- versus high-GI diets[12].

One randomised trial found that breakfast meals with lower GI increased satiety while there was no effect on satiation: energy intake at breakfast was not influenced while energy intake at the following meal was reduced[525]. Other studies of low-GI diets have shown mixed results, and the majority of these do not suggest that the glucose response per se is important for satiation or satiety[243].

Milk protein

A high-protein intake in the first 2 years of life has been associated with the development of overweight in some[1525], but not all studies[762]. In this context, different dietary proteins are apparently not equal. Cow's milk protein, which is the dominant dietary protein after infancy, seems to increase the concentration of insulin-like growth factor-1 (IGF-1) in children, as opposed to meat protein which has no such effect[759]. Other studies indicate that high levels of IGF-1 promote the development of obesity[760]. Casein, which accounts for 80% of milk proteins, has also been shown to increase the expression of sterol-regulatory element binding protein-1[76], a transcription factor which stimulates fat synthesis and possibly increases body fatness[765].

β-Casomorphin-7 is a peptide that results from the breakdown of β-casein A1, but not other caseins, in milk. Studies in satiated rats have shown that this peptide stimulates the intake of dietary fat, but not carbohydrates, and that the effect is inhibited by the opioid antagonist naloxone[1040]. Furthermore, milk proteins increase plasma insulin levels, an effect mainly caused by whey, which constitutes about 20% of milk proteins[1307]. Chronically elevated plasma insulin is often regarded as central in the vicious circle of overweight and obesity[1340]. In epidemiological studies, a high intake of dairy foods has not been associated with overweight, rather the opposite[1408]. This suggests that if milk promotes overweight, some other Western foods may do it even more effectively.

Whole grains versus refined grains

People who prefer whole grains to more refined cereals do not appear to be protected from overweight, or to a very limited extent[601,1070,1779,1849]. In a large controlled trial, the WHOLEheart study, 316 overweight subjects, who consumed less than 30 g of whole grains per day before the study, were randomly allocated to one of three groups: (1) controls (no dietary change), (2) moderately increased intake of whole grains (60 g/day for 16 weeks) or (3) dramatically increased intake of whole grains (60 g/day for 8 weeks, then 120 g/day for a further 8 weeks) (Brownlee IA et al. Abstract, Annual Congress of the American Association of Cereal Chemists, 2008). No beneficial weight change was obtained from whole grains in this study, nor did cardiovascular risk factor levels improve (plasma total, LDL and HDL cholesterol, triglycerides, insulin or glucose). An earlier smaller trial found similar results, including no effect on insulin sensitivity, as measured by the euglycaemic hyperinsulinaemic clamp test[52].

Grains versus no grains

Hypothetically, a number of phytochemicals from cereals, most notably glycosylated proteins and various peptides, can affect weight balance by influencing appetite and energy metabolism[849]. Leptin, the satiety hormone which commands us to stop eating when we are full, is possibly blocked by cereal-derived substances[867], as discussed in Section 4.3. If this is true, it is highly relevant for obesity. This would explain why cereals seem to cause weight gain and excess food consumption in domestic swine[848,1487] and birds[675]. One of the main suspects to interfere with leptin binding is gluten, whose consumption over the last 100 years has increased greatly[141] with acceleration in the last 20 years (G. Svensson, SLU-Alnarp, personal communication).

In our Palaeolithic diet study, waist loss increased with decreasing intake of cereals and increasing intake of fruit, associations which explained 42% of the variation of waist loss among the whole study population ($P = 0.0003$), and 40% in the Consensus group alone ($P = 0.016$)[1049]. In bivariate regression analysis among the whole population, the association between reported cereal intake and waist loss was independent of group assignment, energy intake and carbohydrate intake.

William Banting

In 1863, a Londoner by the name of William Banting published a 25-page pamphlet with the title 'Letter on corpulence, addressed to the public'[109]. He wrote it after having overcome obesity through a diet that has a lot in common with a Palaeolithic diet (but is usually described as a low-carbohydrate diet).

From the age of 30 until he was 65 years old, Banting gradually gained weight until he weighed 91.7 kg. Since he was only 165 cm tall, his final BMI was 33.6 kg/m^2, and his abdomen was so large that he could not bend down to tie his shoes. Due to pain in his ankles and knees, he was forced to go downstairs backwards. The fact that he was an undertaker may have been a contributing factor in why he was particularly motivated to do something about the issue.

Just before his 40th birthday, he had started his long fight against his weight. On the advice of one of the many doctors he consulted, a surgeon and friend, he started rowing on the banks of the Thames River a few hours in the morning. 'It is true', he writes, 'I gained muscular vigour, but with it a prodigious appetite, which I was compelled to indulge, and consequently increased in weight, until my kind old friend advised me to forsake the exercise.' Banting is not the only person who found it difficult to lose weight *only* through increased physical activity[526].

His friend died soon afterwards, and Banting consulted 'other high orthodox authorities'. He was thankful for their efforts but confessed with increasing frustration that neither their cures nor their encouragement to eat less was of any help.

When Banting approached the age of 65, his obesity had, as I suspect from his account, caused diabetes with slow-healing abscesses and reduced vision and hearing. Two of the abscesses developed into 'rather formidable carbuncles, for which I was ably operated upon *and fed into increased obesity*'.

The loss of hearing led Banting to consult two ear surgeons. He recounts that the first surgeon 'made light of the case, looked into my ears, sponged them internally, and blistered the outside, without the slightest benefit. ... He soon after left town for his annual holiday, which proved the greatest possible blessing...'.

This is when he met his saviour, the second ear surgeon, William Harvey. The doctor's assessment that the hearing loss was due to fatty tissue in the throat that obstructed the Eustachian tube was probably false but his linking the symptoms with obesity may have been correct. Today, we have evidence that high blood sugar can cause poor hearing[914,915], even if the issue has barely been studied and the mechanism is unknown. We know more about impaired vision: the concentration of sugar in the tissues absorbs water that causes a swollen cornea, which refracts the light rays incorrectly[556,1063,1477].

Now came the sensational part. Dr Harvey's diet gave Banting his sight back in addition to improving his hearing and reducing his weight. Over the course of 12 months, he lost 21 kg and went from being obese to being just over the threshold for normal weight (BMI 25.9). Half a year later he was precisely on the border with a BMI of 25.

His diet consisted largely of meat or fish, morning, noon or night. A small amount of fruit was permitted while the intake of vegetables was apparently not restricted. The foods that he was ordered to avoid as much as possible were: 'Bread, butter, milk, sugar, beer, and potatoes, which had been the main (and, I thought, innocent) elements of my subsistence, or at all events they had for many years been adopted freely'. Alcohol was permitted and was actually considered advisable according to the rules of conduct, but Banting himself seems to have been very moderate.

His new diet was primarily rich in protein, but also low in fat *and* with a low glycaemic load. Today, we know that almost all types of bread and potatoes have a high GI, even worse is the maltose in beer. When Banting wrote the fifth edition of the book, he had come to the conclusion that parsnips, red beets, turnips and carrots also made it difficult to keep a stable weight. It is worthwhile to note that all of these have approximately the same GI as potatoes, but a higher water content why the glycaemic load will be limited. It is plausible that Banting belonged to a group of people who are particularly sensitive to carbohydrates, at least at this recent stage after reversion of lifestyle. Banting did not restrict the amount of food, instead he could now 'confidently say that *quantity* of diet may be safely left to the natural appetite, and that it is the *quality* only which is essential to abate and cure corpulence' (as stated in the fifth edition). He was surprised that he could achieve such a marked weight loss by 'exchanging a meagre [diet] for a generous [one]'.

From our perspective, his story does not appear to be particularly notable. Instead, the strange thing is that 140 years after it was published, his argument has not achieved full impact, and Banting's most important experiences are not always made clear. When the story is told, these days it is often wrongly described as being equal to the high-fat Atkins diet. Unfortunately, many people spend more time reading various interpretations of the book than they would need to share Banting's own words. It takes little more than an hour.

4.6 Insulin resistance

Insulin is an anabolic (biosynthetic) hormone that facilitates the storage of glucose, fat and protein in the body. Insulin resistance means that the receiving tissues do not react sufficiently sensitively to the hormone signals. Despite considerable efforts, the underlying mechanisms remain elusive, and for many of the components of the disorder it is unknown if they are causes, consequences or innocent bystanders[1625,1630]. In order to overcome the resistance to insulin in the tissues, the pancreatic β-cells produce more insulin, which leads to higher circulating levels of serum insulin (hyperinsulinaemia). A condition that is associated with insulin resistance is the metabolic syndrome with abdominal obesity, hypertension, dyslipidaemia and reduced glucose tolerance. The consequences – and the impact of diet on public health – are probably even more significant.

Prevalence studies

Insulin sensitivity is by all appearances higher among traditional people than among Westerners, but only as long as they maintain their ancestral-like lifestyle. After transition to a Western lifestyle they generally have a lower insulin sensitivity than people of European origin, as discussed below. Three populations of hunter-gatherers in South America and Africa have all shown a similar pattern for oral glucose load, with an insulin response only 40% of that seen in Westerners[832,1213,1702]. The metabolic syndrome does not seem to exist on Kitava. Fasting levels of serum insulin decreased with age instead of increasing as in Sweden and, in the age group 40–65 years, the average in Kitava was 1 SD below that of Sweden (Figure 4.19)[1048]. All inhabitants were lean with no increased waistlines (Figures 4.11–4.14), and the leptin and blood pressure levels were low (Figures 4.19, 4.24

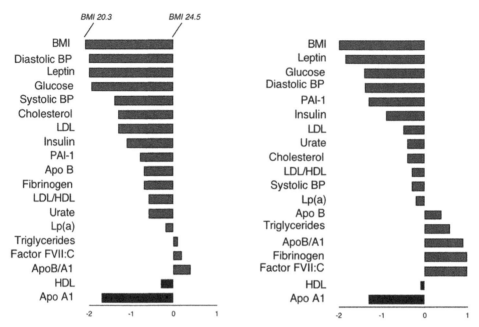

Figure 4.19 Risk factor levels among 40–65-year-old men and women on Kitava in relation to Sweden, expressed in number of standard deviations from the Swedish average (Z scores). The longer the bars, the more Kitava deviated from Sweden. The bars to the left of the zero line indicate a lower level on Kitava. Grey means that it is better and black means that it is worse to be to the left of the zero line. (Adapted from References 1045, 1047, 1048, 1051 and 1053.)

and 4.25)[1045,1046,1048,1051,1053]. In our Western societies, insulin covaries with other risk markers for cardiovascular disease, but not on Kitava, which is an additional indicator that insulin sensitivity is universally high.

Decreasing insulin sensitivity with increasing age is typical in the West[598], but probably cannot be considered to be a part of normal biological ageing[115,1048,1333,2011]. The fact that this process is considered a part of normal biology is due to the difficulty in finding a reference population that is unaffected by a Western lifestyle.

Box 4.1 Average cardiovascular risk factor levels among hunter-gatherers (40-year-old men).

- 40% insulin response with oral glucose load compared with Westerners
- BMI 20 (25 in Sweden)
- No excess weight, trim waistline
- Blood pressure 105/65 (130/80 in Sweden)
- S-cholesterol 3 mmol/L (6 in Sweden)

When humans switch from an ancient to a Western lifestyle, they experience increased waistlines, reduced insulin sensitivity, higher blood pressure and a host of related disorders and diseases. There does not seem to be any ethnic group that can avoid this fate after urbanisation. Furthermore, nothing seems to indicate that this should be unique for our species. A number of other mammals, including monkeys, dogs, cats and rats become overweight and resistant to insulin when they are overfed[421,512,1238,1537]. The pattern of reaction obviously developed long before the common ancestor of these species lived roughly 100 million years ago.

Historically, there has been some awareness of the metabolic syndrome of abdominal obesity in Italy since the eighteenth century (Morgagni, 1765)[679]. The association between abdominal obesity, diabetes and hypertension was independently described in 1921 by Hitzenberger, Austria, and in 1923 by Kylin, Sweden[967], and in 1956 by Vague in Marseille, France, who also noted the increased risk of atherosclerotic disease with abdominal obesity[1846]. Reaven defined the syndrome in modern terms in 1988[1478]. The association with stroke may have been recognised already before 1920[714]. Hippocrates noted, 24 centuries ago, that 'Those who by nature are somewhat stout die sooner than those who are lean'[288].

Attempts to explain

Several hypotheses have been presented to explain the widespread occurrence of insulin resistance. Most of these take into account the evolutionary history of humans and the mismatch between ancient genes and present environments.

The thrifty genotype

In 1962, the geneticist Neel formulated the hypothesis of a 'thrifty genotype', a concept of an economical and efficient metabolism that was set out to explain why diabetes was so common despite the disease's negative impact on fertility and survival[1279,1280]. Neel looked for a selective advantage that outweighed the disadvantages and thought he found one in the idea that the genes that currently cause diabetes provided protection against starvation in the past. The rapid insulin response was assumed to make fat storage more efficient during cycles of calorie surplus/deficit (feast and famine), and modern humans developed diabetes as a result of the constant calorie surplus.

Despite the lack of a mechanistic model to support the hypothesis, the impact of this idea has been exceptional[1379]. It is sometimes presented almost as an axiom that modern humans become overweight and insulin resistant because they have a constant surplus of food for the first time in their development.

However, there are plenty of examples of contemporary hunter-gatherers who stay lean despite a surplus of food, and the average time to collect food is usually 2–3 hours/day[685]. Our findings from Kitava do not agree either with this hypothesis about a thrifty genotype. There is always an excess of food that rots away. Yet, we do not find any people who are overweight or have developed insulin resistance.

Insulin resistance has actually been suggested as beneficial for weight stabilisation, rather than weight gain, by means of the reduced amount of glucose transported to the liver, and the fat tissues reducing the conversion of glucose to fat[209]. For young adults who have become somewhat overweight, insulin resistance can be a potential way to counter additional fat storage[1806]. Among adult Pima-Indians, it is also the most insulin-sensitive people who gain the most weight in prospective studies[1752]. Results from other studies have been divergent[66].

The lack of a weight-regulating mechanism is not biologically plausible either. An animal or human with the characteristic of eating until they become fat and clumsy when they land in an ecological niche with a surplus of food will be evolutionarily disadvantaged compared with those that keep trim. The fact that wild animals generally maintain a stable weight from year to year does not seem to be dependent on regular shortage of food.

The view that a lack of food is necessary to counteract weight gain and insulin resistance (the hypothesis of the 'thrifty genotype') is not credible. Moreover, the hypothesis is not consistent with the fact that persons of European descent seem to be more insulin sensitive than other ethnic groups, i.e. more resistant to urbanisation (see below under 'The non-thrifty genotype').

However, it could explain the exceptional insulin resistance that characterises certain ethnic groups such as Micronesians and North America's Pima Indians[909,1039]. According to one hypothesis, their forefathers should have been the ones who survived long boat rides in the South Pacific as well as journeys across Arctic regions. In this case, it would be an example of a genetic bottleneck.

The carnivore connection

An alternative explanation for human's general tendency for insulin resistance was presented by Brand Miller and Colagiuri[206,209]. They correctly point out that there is no strong evidence of periodically recurring famine being particularly common among hunter-gatherers[151], and that death from famine is not the result of empty fat deposits, rather empty supplies of 'lean mass' (i.e. primarily musculature)[1366].

Instead, their hypothesis is based on the assumption that for approximately 2 million years Palaeolithic hunter-gatherer diets were periodically very rich in protein and had a low percentage of carbohydrates. The lack of carbohydrates would then play a greater role than famine in the selection of genes for insulin resistance. A metabolism with a tendency for insulin resistance, in their view, is a way to prevent dangerously low blood sugar levels with a protein-rich and carbohydrate-poor diet. Insulin resistance in the peripheral tissues facilitates the redirection of glucose from muscles to foetus, mammary glands and brain, which are more sensitive to low blood sugar. Humans have a limited capacity for gluconeogenesis (generation of new glucose) and insulin resistance in the liver, which should have allowed for increased gluconeogenesis with a high-protein intake.

High insulin sensitivity would have been a risk with a high-protein intake and a low carbohydrate intake. Today, a constant supply of high glycaemic load foods exposes the disadvantages of insulin resistance.

In addition to explaining humans' general tendency for metabolic syndromes, the carnivore connection hypothesis could explain the particularly low insulin sensitivity among Pima Indians, Micronesians and Australian Aborigines, whose forefathers are thought to have lived in an environment dominated by wild fish and shellfish.

Even this hypothesis has its weaknesses. It does not explain why Europeans have a higher insulin sensitivity than other ethnic groups. The suggestion that this is due to reduced selective pressure is not convincing, the time period is too short, particularly in northern Europe. There is also a question as to whether a lack of carbohydrates was common during the Palaeolithic era[1227,1972].

The non-thrifty genotype

After transition to a Western lifestyle, ethnic groups of non-European origin seem to have a greater tendency for insulin resistance and type 2 diabetes regardless of their BMI[9,65,205,351,607,628,864]. It appears increasingly obvious that we, who are the descendants of Cro-Magnon, the European humans from the Ice Age 35 000 years ago, have a higher resistance against the modern lifestyle than many other ethnic groups.

It has been well documented that widespread and lasting periods of famine were common in Europe after the development of agriculture[213,574,641,1228], which according to the thrifty genotype hypothesis should benefit people with an efficient metabolism. Hence, according to the hypothesis, today's Europeans should have at least an equally high rate of diabetes as other ethnic groups. But that is not the case.

Allen and Cheer, physical anthropologists in New Zealand, considered the differences in the prevalence of diabetes among the world's various ethnic populations from this perspective[39]. The focus of their analysis is the European population, the one that, in analogy with Neel's hypothesis, should be called the 'non-thrifty genotype'. The authors point out that the focus of most thinking has been on how the non-European population's predisposition was selected to continue, instead of on what made the Europeans' low sensitivity for type 2 diabetes get selected. Thus, in mainstream research, Europeans are considered the norm rather than the exception.

In addition to pointing out that the Europeans' 'non-thrifty genotype' is noteworthy, Allen and Cheer also developed an explanatory model for this phenomenon. They dismissed famine as a selection factor, and therefore they had to find a new mechanism. The idea that the deviation could have developed by pure chance and then be spread throughout Europe via a genetic bottleneck is not very probable. A more credible idea is that high insulin sensitivity brought with it metabolic advantages in a new ecological niche. It is difficult to see any advantage during the period when wild game hunters lived in a subarctic climate, since the selective pressure probably would have fostered insulin resistance at least equally as much as during evolution on Africa's savannahs.

In their search for relevant environmental factors, Allen and Cheer decided to look into cow's milk. They noted a negative, international correlation between

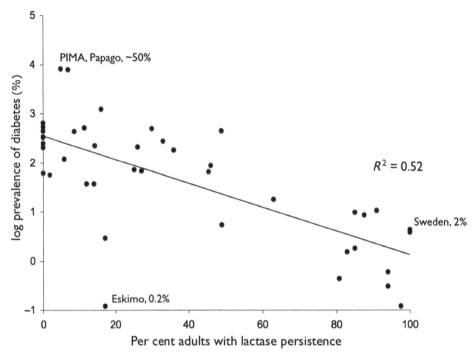

Figure 4.20   The prevalence of diabetes (%, log transformed) in relation to the percentage of persistent lactase activity in various populations. The latter may represent the length of time that dairy products have been a staple food. African populations have been excluded due to limited influence of Western food. (Modified from Reference 39.)

the percentage of adults with persistent lactase activity (lactose tolerance) and the prevalence of type 2 diabetes. In Europe, lactose tolerance is the dominant variant, particularly in the northern part of the continent. However, in populations of a non-European background, lactose intolerance is the norm.

Type 2 diabetes therefore appeared to be most common in populations with a high percentage of lactose-intolerant persons and vice versa. In a slightly modified analysis of Allen and Cheer's material, I excluded African populations (since many people there do not afford a modern lifestyle), and took the logarithm of diabetes prevalence to achieve a normal distribution (Figure 4.20). The international variation of lactose tolerance then explains as much as 52% of the variation in the prevalence of diabetes. Such a strong correlation clearly cannot be dismissed.

The hypothesis about the 'non-thrifty genotype' postulates that when the early cattle herders could survive the winters in Europe's barren ecological niche, thanks to their ability to digest lactose as adults, it was at the expense of diabetes, due to the strong insulin response to milk[499,566]. Natural selection would then favour high insulin sensitivity. In a surplus society, this high degree of sensitivity provides a certain protection against a calorie-rich diet and low physical activity.

The hypothesis is supported by several animal studies suggesting that milk causes insulin resistance, lipotoxicity and glucose intolerance, as discussed below and in

Section 4.4. On the other hand, a cohort study of overweight persons in the USA found that the intake of dairy products was negatively associated with insulin sensitivity[1408]. Confounding factors cannot be ruled out, such that people who drink milk rather than soft drinks may have a healthier lifestyle. Nevertheless, it is plausible that non-milk beverages are in some aspects worse and that milk can have a preventive effect in populations with poor eating habits such as the Americans. It should be noted that all of the theoretically beneficial components that the authors discuss[1408] can be obtained from a Palaeolithic diet, which suggests that no benefit can be expected if milk is added to such a diet.

Allen and Cheer's hypothesis is the first serious attempt to explain what promoted a relatively high insulin sensitivity among Europeans. Explanations based on the 'thrifty genotype' hypothesis are contradicted by the absence of diabetes and insulin resistance among non-Western populations with regular food surplus. It is also highly doubtful whether decreased rates of famine in the last centuries is a sufficient selection factor behind the variable tendency for diabetes between different ethnic groups, as has been suggested[415]. The effects on fertility and survival are simply too small[290,450].

The thrifty phenotype

There are other attempts to explain man's general tendency for insulin resistance or to explain the ethnic differences. One of them, the 'thrifty-phenotype' hypothesis, is based on the finding in many studies that persons with a low birth weight have an increased risk for insulin resistance as adults[645]. A possible mechanism is foetal malnutrition: animal experiments suggest that a protein intake that is too low during pregnancy may be an explanation[1367]. One study indicates that a low intake of the amino acid taurine during pregnancy can be a cause[536]. Taurine is supplied primarily from meat and fish and is missing from most vegetables, which is why vegans have an extremely low intake[1728]. Although fetal programming may be somewhat relevant, it is probably not a major cause of insulin resistance or the metabolic syndrome[391].

Associated abnormalities

The relatively low insulin sensitivity which characterises most people in the Western world, compared to traditional populations, starts to develop early in life, in parallel with the development of abdominal fat accumulation, increased blood pressure and atherosclerosis[1659,1660,1715]. When the body's organs and tissues become insulin resistant, the release of insulin from the pancreas increases, which is reflected in higher insulin levels in the blood, in particular after carbohydrate-rich meals. This compensatory hyperinsulinaemia allows a normal level of glucose tolerance to be maintained for long periods of time. However, one or several of the anomalies in Box 4.2 are usually already initiated, although insulin resistance is not a proven cause of any of them.

Box 4.2   Anomalies linked to insulin resistance.

Diabetes type 2
Metabolic syndrome
Lipotoxicity (ectopic fat deposition)
  Fatty liver
Cardiovascular disease
  Atherosclerosis
Gout
Obstructive sleep apnoea syndrome
Enhanced tissue growth
  Increased stature
  Early puberty
  Acne
Benign prostatic hyperplasia
Cancer
Infertility
Kidney failure

Diabetes type 2 *(see also Section 4.4)*

A commonly held view is that insulin resistance plays a causal role in the early development of type 2 diabetes[862]. Most persons at risk of type 2 diabetes are insulin resistant and overweight or obese with an increased waistline and the same is true for people with glucose intolerance or other components of the metabolic syndrome. Resistance to the insulin-mediated transport of glucose from the outside to the inside of cells (glucometabolic insulin resistance) is counterbalanced by high levels of insulin circulating in the blood (hyperinsulinaemia). When the β-cells of the pancreas after some time (years-decades) fail to produce enough insulin, type 2 diabetes is thought to develop, and the abnormally high insulin levels drop to normal or low levels, because of inability to meet the requirements, and as a consequence blood glucose increases.

   However, the significance of insulin resistance as the fundamental driving process in type 2 diabetes is not confirmed[862]. Some studies in humans suggest that the early stages of glucose intolerance are associated with disturbances in β-cell function (and modest insulin resistance), while more marked insulin resistance is seen in later stages[1854]. Although various strains of genetically modified mice which lack specific insulin receptors can become insulin resistant, they do not develop diabetes, sometimes not even glucose intolerance[229].

Metabolic syndrome

Abdominal obesity, high blood pressure, impaired glucose tolerance, high triglycerides and low HDL cholesterol occur so often together that they are collectively called the metabolic syndrome (also called syndrome X or the insulin resistance syndrome)[366,1097]. In this book, each of these four conditions has their own sections (4.4, 4.5, 4.7 and 4.8).

Lipotoxicity (ectopic fat deposition)

In recent years, the deposition of fat in the wrong places (heart, liver, pancreas, skeletal muscle, arteries, etc.) has been intensely discussed in connection with, or as a cause of, insulin resistance and potential organ damage[15,50,1229,1428,1754,1840]. As long as the excess fat is stored in the fat cells (adipocytes), it does not appear to cause any great damage. Even within other types of cells there is normally a small number of triglycerides that act as a fuel reserve in addition to other functions[602]. These triglycerides are located in lipid droplets in the cytoplasm, the fluid inside the cells. But in the case of lipotoxicity, an abnormally high concentration of triglycerides in these cells is thought to result in the formation of potentially harmful fatty acid derivatives and accelerated cell death (apoptosis).

Hypothetically, lipotoxicity in skeletal muscle and liver is the prime cause of whole-body insulin resistance, while lipotoxicity in the liver, heart, arterial walls and kidneys may cause specific failure of these organs[1839,1917]. Another possible consequence could be osteoporosis, although this has been much less discussed[21,1381].

The satiety hormone leptin apparently plays a central role in lipotoxicity. Leptin is produced in fat cells and has been shown to suppress appetite and also stimulate energy expenditure, leading to weight loss[1840,2003]. The absolute level of leptin in Sweden is just over 3 times as high as on Kitava, which corresponds to the anticipated level based on their low BMI[1048]. Hence, it is not a lack of leptin that makes Westerners overweight with increased waistlines, instead leptin increases alongside with being overweight. It has been suggested that leptin increases to protect the heart, pancreas, liver and other internal organs from the lipotoxicity of lipid overload during times of caloric excess[1841]. If this is correct, the low leptin levels on Kitava, where food is always abundant, potentially reflect a more finely tuned protective mechanism.

Roger Unger, the US scientist who coined the term lipotoxicity, has proposed that insulin resistance is a secondary phenomenon that protects against the double burden of fat and glucose overload inside the cells of various organs, including the insulin-producing β–cells[1838]. Along similar lines of thinking, leptin has been suggested to prevent atherosclerosis[738,929,1975], although the opposite has also been claimed[144,293,1759].

Fatty liver (liver steatosis)

In the old days, when patients were diagnosed with fatty liver, the doctors usually suspected alcohol in excess. Today, the Western lifestyle is considered a prime cause. In people who do not regularly drink an excess of alcohol, ectopic fat deposition in liver cells is now called non-alcoholic fatty liver disease (NAFLD). The afflicted cells are the hepatocytes, the liver cells that are responsible for nutrient processing, carbohydrate storage (in the form of glycogen) and neutralisation of harmful substances, among other things. The prevalence of NAFLD is approximately 20% in the general population and 75% in obese people[1842]. Even in obese children the condition is rather common[1513]. In dairy cows, 40–50% have fatty liver in the first four weeks after calving[187].

Although fatty liver typically does not seem to impair liver function in humans, NAFLD is today the most common cause of increases in liver enzymes and a common cause of concern for patients and physicians. On liver biopsy, there is sometimes inflammation and signs of hepatocyte injury, and then the condition is termed non-alcoholic steatohepatitis. The most advanced and serious stages are fibrosis and cirrhosis.

When symptoms are present, fatigue is a common feature of NAFLD[1294]. Virtually everyone with NAFLD is characterised by insulin resistance, but it is not established which of the two is the cause and which is the effect, or if they are both caused by something else[941,1842].

Cardiovascular disease

Insulin resistant people are at increased risk of cardiovascular diseases, such as ischaemic heart disease, stroke and heart failure[829,893,1024]. The suggested mechanisms include well established factors such as high blood pressure, impaired glucose tolerance and dyslipidaemia, but also reduced fibrinolysis[514], endothelial dysfunction[67], atherosclerosis[190,780], and, again, lipotoxicity[1386].

Atherosclerosis

Hyperinsulinaemia and insulin resistance have long been suspected of causing atherosclerosis[190,780,1731]. The hypothesis of lipotoxicity is highly relevant to the atherosclerotic process, which is characterised by lipid overload of macrophages in the arterial wall (see Section 4.3). Another decisive feature in the development of atherosclerosis is excessive cell growth, a phenomenon that is discussed below in association with insulin resistance. Down-regulation of retinoid receptors and other nucleus receptors are only some of the many plausible mechanisms with regard to atherosclerosis[95,301,770]. Activating the retinoid receptors retards the development of atherosclerosis among genetically modified mice with a lack of apolipoprotein E[301].

Gout

The most common form of gout results from the deposition of urate crystals in single joints. The risk of gout increases with a high serum urate level, which is often due to insulin resistance[1969]. Individuals with the metabolic syndrome are clearly overrepresented, and the serum urate correlates with waist circumference, weight, blood sugar, serum insulin, blood pressure and blood lipids among West-erners[298,300,1932].

On Kitava, urate levels were not significantly lower than in Sweden, but they did not increase with age as they do in Western populations[1047]. Similar comparative studies of traditional populations have not been published, but an uncontrolled study of hunter-gatherers in Namibia suggests that they had considerably lower levels than Westerners[1817]. In the Tokelau Island Migrant Study, Micronesians had an increased occurrence of gout and higher urate values after migration to New Zealand[1452].

Elevated urate levels have proven to be a risk factor for myocardial infarction in some studies, but it is unclear if this remains the case after adjusting for other risk factors[508,1196,1501,1902]. It is possible that the rise in urate is secondary to other disturbances, and it has been suggested that urate actually has a beneficial antiox-idative effect[135,1164,1533,1905], which could prevent the oxidation of LDL and thereby atherosclerosis. High levels of uric acid are possibly more harmful for people with established ischaemic heart disease than for healthy people[100].

Obstructive sleep apnoea syndrome

Obstructive sleep apnoea (arrested breathing due to unstable upper respiratory passageways) is considerably more common among patients with insulin resistance, possibly even in the absence of overweight[796]. The condition is associated with an increased risk for ischaemic heart disease, stroke, heart failure and hypertension[1117]. The first two cases in Papua New Guinea, both among patients with hypertension, were described in 1990[116].

Enhanced tissue growth

There is considerable evidence to suggest that disturbances associated with hyper-insulinaemia and/or insulin resistance can affect several different types of tissues and organs in the form of excessive growth, and that high insulin levels contribute to this[330]. This has bearing not only on cancer, an evident case of enhanced tissue growth, but also on myopia, acne and increased body stature, as outlined by Loren Cordain at Colorado State University[333,334,337].

Insulin inhibits the synthesis of one of the proteins that binds to insulin-like growth factor-1 (IGF-1), insulin-like growth factor binding protein-3 (IGFBP-3)[90,552,1270]. This results in more free IGF-1 being available to exert its mitogenic effects, i.e. to stimulate cell division (mitosis) and cell growth in different body tis-sues. This effect is partly direct[518], and partly indirect through the down-regulation (reduced occurrence or activity) of retinoid receptors in the cell nucleus[502,1066]. These retinoid receptors normally inhibit cell growth when activated by natural or synthetic retinoids, and medication with this effect is used in the treatment of ma-lignant diseases, primarily certain types of leukaemia and breast cancer[1653,1760,1778].

In this way, hyperinsulinaemia may potentially contribute to unregulated cell growth. The mechanisms in question may hypothetically be involved in such varied conditions as increased body size, early puberty, acne, nearsightedness and certain forms of cancer. Although the relationships are complex and open for debate, they seem to open up a new chapter in our understanding of how Western lifestyles influence modern, human health problems. On top of that, genetic factors are significant in terms of which tissues are affected in a particular individual.

Increased stature

The above reasoning can be applied to body height (see Figure 4.22). It is well known that free IGF-1 stimulates the growth rate during puberty[857], and that high levels of IGF-1 are associated with increased stature while low levels are associated with reduced body height[1523]. Treatment with IGF-1 results in increased height[252]. Blocking retinoid receptors in the growth zones of the long bones causes increased body length in rats[389]. Since hyperinsulinaemia has important effects on key mechanisms in growth regulation, insulin resistance is expected to contribute to increased body height.

Young Swedish men not only are increasing in weight but are also becoming taller (Figure 4.21) (www.pliktverket.se). During the 1980s, the increase in body height seemed to level off, but since then it has gradually continued to rise in Sweden. Unfortunately, after 2000 the data are not reliable since height is no longer measured in all Swedish men. In other northern European countries, the increase in height that has been present during the twentieth century is thought, by

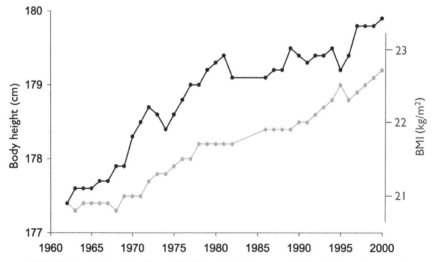

Figure 4.21 Body height (black) and BMI (grey) of 18-year-old Swedish male conscripts between 1962 and 2000. The increase in height from 1980 to 2000 is highly statistically significant ($P = 0.0006$). (Adapted from www.pliktverket.se.)

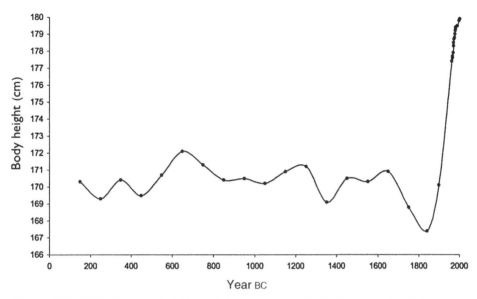

Figure 4.22 Estimated body height of adult European men in the time period 150–1650 (Adapted from Reference 935), and in Sweden in 1840–2000 (Adapted from www.pliktverket.se).

some researchers, to have levelled off around 1980–1990, but there is limited data after 1990 to support or refute that notion.

Previously, secular trends of increased body height in the twentieth century have been attributed exclusively to improved nutrition, in particular increased protein intake and less famine[890,1517]. This was called into question already in the 1960s by Ziegler, who showed that the increase in the population's height in England, Japan, Holland, Sweden, Norway, Denmark, USA and New Zealand was strongly correlated to increased sucrose consumption, but not to protein intake[2005,2006]. Even observations among Canadian Eskimos point in the same direction. For a 30-year period (1938–1968), body height increased by 4.6 cm among men and 2.9 cm among women, while the onset of puberty moved down 2.0 years. During the same period, there was a sevenfold increase in sucrose consumption, while protein intake diminished by 60%[1587]. Today, it is generally acknowledged that the growth in height is inhibited only by a protein consumption that is far below what is common in the Western world[217,608]. The importance of protein consumption for the rate of growth is often overestimated in the general discussion. Therefore, the fact that cow's milk promotes growth in body height among today's Western children[180,760,1010,1942] probably cannot be attributed to optimised protein consumption. Instead, the findings add to the notion that milk is a cause of insulin resistance and/or that milk-derived peptides have endocrine-disrupting properties.

Thus, there is evidence that milk proteins enhance linear growth in humans, partly through the stimulation of IGF-1, and even in situations where nutrient intake is adequate[760,1316,1942]. This could, to a large extent, explain the tall stature of northern Europeans as well as the secular trend for increasing height in populations with increasing intake of dairy products. In 1966, Takahashi suggested that milk was the most effective way to increase the height of the Japanese population[1757]. Preliminary data from a Danish research group suggest that casein has a stronger IGF-1-stimulating effect than does whey[760]. Another study from the same group found that high intakes of skimmed milk, but not meat, increased serum IGF-I and IGFBP-3 in 8-year-old boys[762].

It is primarily the size of the lower extremities that begins to grow in populations that switch to Western dietary habits, while their seated height remains almost the same[1764]. Today's young Japanese have the same relationship between leg length and body height as Europeans, as opposed to Africans who have relatively long legs.

A partial cause of increased adult stature is enhanced foetal growth. In a Turkish study of 60 unusually large (heavy and tall) infants, serum levels of IGF-1 and leptin were considerably increased, compared to infants of normal birth size[936]. Since leptin apparently stimulates chondrocytes of skeletal growth centres[1146], the high circulating leptin levels in Westerners may contribute to their increased stature. In addition, the intima-media part of the carotid artery was considerably thicker, as a sign of early atherosclerosis.

Pigs grow fast and become big, fat – and long – if they are fed today's concentrated feeds. One of the potential reasons is the increased insulin resistance, but the question has not been sufficiently investigated yet[1179]. In our own experiments, pigs that were fed a grain-free Palaeolithic diet became shorter and thinner than pigs raised on traditional feed[848].

These observations shed new light on the short stature of traditional populations such as the Kitavans, Trobriand Islands, Papua New Guinea (Table 4.8). It is obviously a mistake to regard this as a sign that their diet is not optimal. The diet on Kitava is rich and varied, and with sufficient protein [1055]. A more probable interpretation is that Westerners are abnormally tall. If you want your children to become basketball-players, raise them on Western food. Or, contrariwise, if they

Table 4.8   Height (cm, mean ± standard deviation) in Kitava, Papua New Guinea, and Sweden in different age groups[1130].

Age (years)	Height (cm)	
	Kitava	Sweden
Males		
20–39	162 ± 6	180 ± 6
40–59	161 ± 5	178 ± 6
60–86	161 ± 5	175 ± 6
Females		
20–39	150 ± 5	168 ± 6
40–59	150 ± 5	163 ± 6
60–86	150 ± 4	163 ± 6

thrive on a Palaeolithic-like diet, don't worry about their physical health if they are slightly shorter than their classmates.

Early puberty

The connection between insulin resistance and enhanced tissue growth is also relevant for the timing of puberty[788]. In Western Europe, mean age at menarche has decreased from 1920 and onward, while at the same time stature has increased[1356]. Young people with elevated levels of insulin and free IGF-1 reach sexual maturity at a younger age than other young people[789,1807,1966], and supplying IGF-1 also accelerates puberty in rhesus monkeys[1951]. In addition, the increase in leptin levels that accompanies overweight and abdominal obesity is predictive of early puberty in both sexes[1629].

Early-onset puberty, like insulin resistance, is particularly common among ethnic minorities of non-European origin[1456,1882], further emphasising their apparent increased vulnerability to the Western lifestyle. In a Swedish study of 107 adopted girls of Asian Indian origin, the median age of their first menstruation was 11.6 years, compared with the Swedish average of approximately 13 years[1456]. Five of the girls started menstruating before the age of 9 years, the youngest being 7.3 years.

Among hunter-gatherers and traditional horticulturalists, the average age of first menstruation is 15 years or slightly more[1968]. This figure is also valid for the Trobriand Islands (W. Schiefenhövel, unpublished data), where food is rich and abundant. Hence, inadequate nutrition is no plausible explanation for the late occurrence of first menstruation in traditional people. Instead, we should shift focus and increase our knowledge of the apparent relationships between Western lifestyles, endocrine disruption and early puberty.

Myopia

Another condition with excessive tissue growth that is mediated by retinoid receptors is myopia (nearsightedness), a disease that is due to the eye growing too long, resulting in the focus point of the image landing too far in front of the retina. In 2002, Loren Cordain proposed the idea of a causal connection between insulin resistance and myopia[334].

The prevalence in modern society varies between 13% and a staggering 90%, and most studies point to an increase in many countries[149,815,1706,1868]. Among roughly 1000 children studied in Gothenburg at the age of 12–13 years, 50% were myopic (≥ 0.5 D, i.e. at least 0.5 diopters negative refraction error). In total, 23% were considered in need of glasses (≥ -0.75 D). In contrast, a study of Danish conscripts found a decreasing prevalence, from 14.5% in 1964 to 12.8% in 2004[815].

Although myopia clearly depends on genetic factors, these are obviously insufficient to act as the sole cause for such widespread presence among the earth's different ethnic populations[284]. During human evolution, clear distance vision was highly required for escape from predators, location of food and social interaction[1289]. Any gene or genes capable of eliciting myopia without the additional help of environmental factors would be rapidly eliminated by natural selection. In addition, reduced selection pressure due to glasses has existed for a negligible number of years.

A prevalence of myopia of 0–2% has been recorded in several studies of hunter-gatherers[748,1674,1863,1991]. A host of other studies have documented an explosive increase after transitioning to a Western lifestyle[334]. Non-European ethnic groups seem to be at increased risk for myopia[91,1172], in parallel to a higher degree of insulin resistance[9,65,351,607,628,864].

Myopia does not appear to affect other free-ranging mammals[839,1895]. In contrast, the disease is not entirely uncommon among today's domesticated dogs, and an often-afflicted breed is the Labrador Retriever[1262], which also seems to have a high tendency for becoming overweight[1946] and developing atherosclerosis[1072] and diabetes[272].

Much evidence suggests that reading at close range during childhood can be a partial cause of myopia[1261]. This creates a fuzzy image on the retina (form deprivation), which signals the sclera to grow in an attempt to correct the eyeball's size in relation to the image. Form deprivation in animal experiments has also been shown to lead to myopia[1325,1474,1811], and it is probably the same case for humans[1217].

However, there are examples of urbanised, illiterate populations with a very high prevalence of myopia and, conversely, non-urbanised ethnic groups who despite an 8-hour school day, have a very low prevalence[334]. The fact that domestic dogs are affected also indicates that form deprivation is not the only environmental factor.

The chemical messengers that translate the retina's image onto the appropriate growth of the sclera, have proven to be locally synthesised retinoids in the retina and sclera[173,1214]. Based on the above-mentioned reasons (see Enhanced tissue growth), hyperinsulinaemia may hypothetically lead to reduced activity in the eyes' retinoid receptors, which intensifies the growth of the sclera. Additional support for this relationship is that myopia has been associated with increased stature and earlier puberty in most studies[334,903,1344,1584,1773].

Gardiner observed some of these connections in the 1950s[567], and he suspected that modern dietary habits, including highly refined carbohydrates and a low intake of 'animal' protein, could contribute to both myopia and accelerated growth[568,569]. In a 1-year controlled study with dietary modification, which included increased 'animal' protein consumption, he noted a slowed progress of myopia, compared with a control group that did not receive any recommendation regarding dietary changes[570]. Gardiner suspected milk protein to be beneficial, but he did not clearly distinguish between protein from milk and meat. A subsequent trial also found slowed progression of myopia by increased intake of protein and reduced intake of carbohydrate[1891]. In animal trials, refraction changes in the direction of myopia appeared with a diet rich in sucrose and low in protein, which was shown in rabbits[571] and rats[114].

In summary, these studies indicate that a diet that worsens insulin sensitivity can contribute to myopia.

Acne

Loren Cordain has also unravelled the likely relationship between hyperinsuli-naemia and acne (acne vulgaris)[337], a condition which afflicts more than 80% of Westerners[1690]. The disease is caused by excessive production of sebum which collects and forms blackheads (comedones) and, in more advanced forms, inflam-mation[1781]. It is well known that stimulating the retinoid receptors counteracts this process, a principle that is used in local treatment with tretinoin in skin creams or oral treatment with isotretinoin (13-*cis*-retinoic acid). In addition, hyperinsuli-naemia contributes to high level of the male sex hormone, which in turn accelerates growth of sebaceous follicle via IGF-1[806]. Therefore, it is appropriate to assume that insulin resistance can be a contributing factor for acne by inhibiting the body's ability to limit follicular cell proliferation.

There is additional support for the hypothesis in that IGF-1 treatment creates acne as a side effect[922], as well as the fact that adult women with acne are often insulin resistant and have elevated levels of IGF-1[25,26]. The male sex hormone raises the concentration of IGF-1[734], and anabolic steroids cause acne through increased sebum production[1606].

In sharp contrast to Western countries, we found acne to be non-existent on Kitava or among the Aché, hunter-gatherers in Paraguay[337] (Figure 4.23). On Kitava, 1200 individuals were examined, of which 300 were between the ages of 15 and 25, while the Aché population was made up of 115 individuals and a few young people. Even if our methods do not permit exact comparisons, we are certain that acne is remarkably less common than in Western populations. Sporadic information from other traditional populations points in the same direction[134,547,1385,1588,1720].

The earlier view among dermatologists, that diet has no or little influence on acne, may need to be reconsidered, and it appears logical to test the hypothesis with a Palaeolithic diet.

Benign prostatic hyperplasia

The Swedish urologist, Jan Hammarsten, noticed early on that abdominal obesity and diabetes were more common among men with benign enlargement of the prostate gland (prostatic hyperplasia) than in other men[657]. The association has since been confirmed in systematic studies, which have shown that both the size of the gland as well as its growth rates correlate to several variables within the metabolic syndrome (including serum insulin)[654,655]. It is also known that retinoid receptors regulate the growth of the prostate gland[634], which suggests that insulin resistance can exert an effect by down-regulating these receptors according to the guidelines given above. α-1 receptor blockers, such as doxazosin, not only stop further enlargement of the prostate, but also improve insulin sensitivity and reduce blood pressure, which points in the same direction[554].

Barss observed one case of acute urinary retention (obstructed urination) on Kiriwina, Trobriand Islands, around 1980[121]. The man refused treatment, why the cause could not be determined. His relatives revealed to Barss that they knew of

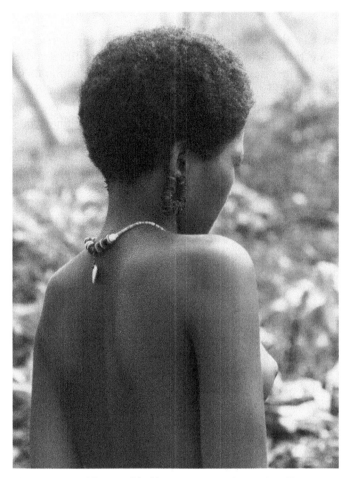

Figure 4.23 A 16-year-old Kitavan girl without any sign of acne, just like all other examined inhabitants. (Photo courtesy of Göran Burenhult.)

up to nine other men who died from acute urinary obstruction, but this is not consistent with Jüptner's, Schiefenhövel's or my experience. If the information is correct, one conceivable cause is the so-called 'rebound phenomenon' after long-term use of areca nuts (in betel chewing), whose alkaloid arecolin has a well-known parasympathomimetic effect[509,1305].

In other areas of Milne Bay Province (the province to which the Trobriand Islands belong), Barss noted a high prevalence of prostatic hyperplasia, where the patients often presented with urinary retention[121]. Prostate cancer was, however, uncommon in these areas. He did not address lifestyle factors, but it is well known that large sections of the area's population changed their eating habits in a more Western direction.

Benign enlargement of the prostate gland is very common in domestic dogs, in particular in those who are overweight, and the process often begins early in life[87,160,216].

Cancer

Cancers of the breast, prostate and colon/rectum, the most common forms of cancer in developed societies, are widely suspected to be linked to insulin resistance[858,1496,1805]. This could explain the high degree of worldwide covariation between these three forms of cancer[1084]. One of the suggested mechanisms is disruption of the insulin–IGF axis[1496]. A high plasma concentration of IGF-1 is a strong risk factor for prostate cancer in Sweden[1964], Greece[1145], USA and China[297]. Women who reach their maximum height before 12 years of age have an increased risk of breast cancer[1025], and women who develop breast cancer before menopause are taller than average and have an increased presence of acne as adults[549,1247]. Children who are treated with growth hormones potentially have an increased risk for epithelial cell cancer later in life[1751]. It is hoped that medications that activate retinoid receptors can also treat epithelial cell cancer[1435,1745,1974].

Other studies have confirmed, by way of additional mechanisms, the connection between insulin resistance and cancer of the breast[549,573,869,1729,1747,1901], prostate[653,1824], colon/rectum[313,626,820,1597,1805] and other organs[142,275].

Infertility

It is generally accepted that infertility can be caused by both obesity and insulin resistance, and weight loss is an established treatment for obese women who fail to become pregnant[1283,1393]. It has even been discussed if obese women should be denied medical treatment to improve ovulation rate and achieve pregnancy until they have reduced their body weight[102,1283].

Polycystic ovary syndrome (PCOS) is a very common cause of infertility[1393]. Many studies have shown reduced insulin sensitivity and high IGF-1 in PCOS, in particular when overweight is present. Metformin, an anti-diabetic drug which improves insulin sensitivity, is commonly used to treat PCOS[413]. PCOS is associated with obesity, the metabolic syndrome, gestational diabetes and various cardiovascular risk factors[413,942]. Acne is often a dominant symptom in PCOS[507], and over the long term, there is a risk of developing cardiovascular disease[1940]. Both acne and cardiovascular risk factors within the metabolic syndrome can be improved after adjusting the diet or using medication in order to control hyperinsulinaemia[1009].

Polycystic ovaries seem to be particularly common among non-European women, even in the absence of overweight[830]. In a British survey, 110 of 212 (52%) randomly selected women of Asian Indian descent had polycystic ovaries detectable with ultrasonography[1521]. Among women of northern European origin, PCOS is significantly less common, which, again, highlights the apparent ethnic differences in resistance to the Western lifestyle.

Infertile women without PCOS, and infertile men, are more often overweight or insulin resistant than individuals without disturbed reproduction[1393]. Impotence in elderly men appears to be related to insulin resistance and the metabolic syndrome[416,706].

Kidney failure

Chronic progressive kidney failure is prevalent in Western countries[1020]. The most common causes are high blood pressure and diabetes, and much evidence suggests that even 'normal' Western levels of blood pressure and glucose increase the risk[1862]. Insulin resistance and lipotoxicity seem to be linked to chronic kidney failure, but the exact mechanisms are not known[1750,1829,1917,1962]. There are probably several different mechanisms involved, as illustrated by the various microscopic changes in the tubules, glomeruli, arterioles and interstitial tissue of the kidney.

Relevant dietary factors

Conventional wisdom holds that the dietary factors that improve insulin sensitivity are largely the same factors that benefit the prevention and treatment of type 2 diabetes and overweight (see Sections 4.4 and 4.5)[1142,1480]. However, the links between diet and insulin sensitivity are largely unexplored and there is much uncertainty about the role of individual dietary factors. In our mind, insulin resistance is a rather straightforward condition, while in the laboratory it is quite elusive. The gold standard laboratory method, the hyperinsulinaemic–euglycaemic clamp, is time-consuming, costly, labour-intensive and artificial, and most studies have used simpler methods (such as the HOMA-IR based on fasting glucose and insulin) that are even less precise and may relate to other metabolic events.

Although studies of glucose tolerance do not automatically translate into insulin sensitivity, the preventive dietary factors that are discussed in Section 4.4, all need to be considered. Long-term *calorie restriction* apparently leads to exceptionally high insulin sensitivity in humans and monkeys[529,618]. Generally, a *reduced waistline also* results in improved insulin sensitivity[1480], and calorie restriction is apparently the most evidence-based method to achieve this (see Section 4.5). In our short-term trial of a *Palaeolithic diet* in people with ischaemic heart disease and high blood sugar, we found insulin sensitivity to improve slightly more on a Palaeolithic diet, compared to a Mediterranean-like traditional diet, but this was fully explained by the larger waist loss in the Palaeolithic group[1049]. There was no relationship between change in glucose tolerance and change in insulin response to ingested glucose, although this could partly be due to a low precision in our methods of assessing insulin sensitivity.

The isolated impact of *total fat* intake and dietary *fat quality* on insulin sensitivity has not been determined. In a large number of experiments in rats and mice, high-fat diets have consistently resulted in insulin resistance[235,276]. In dogs, even a moderate increase in dietary fat (at fixed caloric intake) has caused abdominal obesity and insulin resistance[907]. However, the lack of standardisation with respect to other dietary factors (e.g. grains and milk proteins) makes it premature to state that a high-fat diet is sufficient to cause insulin resistance. With regard to dietary fat quality, there is some support for a beneficial effect in humans from substituting saturated fat with monounsaturated[1866] or polyunsaturated fat[1744], although other dietary factors have not been fully controlled for.

In recent years, the notion that a high *glycaemic load* causes insulin resistance has been intensively discussed, but there is surprisingly little support from published studies to date. The longest intervention trial actually found an improved insulin sensitivity with a *high*-glycaemic index, low-fibre diet in healthy young men[905]. Other studies have shown mixed results but do not indicate a major role of dietary carbohydrate (glycaemic index or glycaemic load) in the causation of insulin resistance[162,455,913,1035,1173,1480,1628,1960].

As already mentioned, the excess accumulation of fat inside the cells of various organs is now increasingly regarded as part of the insulin resistance syndrome, even in the absence of overweight. The best diet to avoid this problem is not known but calorie restriction and a narrow waistline can always be recommended. One study compared a very low-fat (16 E% fat) diet with a high-fat (56 E% fat) diet and changes in liver fat accumulation (fatty liver) using proton spectroscopy in 10 women with obesity[1927]. During 2 weeks, liver fat decreased by $20 \pm 9\%$ during the low-fat diet and increased by $35 \pm 21\%$ during the high-fat diet ($p = 0.042$ for difference between the groups). Fasting serum insulin decreased in the low-fat group and increased in the high-fat group ($p = 0.005$ for group difference). Dietary fat was mainly reduced in exchange for carbohydrate, but differences in food choice were not reported. A similar but non-controlled trial in 13 subjects, with mean BMI 33, who lost 6 kg of total weight and 4 cm of waist circumference on a low-fat (25 E%) diet found significant decrease of intracellular liver fat[1580].

In contrast, another non-controlled study of 10 healthy volunteers found reductions in liver fat during 10 days of carbohydrate restriction[747]. All subjects lost weight, but this was not correlated with liver fat loss. In mice, a methionine- and choline-deficient diet causes fatty liver irrespective of the amount of fat (5% compared with 20%), but this animal model may not be representative for humans[986].

Dietary *fructose* (at very high levels) causes insulin resistance in animal experiments, but available evidence suggests that fruits are safe, in particular for humans[487]. One short-term study in healthy men (age 33 ± 3 years, BMI 27 ± 1) suggests that not even *sucrose* (table sugar), which is made up of fructose and glucose, would suffice to cause insulin resistance as long as calories are not consumed in excess[181].

The effect of *cow's milk* on insulin sensitivity is complex. Two components of milk have been shown to contribute to insulin resistance in animal experiments: lactose in calves[777,778,1375] and casein in rats[377,993,1808]. The expected culprit in lactose would be galactose rather than glucose, and a proposed mechanism is based on the fact that insulin increases extra-hepatic uptake of galactose in competition with glucose without stimulating insulin release[1616]. In humans, when galactose is absorbed together with glucose (as ingested monosaccharides or from digested lactose), the serum galactose response is depressed whereas serum glucose and insulin levels are raised. Another possible mechanism related to lactose could be galactosylation of glucose transporters at the cell membranes leading to insulin resistance[246,1996].

The metabolic effects of casein and other types of protein have been compared in a series of experiments in rats fed high-fat diets[993]. Three groups received a high-fat diet and a fourth group received a low-fat diet. All of them received normal grain-based rat feed (chow). The fat-rich diet caused insulin resistance if, and only if, it was combined with casein or soya protein, but not in combination with fish protein. There was no difference in weight gain among the different groups. One might suspect that meat protein would have produced the same results as with fish protein, since rats are omnivores[1102], but this has not been studied. A human 4-week trial found that a cod protein diet improved insulin sensitivity and β-cell function, as measured by the hyperinsulinaemic–euglycaemic clamp, compared with a diet containing lean beef, pork, veal, eggs, milk and milk products, with no specification of the proportion of milk or meat proteins[1365].

Another aspect of casein and insulin sensitivity relates to β-casomorphin-7, a peptide derived from β-casein A1. This peptide is an agonist to the μ-opiod receptor, meaning that it binds to the receptor and activates it[1777]. Such activation is thought to result in insulin resistance by way of cross-talk between the μ-opioid receptor and the insulin receptor signalling cascade[561,1027]. It has been proposed that the much higher prevalence of type 2 diabetes in African Americans than in US whites is partly caused by different molecular variants (single nucleotide polymorphisms, SNPs) of the μ-opioid receptor[561].

Dietary protein stimulates the release of insulin, and milk protein is no exception[1364]. In particular, the whey fraction of milk contains the responsible protein(s)[548,1307]. It is not known if this affects long-term insulin sensitivity. The insulin response to dietary protein is at least as high as with a corresponding amount of carbohydrates, but glucagon, the hormone that raises blood glucose, also increases which makes the net effect difficult to determine[210,1594]. In a 1-week study in children, a high intake of milk, but not meat, resulted in markedly increased fasting serum insulin and decreased insulin sensitivity calculated from fasting glucose and insulin (HOMA-IR)[761].

In some animal experiments, casein contributes to fat overload and lipotoxicity in the liver, clearly suggesting that milk contributes to fatty liver[76,1804]. However, in another study, rats fed a diet with 50% milk protein for 6 months did not develop fat overload in liver or kidneys, while a control group fed 14% milk protein and 85% more corn starch and sucrose did develop such alterations[969].

The role of *cereals* for insulin sensitivity is open to question and scarcely studied from an evolutionary perspective. Cereals are a major source of starch in Western societies but, although this causes hyperinsulinaemia, it may not be an important cause of insulin resistance, as already discussed. Most studies focusing on cereals have compared whole grains with more refined ones, while there is a paucity of data on high versus low intakes of cereals. A controlled trial of whole grains found no effect on insulin sensitivity as measured by the hyperinsulinaemic–euglycaemic clamp test[52]. A similar short-term study found that cereal fibre improved insulin sensitivity[1913]. This is in line with findings in epidemiological studies but, as usual in such studies, the role of confounding factors is uncertain[8,1142].

Gluten exorphins, opioid peptides derived from wheat gluten, stimulate the pancreatic release of insulin in rats and dogs, an effect which is inhibited by naloxone[553,1602]. The relevance of this for insulin sensitivity is unknown.

Possibly, other endocrine disrupting phytochemicals from grains (and beans) are more significant. The concept of endocrine disruption, i.e. disturbance of hormonal function by exogenous substances, is widely used among researchers of environmental toxicology. A large observational study found a very strong, gradual increase in risk of type 2 diabetes with increasing serum concentration of endocrine-disrupting persistent organic pollutants[1004]. The included pollutants dioxin and polychlorinated biphenyls are known to inhibit insulin action at the cellular level. It is also entirely relevant to consider endocrine disruption for food-derived phytochemicals which interfere with hormonal action, such as glycoproteins in wheat.

There are many indications that cereals and beans affect glucose metabolism by means of their glycoproteins. The best studied of these is wheat lectin (WGA), a highly stable substance which escapes digestion in the gastrointestinal tract[1848]. Thus, it passes the gut barrier and enters the bloodstream intact[1461], and thereafter it binds to several hormone receptors including the insulin receptors and other tyrosine kinase receptors (the IGF-1 and EGF receptors)[1900]. The binding of wheat lectin to the insulin receptor is strong and long-lasting with high molecular efficiency, suggesting that it may hinder insulin to exert its effects for many hours[353,354,705,1073,1459,1640,1641]. Hence, it is theoretically capable of causing insulin resistance. Further, wheat lectin increases glycolysis (metabolic breakdown of glucose)[1986] as well as fat storage[544], but in contrast to insulin, which has the same effects, it does not seem to stimulate protein synthesis[1460], which is relevant since loss of muscle mass (sarcopenia) has been suggested to worsen insulin sensitivity[503]. Rats that were fed Turkish beans (*Phaseolus vulgaris*) quickly lost 30% of their skeletal muscle mass, which is thought to be an effect of its lectin, phaseolus vulgaris agglutinin (PHA)[1348].

Plant lectins including the wheat lectin bind to pancreatic islet cells[1439], and the lectin from *Agaricus bisporus* (the common edible mushroom) stimulates calcium uptake by, and insulin release from, rat islet cells. Intraperitoneal injection of *Robinia pseudoacacia* lectin in mice produces hypoglycaemia for the first few hours, followed by reactive hyperglycaemia. In this animal model, liver glycogen falls and then rises in step with blood glucose, and skeletal muscle glycogen falls after 3 days[544].

Insulin resistance refers to a low response to insulin-stimulated glucose uptake in the cells, but not to other actions of insulin such as the formation of fat. It has been proposed that insulin resistance is a protective mechanism that reduces lipotoxic damage to non-adipose tissue by keeping glucose outside of the cells[1838]. In that perspective, the finding that wheat lectin stimulates not only the breakdown of glucose, but also the formation of fat seems worrying[1986].

A number of additional dietary factors have been discussed in relation to insulin resistance. *Salt restriction* paradoxically reduces insulin sensitivity in several studies, in particular among salt sensitive men[435,1198,1345,1416]. Many of the relationships between sodium intake, insulin resistance, hypertension and cardiovascular disease are complex, counterintuitive and confusing. A parallel paradox exists with regard to the renin–angiotensin system, which can be described as 'down-regulated' in most Westerners, in sharp contrast to traditional populations like the Yanomamo hunter-gatherers. They consume a small fraction of the sodium of Westerners, are 'abnormally' insulin sensitive and have exceptionally low blood pressure, suggesting that an activated renin–angiotensin system is not always pathological[473].

In conclusion, available evidence tends to support the idea that an ancestral diet is beneficial for long-term insulin sensitivity. Unfortunately, there is a paucity of studies where physical activity and other lifestyle factors have been matched for.

Box 4.3   Insulin resistance

- Depends on lifestyle for its genetic expression
- Can have wide-ranging effects on health
- Is seen in the majority of Westerners at an early age
- Is less pronounced among northern Europeans
- Awaits a better explanation than the 'thrifty genotype' hypothesis

---

4.7   Hypertension (high blood pressure)

The definitions of normal and high blood pressure are arbitrary and consequently vary between different parts of the world. The classification that best matches the perspective of evolutionary medicine is the one from the USA. In the Seventh Report of the US Joint National Committee on the Prevention, Detection and Treatment of High Blood Pressure (JNC 7), blood pressure needs to be lower than 120/80 mm Hg in order to be classified as 'normal'" (Table 4.9)[295], while most other authorities regard blood pressures below 140/90 as 'normal' (Table 4.10).

With regard to medication the most evidence-based guidelines are those of the British Hypertension Society[1948], which are strictly based on randomised controlled trials, whereas other guidelines are partly based on observational data. The British guidelines do not recommend drug treatment for sustained systolic blood pressures $\geq$160 mm Hg or sustained diastolic blood pressures $\geq$100 mm Hg in the absence of inner organ damage, cardiovascular disease or diabetes, unless there is an estimated 10 year risk of cardiovascular disease of $\geq$20% despite lifestyle advice.

The disadvantage of the US classification (Table 4.9) is that it tends to push doctors to treat most Westerners with antihypertensive drugs even in blood pressure categories for which proof of benefit from drug treatment is lacking. The disadvantage of other classifications, such as that of the European Society of

Table 4.9   Classification of blood pressure levels for untreated US adults[295].

Category	Systolic blood pressure (mm Hg)	Diastolic blood pressure (mm Hg)
Normal	<120	<80
Prehypertension	120–139	80–89
Stage 1 hypertension	140–159	90–99
Stage 2 hypertension	$\geq$160	$\geq$100

Table 4.10 Classification of blood pressure levels for untreated European adults[1130].

Category	Systolic blood pressure (mm Hg)	Diastolic blood pressure (mm Hg)
Optimal	<120	<80
Normal	<130	<85
High normal	130–139	85–89
Hypertension		
Grade I (mild)	140–159	90–99
Grade II (moderate)	160–179	100–109
Grade III (severe)	180–209	110–119

Hypertension and the European Society of Cardiology (Table 4.10) is that they conceal the increased risk with an average Western blood pressure, compared to a low level. Possibly, it is difficult for many experts to accept the fact that the majority of the population have an abnormally high blood pressure[1043].

This chapter deals with primary (essential) hypertension, the common form of high blood pressure. Secondary hypertension, which is usually caused by endocrine or renal disease, is not considered. When the heart pumps the blood along the blood vessels, these dilate or contract in order to keep the pressure constant. For reasons essentially unknown, the blood vessels tend to lose some of their flexibility with advancing age, either because of structural wall changes or because the tiny muscles inside the walls force them to contract. As a result, the heart must pump more forcefully, thereby increasing the blood pressure. Sometimes this higher pressure can damage smaller vessels (arterioles) of inner organs but usually the relationship between hypertension and organ failure remains obscure. It is very difficult to determine the impact of individual dietary factors (or other lifestyle factors). Most studies only run for a short time, and structural changes in the blood vessels that are significant for blood pressure often require months or years to develop (or to diminish).

Prevalence studies

Among US adults (age ≥ 18 years), the estimated prevalence of hypertension (systolic ≥140 and/or diastolic ≥90) in 2004 was 21.2% in whites, 29.2% in African Americans, 19.6% in Hispanics or Latinos and 25.4% in American Indians or Alaska Natives[1531].

These figures are in sharp contrast with the situation among hunter-gatherers and similar ethnic groups. Many studies have convincingly shown that hypertension is very rare among such populations, and that the average blood pressure is low compared to the Western world[118,126,434,576,690,816,821,868,885, 1051,1086,1109,1132,1139,1350,1369,1453,1631,1634,1669,1711,1814,1818,1937]. Table 4.11 shows average blood pressure in middle age among hunter-gatherers, traditional horticulturalists in Kitava, Trobriand Islands, and in Sweden.

Table 4.11   Blood pressure at age 40–60 years among hunter-gatherers, on Kitava and in Sweden (mm Hg, mean ± standard deviation).

Population	Men	Women
Bushmen[868]	108/63 ± 11/7	118/71 ± 13/6
Yanomamo[1350]	104/65 ± 8/8	102/63 ± 14/12
Xingu[126]	107/68 ± 20/11	102/66 ± 23/11
Kitava[1051]	113/71 ± 13/7	121/71 ± 16/8
Sweden[1051]	134/92 ± 15/10	126/86 ± 16/11

In the Kitava study, we measured blood pressure in 272 people aged 4–86[1051]. Compared to Westerners, the most marked difference was seen for diastolic blood pressure that was low in all age groups, with an average of 70 mm Hg (Figures 4.24 and 4.25). Among adults, diastolic blood pressure did not increase with age, and all the subjects examined who were over the age of 40 fell below the Swedish median. In the same age group, 83% of men and 61% of women had diastolic pressure below the 10th percentile in Sweden. The Swedes were made up of randomly selected residents of the city of Söderhamn. Both populations were examined using an identical methodology, with the subject sitting with the arm parallel to the sternum, which makes the comparisons reliable[1054,1776]. Systolic blood pressure also differed, although less markedly, and there was significant overlap between Kitava and Sweden (Figures 4.26 and 4.27). This overlap was most pronounced

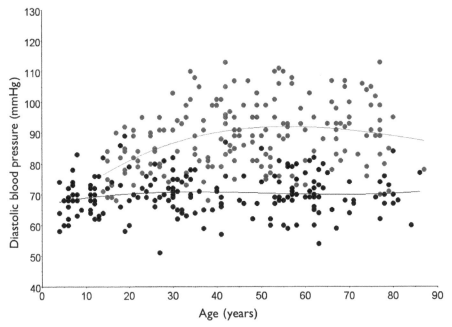

Figure 4.24   Diastolic blood pressure among males in Kitava, Trobriand Islands, Papua New Guinea (black) and Sweden (grey).

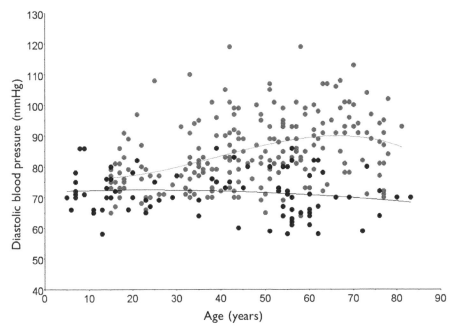

Figure 4.25 Diastolic blood pressure among females in Kitava (black) and Sweden (grey).

among women, where the Kitavans did not have lower blood pressure than the Swedes until after the age of 60.

There is no doubt that high blood pressure is a disease of modern civilisation, and that blood pressure does not rise in traditional populations before middle age. However, the extent to which blood pressure rises after middle age in traditional populations is not clear. On Kitava, after the age of 40, there was a significant increase of systolic blood pressure among men ($r = 0.12$; $P = 0.0005$; $n = 92$) and women ($r = 0.12$; $P = 0.01$; $n = 46$). On average, the systolic pressure among the 15 men who were over the age of 75 was 133 mm Hg (min 100, max 162). This was significantly ($P = 0.002$) higher than among the 31 men who were between the ages of 60 and 74, whose average blood pressure was 115 mm Hg (range 84–166). No previous study of traditional populations had included so many different ages as the Kitava study. In addition, the accuracy of our age estimates was unusually high.

However, the findings from Kitava should be seen against a background where the intake of salt and saturated fat was probably not entirely optimal. The estimated sodium intake (primarily sea salt for cooking food) was 40–50 mmol/day, which is higher than what was typical during evolution (see Chapter 3).

Effects of urbanisation

When aboriginal populations transitioned to a modern lifestyle, without any known exceptions, their blood pressure rose and then displayed the same clear

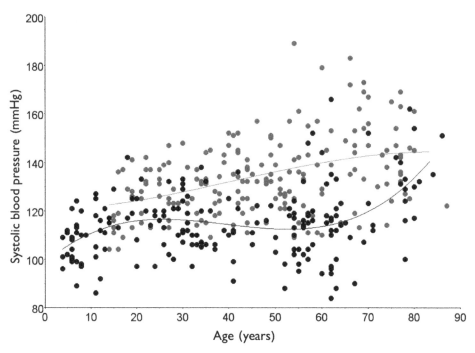

Figure 4.26   Systolic blood pressure among males in Kitava (black) and Sweden (grey).

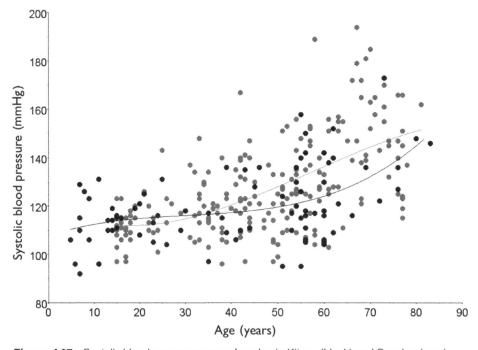

Figure 4.27   Systolic blood pressure among females in Kitava (black) and Sweden (grey).

relation to age as among Westerners[22,44,352,457,472,521,576,690,816,885,1086,1108,1220, 1271,1437,1453,1632,1770,1795,1814,1890,2010,2012].

In a migrant study in Kenya, two groups of ethnic Africans were followed for two years[1437,1438]. One had moved to the city while the other remained in the original environment. A gradual increase in blood pressure was noted in all of the migrants, where the entire normal distribution curve shifted upwards, but not among the non-migrants. Hence, almost everyone in this group eventually developed a higher blood pressure than if they had maintained their original lifestyle. This can be interpreted to mean that essentially all Westerners have a higher blood pressure than they would if they had a biologically optimal lifestyle. Other migration studies came to the same conclusion[176,478,695,1265,1559].

Risks with hypertension

Hypertension is a well-established cardiovascular risk factor in the Western world, and numerous studies suggest that 'the lower the better' down to very low levels[1023]. However, most people who experience myocardial infarction or stroke have average or only mildly elevated blood pressure (often around 150/90 mm Hg) before becoming ill. This is explained by the fact that the increase in risk is very modest from very low to modestly elevated blood pressure. It is only with very high blood pressure that the risk increases sharply. Figure 4.28 shows how the risk varies with blood pressure among healthy people with an average cholesterol level. Since blood pressure categories are not evenly distributed in society and the large majority has blood pressure below 160 mm Hg, more than 80% of all patients with myocardial infarction come from the three lowest groups, despite a lower relative risk. Even at 'optimal' pressure (<120 mm Hg), there is still a substantial risk if the subject lives a Western lifestyle.

Two people with the same blood pressure can have very different risk levels depending on age and the presence of other risk factors. Take, for example, two middle-aged men who both have a blood pressure of 160/100. One is a 45-year-old, non-smoker with a 5 mmol/L cholesterol level and a normal ECG, who is only moderately overweight (BMI 27). The other is a 65-year-old smoker with a cholesterol level of 8 mmol/L, who is borderline obese (BMI 30) and has signs of ischaemic heart disease on the ECG. The probability of a myocardial infarction per year is only 0.2% for the first man versus just over 10% for the second one.

Relevant dietary factors

There are several dietary factors which may explain the low blood pressure in non-Western populations, and an ancestral diet fits well into the prevailing concepts of dietary treatment of hypertension. There is widespread agreement that weight management, fruits and vegetables, salt restriction, regular physical activity and alcohol moderation are beneficial for prevention and treatment of high blood pressure (Table 4.12)[58,295,643,1130].

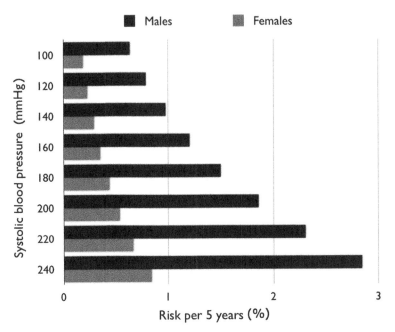

Figure 4.28 Risk of death due to cardiovascular disease in the next 5 years, depending on systolic blood pressure, among healthy non-smoking Westerners aged 50 and with serum cholesterol 6 mmol/L. (Adapted from www.riskscore.org.uk.)

Weight management

Preventing and treating excess weight and obesity, particularly abdominal obesity, is crucial for optimal blood pressure. For overweight or obese people, weight loss of as little as 5 kg can significantly lower blood pressure, although the ideal would often be to obtain a BMI below 25, and sometimes even below 20. The relevant dietary factors for weight loss are discussed in Section 4.5.

Table 4.12   Lifestyle interventions for blood pressure reduction.

	Recommendation	Expected reduction in systolic blood pressure
Weight reduction	Maintain ideal BMI (20–25)	5–10 mm Hg/10 kg weight loss
DASH eating plan	Fruits, vegetables, low-fat dairy products, less saturated fat	8–14 mm Hg
Dietary sodium restriction	Less than 100 mmol Na/day (<2.4 g Na or <6 g NaCl)	2–8 mm Hg
Physical activity	Regular aerobic physical activity, e.g. brisk walking, 30 minutes most days	4–9 mm Hg
Alcohol moderation	Men: 21 units/week; Women: 14 units/week	2–4 mm Hg

Source: From the British Hypertension Society 2004[1948].

Fruits and vegetables

In a month-long study (DASH), 459 healthy people were randomly assigned into one of three dietary models: one rich in fruits and vegetables in combination with lean dairy products (DASH-diet), another one only rich in fruits and vegetables, or a control group[61]. The DASH diet distinguished itself from the other two groups in terms of a very low percentage of total fat (27 E%) and saturated fat (6 E%) (in exchange of protein and carbohydrates). The control group differed from the two other groups by a low intake of potassium and magnesium (corresponding to 25th percentile in USA compared with the 75th percentile in remaining groups). Despite the fact that blood pressure was relatively low even at the starting point (131/85 ± 11/5), it still dropped in the group consuming fruits and vegetables, and even more so in the group with the DASH diet. Among the 133 patients with hypertension, the DASH group achieved a 11/5 mm larger reduction than the control group.

Slightly contrasting results from the PREMIER trial suggest that the DASH diet, when added to a program including weight loss, sodium restriction, increased physical activity and limited alcohol intake, does not lead to further improvement of blood pressure[59].

Several other studies suggest that a high intake of fruits and vegetables reduces the risk of hypertension[1130]. The DASH study has also been pointed out as evidence of the benefits of lean dairy products, but all of the suggested advantages can be obtained with a Palaeolithic diet, while avoiding the risks that may result from long-term milk consumption (atherosclerosis, insulin resistance, etc.).

In a British, randomised, controlled study with an increased intake of fruits and vegetables, a 4 mm lower systolic blood pressure was noted in the intervention group (95% CI 2–6; $P < 0.0001$), and 1.5 mm lower diastolic pressure (95% CI 0.2–2.7; $P < 0.0001$) compared with the control group after 6 months[834]. The study was conducted on 690 healthy subjects between the ages of 25 and 64.

Salt restriction

It has been well documented that Western levels of salt consumption (>100 mmol Na/day) can increase blood pressure and that restricting salt can reduce it, both in humans[305,319,688,997,1338] and animals[485,696,1203]. Even in elderly people, reduced salt intake seems to result in lower blood pressure[60,258]. Chimpanzees which are raised on vegetables and fruits develop high blood pressure if they also receive salt. Piglets which get supplemental salt in their food develop high blood pressure after only 3 weeks[328]. Not even so-called spontaneously hypertensive rats develop hypertension if the amount of salt in their food is brought down to the level of free-ranging rats[1758,1799].

In the previously mentioned DASH study, blood pressure was studied at three different levels of salt intake, 145, 105 and 65 mmol Na/day, together with a DASH diet or a control diet[1554]. There were six different groups, either with or without a DASH diet and at the three different salt levels, who showed a gradual drop in blood pressure, the lower the salt intake. The DASH diet reduced blood pressure regardless of salt consumption. The results were the same for people with normal blood pressure[1877].

In the Trials of Hypertension Prevention (TOHP I and II), 3126 individuals aged 30–54 years with prehypertension were randomised to sodium restriction or control group. The risk of a cardiovascular event (myocardial infarction, stroke, coronary revascularisation or cardiovascular death) was 25% lower among those in the intervention group (relative risk 0.75; 95% CI 0.57–0.99; $p = 0.04$), adjusted for trial, clinic, age, race and sex.

The effect of salt on blood pressure is also supported by epidemiological studies[287,996]. However, in the large, international, epidemiological INTERSALT study, which included 10 020 men and women in 32 countries, there was no relationship between blood pressure and sodium consumption in the interval of 100–250 mmol Na/day, but certainly at lower intake levels (Figure 4.29)[795]. Thus, there may be a threshold effect so that salt intake must be less than 100 mmol/day (<5 g common salt/day) to achieve a significant drop in blood pressure. In the DASH-sodium trial, blood pressure dropped more between 105 and 65 mmol/day than between 145 and 105 mmol/day[1554]. A traditional tribe in Melanesia with a high salt intake from

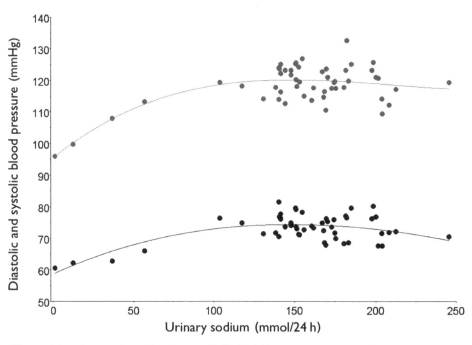

Figure 4.29 Systolic (above) and diastolic (below) blood pressure in relation to urinary sodium excretions (an estimate of salt intake) in the INTERSALT study. (Adapted from Reference 795.)

seawater, but otherwise with their original dietary habits, had higher blood pressure than their neighbours who did not use seawater to prepare their food[1369]. In contrast, the Kuna Indians, hunter-gatherers of Panama, have low blood pressure despite an estimated salt intake which is comparable to Western populations[1178], suggesting that high salt intake is no prerequisite for hypertension.

One issue that has been thoroughly discussed is salt sensitivity, i.e. individual difference in the effect of salt on blood pressure[344,1092]. Although there is little doubt that such a difference exists, it seems rarely possible to identify individuals who will not benefit from salt restriction[1339]. One problem is that research on salt sensitivity usually involves short-term studies for a week or two, where long-term structural changes to the blood vessel will be overlooked. Even if there are connections between decreased salt sensitivity and insulin resistance[1198,1516], and salt sensitivity is a potential independent cardiovascular risk factor[1242], salt restriction should not be reserved just for certain individuals.

Nevertheless, a lesson from salt sensitivity studies is that the contribution of salt intake to high blood pressure is more likely if the patient is old rather than young, overweight rather than lean, black rather than white, has diabetes or glucose intolerance, or has evidence of reduced kidney function[746]. Furthermore, among people who use medication to treat high blood pressure, salt restriction should be gradually introduced and with monitoring of blood pressure. This is particularly important for those on ACE inhibitors or angiotensin receptor blockers.

Other factors

There is a lot of evidence to indicate that *insulin resistance* and hypertension are causally related[317,383,979,1575], especially in the kind of hypertension that is unresponsive to drug treatment[799,1151]. A recent study in normal-weight hypertensive subjects without the metabolic syndrome (average waist circumference 88 cm) found a 143% increase of the insulin response after glucose intake, compared to subjects with normal blood pressure, indicating insulin resistance in the former group[238]. Hence, dietary changes that improve insulin sensitivity are expected to improve blood pressure (see Section 4.6).

Potassium is one of the nutrients that can be studied in a double-blind fashion, which has also been done. A Cochrane review could not confirm whether potassium supplements can lower high blood pressure and therefore does not recommend them for treating hypertension[418]. More trials enrolling a large number of participants with long periods of follow-up were thought to be necessary to know whether or not potassium supplements can lower high blood pressure. Some studies suggest that the effect is more pronounced in people on a high salt intake[1928].

Randomised controlled trials and observational studies in humans, as well as animal experiments, indicate that a *high protein intake* may prevent the development of hypertension[62,484,697,735,1067,1980], and one of the characteristics of the DASH diet is a high percentage of protein[58]. A trial in 164 subjects with prehypertension or stage 1 hypertension (see Table 4.9 for definitions) found a diet rich in protein to decrease systolic blood pressure by 1.4 mm Hg ($p = 0.002$) in the whole population and by 3.5 mm Hg ($p = 0.006$) among those with hypertension, compared with a high-carbohydrate diet[62]. In the same trial, a similar decrease of blood pressure was obtained by a diet high in monounsaturated fat, suggesting that the high-carbohydrate diet increased blood pressure, rather than the two other diets decreasing it.

The type of protein may also be important. A trial in 60 hypertensive persons found that an increased intake of protein from *lean red meat* during 8 weeks lowered mean systolic blood pressure by 5.2 mm Hg, on average[735]. One half of the group increased their protein intake from 18.6 to 23.8 E% in exchange for carbohydrate from cereals and potatoes, while the other half did not change their protein intake. Both groups had a fairly low fat intake at approximately 31 E%. In an epidemiological study of 11 different middle-aged populations in separate parts of China, 56% of the geographic variation in blood pressure was explained by an inverse association with the urinary excretion of 3-methylhistidine[1067], which is a good marker of the consumption of meat protein[1672]. Thus, blood pressure was lower in areas with a high meat protein intake.

A number of other dietary factors could be mentioned. A meta-analysis of randomised controlled trials of supplemental *dietary fibre* (soluble or insoluble) found a small blood pressure lowering effect, but after adjustment for possible publication bias the effect was no longer statistically significant[2034], and in the largest trial there was no beneficial effect[694]. A Cochrane review found no strong evidence of a causal association between *magnesium* supplementation and blood pressure reduction[419]. In the very large randomised placebo-controlled Heart Protection Study, supplementation with *vitamin C, vitamin E* and β-*carotene* had no effect on blood pressure over 5 years[5]. Increased *fish* consumption has been suggested to reduce blood pressure[111,140], but it is doubtful whether this is due to the fatty acid composition, since the addition of omega-3 fat in realistic doses does not seem to affect blood pressure[305]. Studies of *coffee* have shown conflicting results[651].

4.8   Dyslipidaemia (blood lipid disorders)

Dyslipidaemia involving primarily high serum levels of total and LDL cholesterol, low HDL cholesterol and high triglycerides are well-documented cardiovascular risk factors (see below). However, the onset of atherosclerosis also seems to require other contributing factors such as the increased endothelial permeability of blood vessels, oxidative modification of LDL particles, and the blood's increased tendency to clot (see Section 4.3).

The picture in terms of blood lipids among aboriginal populations is not as consistent as it is in terms of their lack of overweight, abdominal obesity and high blood pressure. There are examples of populations with a very low prevalence of ischaemic heart disease despite blood lipid levels that would be considered high risk in the West.

Prevalence studies

Serum cholesterol

The average serum cholesterol is 2.8–3.5 mmol/L among hunter-gatherers and other traditional populations living off shore[118,223,320,393,1098,1131,1137,1139,1369, 1403,1669,1819], which corresponds to half of the northern European levels. Hypercholesterolaemia (serum cholesterol above 5 mmol/L) does not seem to develop in these populations.

However, in several cases, other aboriginal populations have shown an average serum cholesterol of 5 mmol/L or higher, i.e. fully comparable with Westerners. This applies to populations in the South Pacific with a high intake of coconut[785,1451] and Eskimos with a high total fat intake[454]. This in combination with a low occurrence of cardiovascular disease highlights the significance of other contributing factors.

On Kitava, total and LDL cholesterol levels among men were somewhat lower than among Swedish men (Figures 4.30–4.33), and close to today's Japanese, while women had levels comparable with Swedish women, especially below 60 years of age[1051]. Hypercholesterolaemia was not an unusual condition (Table 4.13). The primary cause is possibly the high intake of saturated fat from coconut[1055]. One would expect an even higher level of serum cholesterol due to the high intake of saturated fat, and since the two major fatty acids in coconut, 12:0 lauric acid and 14:0 myristic acid, are considered to have a stronger cholesterol-raising effect than 16:0 palmitic acid, which is the dominant fatty acid in Western countries[139].

Traditional cattle-herding nomads are a special case: East African nomads (with the exception of the Masai, see below) have had serum cholesterol levels that match those of Westerners[1633].

HDL cholesterol and triglycerides

Traditional populations do not have 'better' HDL cholesterol and triglyceride levels than Westerners[320,931,1051,1131,1608,1669,1819,1926] (Figures 4.34, 4.35, 4.38 and 4.39). Healthy dietary habits do not always seem to have the desired effect on HDL and triglycerides. Hence, it is unclear whether 'dyslipidaemia' in ancestral populations should be classified as such, so that, for example, the traditional South Pacific diet would be less healthy than a typical hunter-gatherer diet. If this is the case, other

Table 4.13 Approximate prevalence of hypercholesterolaemia (high serum cholesterol, i.e. >5 mmol/L) among male hunter-gatherers, on Kitava and in Sweden.

	Age 30–50 years	Age 50–70 years
Hunter-gatherers	0%	0%
Kitava	50%	50%
Sweden	70%	>90%

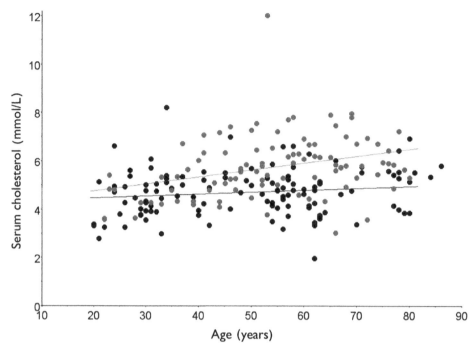

Figure 4.30   Serum cholesterol (total cholesterol) among males in Kitava, Trobriand Islands, Papua New Guinea (black) and Sweden (grey). (Adapted from Reference 1051.)

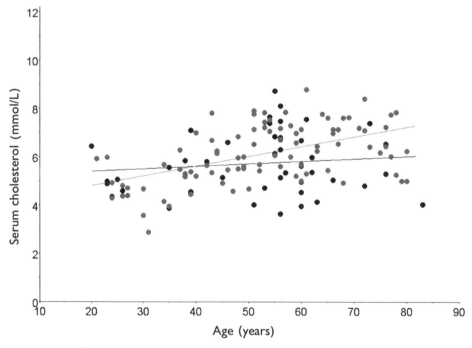

Figure 4.31   Serum total cholesterol among females in Kitava (black) and Sweden (grey). (Adapted from Reference 1051.)

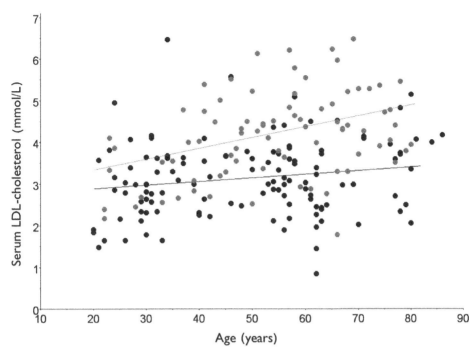

Figure 4.32 Serum LDL-cholesterol among males in Kitava (black) and Sweden (grey). (Adapted from Reference 1051.)

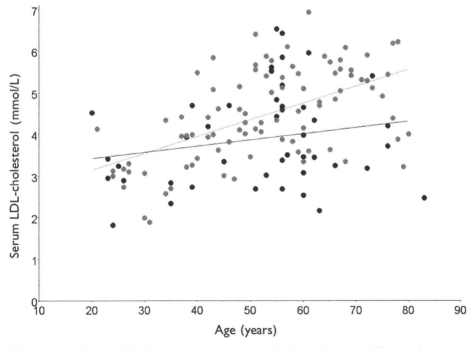

Figure 4.33 Serum LDL-cholesterol among females in Kitava (black) and Sweden (grey). (Adapted from Reference 1051.)

lifestyle factors seem to be contributing to a beneficial net effect among the Pacific populations (Figures 4.36–4.38, Table 4.14).

Effects of urbanisation

Serum cholesterol

When traditional populations become urbanised, the cholesterol levels, both total and LDL cholesterol, rise to Western levels, if they weren't there already[1041]. In Sweden, the vast majority have hypercholesterolaemia (serum cholesterol >5 mmol/L; Table 4.13), and the numbers are roughly the same in the Mediterranean countries, including France[101,253,260,1056].

Among semi-traditional Polynesians, who were forced to emigrate from Tokelau to New Zealand due to a tsunami, serum cholesterol levels rose after the migration, despite the fact that the intake of saturated fat fell sharply due to a reduced intake of coconut[1451,1713]. This clearly shows that other factors are also at work.

The cattle-herding Masai of East Africa should be mentioned in particular. During their traditional nomadic life, the intake of saturated fat from milk has been very high, and they also suffered from significant coronary atherosclerosis, although raised plaques were rare[1140]. Despite this, researchers noted a very low serum cholesterol level (3.5 ± 0.9 mmol/L; average $\pm$ standard deviation; $n = 254$) that did not rise with age. It has been suggested that this would be due to

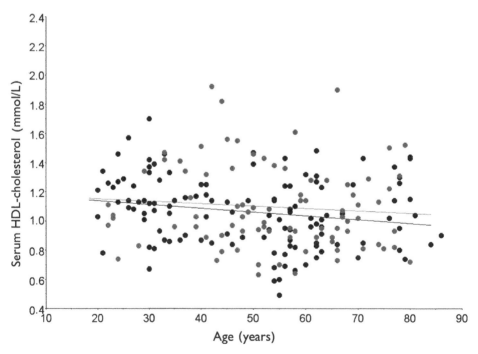

Figure 4.34   Serum HDL-cholesterol among males in Kitava (black) and Sweden (grey). (Adapted from Reference 1051.)

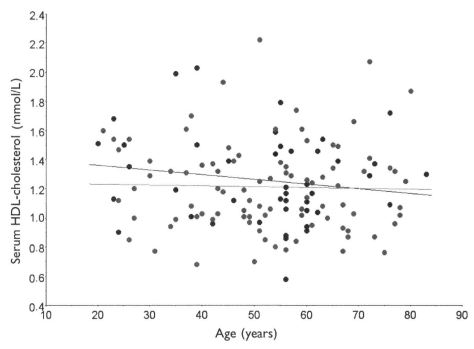

Figure 4.35 Serum HDL-cholesterol among females in Kitava (black) and Sweden (grey). (Adapted from Reference 1051.)

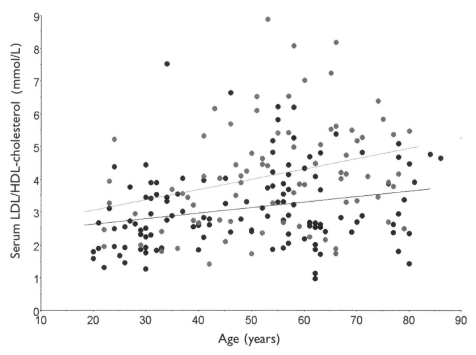

Figure 4.36 Serum LDL/HDL-cholesterol among males in Kitava (black) and Sweden (grey). (Adapted from Reference 1051.)

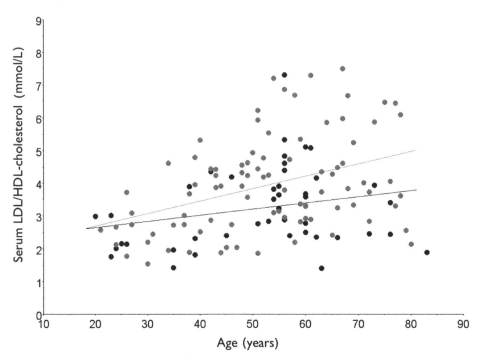

Figure 4.37   Serum LDL/HDL-cholesterol among females in Kitava (black) and Sweden (grey). (Adapted from Reference 1051.)

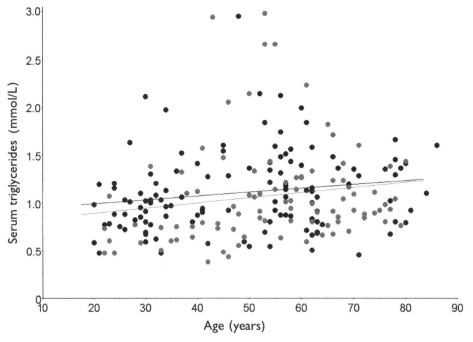

Figure 4.38   Serum triglycerides among males in Kitava (black) and Sweden (grey). (Adapted from Reference 1051.)

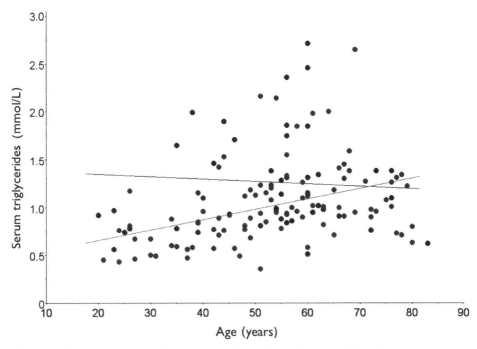

Figure 4.39 Serum triglycerides among males in Kitava (black) and Sweden (grey). (Adapted from Reference 1051.)

an increased ability to suppress cholesterol synthesis in the liver[731]. However, after urbanisation the serum cholesterol levels rose to 5.2 ± 1.2 mmol/L[380]. The usual hypothesis that this may be due to differences in physical activity is doubtful, since men traditionally stop acting as warriors around the age of 25, and later their wives do most of the daily work[1768].

HDL cholesterol

The effects of urbanisation on HDL cholesterol has barely been studied. In an international comparison of 14 countries, a significant negative correlation was

Table 4.14 Total cholesterol, serum HDL cholesterol and triglycerides among men and women aged 40–65 years, on Kitava and in Sweden (mmol/L; average ± standard deviation).

	Men		Women	
	Kitava (*n* = 58)	Sweden (*n* = 52)	Kitava (*n* = 28)	Sweden (*n* = 50)
Cholesterol	4.7 ± 0.9	5.9 ± 1.0	6.1 ± 1.3	6.4 ± 1.0
HDL	1.0 ± 0.2	1.1 ± 0.3	1.2 ± 0.2	1.2 ± 0.3
Triglycerides	1.2 ± 0.5	1.2 ± 0.6	1.3 ± 0.5	1.1 ± 0.4

Source: Adapted from Reference 1051.

seen between population means of HDL and prevalence of cardiovascular disease among men ($r = -0.57$)[1654]. The probable explanation was that the lifestyle-induced metabolic syndrome leads to low HDL[81]. Among women, the relationship was not statistically significant ($r = -24$), but data on this group were only available for 11 populations.

Risks with dyslipidaemia

High total cholesterol

Several observational studies have found that the risk of cardiovascular disease in both sexes increases gradually with rising cholesterol (Figure 4.40). Some studies are ecological studies[999], while most are prospective cohort studies in restricted Western populations[994]. A meta-analysis of 61 prospective cohort studies, mostly in Western Europe or North America, consisting of almost 900 000 healthy adults, found that 1 mmol/L lower total cholesterol was associated with about a half (hazard ratio 0.44; 95% CI 0.42–0.48), a third (0.66; 0.65–0.68), and a sixth (0.83; 0.81–0.85) lower ischaemic heart disease mortality at ages 40–49, 50–69, and 70–89 years, respectively, throughout the main range of cholesterol in most developed countries,

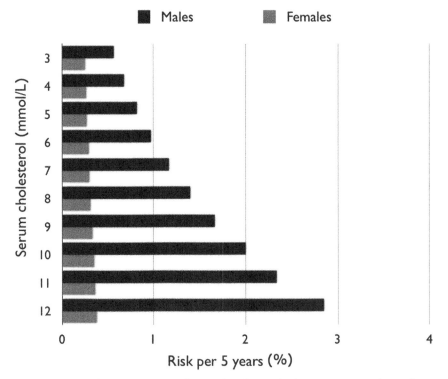

Figure 4.40   Risk of death due to cardiovascular disease in the next 5 years, depending on serum cholesterol among healthy non-smoking Westerners aged 50 and with systolic blood pressure 140 mm Hg (www.riskscore.org.uk).

with no apparent threshold. Even among the residents of Shanghai in the 1980s, where Western lifestyle customs were increasingly being adopted, but where the average cholesterol level was yet very low, the same relation was present[286].

High serum cholesterol is also a risk factor for developing atherosclerosis, both among humans[152,1484] and animals[71,1176,1183,1515,1730,1934]. An optimal cholesterol level is probably below 4 mmol/L (which, after age 40, is seen in only about 2% of Westerners and 20% of Kitavans). It has been well documented that atherosclerosis, even at an advanced stage, can be regressed in animals by means of normalising LDL levels[1118,1820]. There are strong indicators that the same is true for humans[1232,1360,1598,1701,1909].

Smoking, hypertension, abdominal obesity, left ventricular hypertrophy (enlargement of the left main chamber of the heart), glucose intolerance and diabetes are more serious if dyslipidaemia is also present, particularly among patients with known ischaemic heart disease.

Nevertheless, for most individuals, serum cholesterol is of limited value to predict the risk of becoming sick. This is particularly the case for women, as seen in Figure 4.40. Furthermore, as discussed above, there are examples of low-risk populations with clearly 'adverse' cholesterol levels. Therefore, the discussion about sick and healthy populations is also relevant here. Having a cholesterol level of 4.8 mmol/L may result in a highly variable risk for ischaemic heart disease, depending on whether the person is an American citizen[1707], a Chinese person in Shanghai[286], a person from Finland[902] or a resident of Kitava[1051].

A somewhat better indicator can be obtained by LDL cholesterol, apolipoproteins B and A1 (see below), the percentage of small, dense LDL particles and/or the amount of oxidized LDL[780,781].

Low HDL cholesterol

In Western populations, the incidence of myocardial infarction is negatively associated with HDL cholesterol in both sexes, i.e. the higher the HDL level, the better[1952]. The relationship is often clearest when total cholesterol level is below 5.2 mmol/L, such that people with 'good' overall cholesterol may be at much higher risk if HDL is low[10,1708]. The relationship appears to be particularly evident among women[1502], in whom it may also be more independent of total cholesterol than in men[10]. The same relationship between HDL and ischaemic heart disease can be seen among Japanese urban residents[917]. Furthermore, HDL is strongly negatively correlated with the degree of coronary atherosclerosis[1306,1528].

The concentration of HDL cholesterol reflects how efficiently cholesterol is transported out of the vascular wall and back to the liver[355]. This ability is largely hereditary. It is plausible, but speculative, that the low HDL levels, which characterise traditional populations, are due to a lower need to clear the vessel wall of undesired cholesterol.

For now, HDL should be considered a risk indicator similar to heredity or male sex, and there is very little support for the idea that an artificial increase of HDL can reduce the risk of future ischaemic heart disease, at least by using presently available medication[219].

Recently, there has been much discussion about the carrier proteins of LDL and HDL, apolipoproteins B100 and A1 or, for short, apoB and apoA1. It has been suggested that they are better predictors of cardiovascular disease than LDL and HDL but this is still open to debate[792,1893]. The issue is complicated by the fact that these factors are even less 'beneficial' in Kitava than LDL and HDL[1051]. In fact, the ratio of apoB to apoA1 is higher among men and women in Kitava than in Sweden.

High triglycerides

The significance of serum triglycerides on ischaemic heart disease is somewhat unclear. Levels above 2 mmol/L (after an overnight fast) have been shown in some studies to be an independent risk factor for ischaemic heart disease and stroke[92,1578,1763]. After considering the total cholesterol, HDL, abdominal size and blood pressure, which correlate with the triglycerides, the clinical significance appears to be limited, at least in men[92,1578]. Most patients with high triglycerides have abdominal obesity and/or hypertension[93]. Due to the strong variation from day to day, several samples are needed to correctly determine the risk of triglycerides, both before and after intervention. Moreover, the samples must be taken from fasting patients as opposed to total and HDL cholesterol. Furthermore, serum triglycerides increase with a diet that is low in fat and high in carbohydrates, even with one that is apparently healthy (see below) and from a high alcohol consumption, which further complicates the assessment. Measurement of triglycerides in the non-fasting state appear to be a stronger independent risk factor, particularly among women, but there are few studies as yet[108,1317].

Relevant dietary factors

Despite many years of research in the area, there is much uncertainty about the major explanations of the lower prevalence of dyslipidaemia in non-Western populations. *Saturated fat* and *trans-unsaturated fat* raise total and LDL cholesterol, but the effect is usually small and is sometimes outweighed by other, opposing factors[1210]. On average, a 0–4% drop in cholesterol can be expected with outpatient care (as opposed to being 'locked up' in a hospital or laboratory) using a diet from the US National Cholesterol Education Program (NCEP) Step One (total fat <30% of energy intake (E%), a P/S (polyunsaturated/saturated fat) ratio = 1; dietary cholesterol <300 mg/day and reduced energy intake to achieve desired weight.) A drop of 7–15% in total cholesterol can usually be achieved with diet according to step two of the NCEP program (total fat and saturated fat as in step one, P/S ratio 1.4 and dietary cholesterol <200 mg/day)[306]. There is wide individual variation, from no change up to 50% reduction in LDL cholesterol[1586].

Conventional wisdom also holds that a small improvement in blood lipid levels can be achieved from consuming foods that are rich in *soluble dietary fibre*[225].

In contrast, insoluble fibre from wheat bran apparently has no effect[2028]. The benefit of dietary fibre for people with typical Western cholesterol levels has been questioned by a research group who found no effect of soluble fibre from oat bran in a randomised controlled trial[285].

Plant sterols are probably more efficient, as shown in several studies[995,1323], and have also been shown to slow the proliferation of the atherosclerotic plaque in hamsters and rabbits[1327]. It is believed that the intake of plant sterols was often high during human evolution, since the content of plant sterols in corresponding modern plant foods is high[1324]. However, the risk of side effects (possibly including atherosclerosis!) should not be ignored[82,427,431,537,1304,1772,1976,1983] (see also Section 4.1). In my opinion, exclusive consumption of the same plant sterol day after day should be avoided.

A number of studies from David Jenkins research group have shown that ancestral-like *vegetarian diets* based on vegetables, fruits and nuts, but not wheat, can dramatically improve blood lipid levels, actually just as much as drug treatment with statins[822–825,827,828]. The total and LDL cholesterol have dropped on average by 25–30%, compared with a diet that followed US nutrition guidelines. Improvement of blood lipids were obtained even compared to a third, grain-based, lacto-vegetarian diet, suggesting that even whole grains may not be an optimal choice for lipid lowering. The HDL level has not dropped significantly from such diets, but the LDL/HDL ratio has improved.

In an observational study among eight people who lived for 2 years in Bio-sphere 2, Columbia University's environmental experiment (www.b2science.org/), and mainly fed themselves a plant-based low-calorie diet based on root vegetables and greens, and limited their intake of dairy products, meat, eggs and grains, serum cholesterol dropped from 4.7 ± 0.3 to 3.1 ± 0.1 mmol/L[1861]. For the first 16 months, the triglycerides remained stable at roughly 1.3 ± 0.2 mmol/L and then dropped to 0.7 ± 0.1 mmol/L.

Some studies indicate that *calorie restriction* per se lowers cholesterol synthesis in the liver, which leads to reduced circulating levels of total and LDL cholesterol[411,1466], unless cholesterol absorption in the gut is increased in a compensatory manner, as suggested by other studies[1574]. There are, to my knowledge, only two studies where LDL cholesterol among Westerners has been equivalent to the usual level among hunter-gatherers, and both of these has been with long-term strict caloric resitriction[529,1861]. However, in both cases, typical energy-dense Western foods were excluded. Thus, a reduction of food intake without a change in food choices is apparently not sufficient.

With regard to *meat*, it seems evident from the majority of intervention studies that high consumption of lean meat per se (including red meat) does not cause dyslipidaemia[79,304,374,782,887,896,1026,1293,1335,1605,1908]. Therefore, the above findings probably cannot be associated with a low meat consumption. Inversely, a high meat intake is not a prerequisite for low serum cholesterol.

A high *cholesterol intake* has a marginal elevating effect on serum cholesterol in humans, since most of our cholesterol is produced in the liver[303,758,1880]. Therefore, omission of the advice to avoid cholesterol-rich foods such as eggs, shellfish, fish and meat is long overdue. According to a meta-analysis, increasing the cholesterol intake by 100 mg/day should raise serum cholesterol as little as 0.056 mmol/L (95% CI 0.046–0.065)[1911]. If this amount of cholesterol is provided by lean meat (e.g. 60 g venison) as opposed to standard dairy products (e.g. 60 g 17% cheese), the net effect will be a reduction in serum cholesterol, since the cheese provides just over 10 times as much fat and 3 times as many calories.

The effect of *milk products* is complex. *Casein* raises total and LDL cholesterol as seen in some, but not all studies[51,670]. Most of the studies have compared casein with soya protein and in these studies the effect has been small. Two reviews of soya for cholesterol reduction in high-ranked journals state that available evidence does not confirm a clinically important effect, and that the effect appears trivial even at very high doses[409,1553] (dangerously high in my opinion). A recent study in rats found that soya peptides were no better than potato peptides compared with casein[1074], suggesting, again, that casein (which was given to the controls) is by no means neutral.

Diets that are high in *carbohydrate* (>65 E%) and low in fat (<25% E%) but where saturated fat dominates, such as on Kitava, result in slightly decreased LDL but also lower HDL cholesterol and increased triglyceride levels[931,1051]. Short-term studies on Westerners who modify their diet in the same way have achieved the same results[1209]. This effect of carbohydrate on triglycerides and HDL cholesterol is part of the rationale for modern low-carbohydrate diets such as the Atkins diet, and in recent randomised controlled trials, such benefits have usually been obtained by low- or very-low-carbohydrate diets, while LDL cholesterol has generally slightly increased, especially when saturated, rather unsaturated, fat intake has increased[371,446,572,724,1312,1321,1552,1628,1875].

Somewhat along the same line of thinking, a widespread contention is that fat intake should not be reduced too drastically, at least not in exchange for very high amounts of carbohydrate (>60 E%). A reduction of total fat intake below 25 E% does not lower LDL levels more than a moderately reduced fat intake, and the effects on triglycerides and HDL are a matter of concern[400,927,931,1209].

The more typical Palaeolithic diet, with a relatively high percentage of protein (20–30 E%) and a low glycaemic load, is expected to have a more beneficial effect on the triglycerides, than if the carbohydrate intake exceeds 60 E%[1331,1963]. Foods that attenuate insulin resistance can play a significant role in improving HDL and triglyceride levels[18,530], and possibly LDL cholesterol as well[1420]. The same may be true for an increased consumption of monounsaturated fat[623].

4.9   Heart failure

Heart failure is an increasingly common disease with reduced exercise capacity and premature death, usually among older individuals[1287]. The most common symptom is shortness of breath. The more advanced cases have a poor prognosis: 5 years after their first hospital stay for heart failure, only about 25% of patients are still alive, which makes the disease more harmful than most forms of cancer[1725]. Most types of cancer have a higher 5-year survival rate than heart failure, requiring hospital care[1193].

In its typical chronic form, the disease is caused by changes to the microscopic structure of the heart, with abnormal tissue growth (fibrosis) and/or excess growth of cardiac muscle cells; changes that are difficult to distinguish from normal ageing in Western countries[316,584,586,619,973,974]. The primary symptom of many prospective heart failure patients is enlargement of the heart (cardiac hypertrophy), particularly of the left chamber (left ventricular hypertrophy). The process supposedly starts early in life and progresses slowly over several decades.

The risk factors for heart failure are largely the same as for other cardiovascular diseases, but especially important ones include hypertension, obesity and type 2 diabetes[1187,1297,2029,2030] (see Table 4.15). Even a moderately elevated systolic blood pressure slightly above 145 mm Hg is associated with a clearly increased risk[1945]. Therefore, a lifestyle that keeps the blood pressure at biologically normal levels (below 130/80) can be expected to prevent heart failure. Body weight is also significant, with the apparent risk of heart failure increasing with being overweight[891,1427], and particularly with increased waistline[1298] or extreme obesity[1440]. Furthermore, high blood sugar is a risk factor for heart failure even in the absence of overt diabetes[710].

In addition to hypertension, atherosclerosis and ischaemic heart disease were traditionally seen as a major underlying cause of heart failure, but a recent shift of focus has drawn attention to metabolic disturbances at the cellular level[78,1287]. Thus, several studies now indicate that the basic structural and physiological changes behind the failing heart musculature are closely linked to insulin resistance and the metabolic syndrome[72,78,96,430,791,1081,1287,1378] and, hypothetically, lipotoxicity[11,520,1081,1180,1361,1638,1754,1837,1982]. Atherosclerosis and dilated cardiomyopathy, two major suspected causes of heart failure, are both hypothetically linked to lipotoxicity, which lends more weight to this line of thinking.

Prevalence studies

Heart failure among traditional people is largely unknown. In the Kitava study, we found no signs of clinical heart failure, but the population was too small to draw decisive conclusions. Other doctors in the area have not observed the disease (H. Jüptner and W. Schiefenhövel, personal communication). An ECG examination of 161 people, aged 20–86, showed no signs of left ventricular hypertrophy on Kitava[1050]. The normal, age-related, leftward deviation of the heart's electrical axis on the ECG among Westerners was missing[1041], similar to findings among the original inhabitants of New Guinea's highlands[1669]. A possible explanation is a lack of the gradual enlargement of the left ventricle that is seen as part of normal ageing in the West[404,584].

The prevalence of heart failure in developed countries is around 2% among the entire population and 6–10% of people older than 80 years[1135]. Latent, mild heart failure without subjective symptoms is seen in a significant portion of a normal Western population[97,1481].

Table 4.15 Approximate increase in risk of heart failure in various conditions[691,891].

	Risk increase (%)
Overweight	50
Obesity	100
Hypertension	50
Diabetes	100
Smoking	50
Ischaemic heart disease	700

Primary prevention

Foods that prevent or cause heart failure are expected to be similar to the ones associated with high blood pressure, type 2 diabetes, overweight, insulin resistance, atherosclerosis and ischaemic heart disease (see respective sections). Among related preventive factors, only reduced salt intake and weight loss are discussed below, due to a paucity of research in the area.

Salt restriction

Several animal experiments indicate that dietary salt is a contributing factor in the development of heart failure, and that this to some extent is independent of blood pressure[368,550,1008,1241,1470,1799,1994]. Salty food causes cardiac hypertrophy among rats, which was reversed after feeding a low-salt diet[497,1741].

In several epidemiological studies in humans, urinary sodium excretions (a measure of salt intake) correlate with the size of the heart[182,965,1031,1596]. In a Swedish study on patients with hypertension, heart size was not affected by mild salt restriction in combination with weight loss[505]. However, a more pronounced reduction in salt intake produced a clear effect on the size of the left ventricle in a similar study[853]. Further, regression of left ventricular hypertrophy was achieved in dialysis patients with the help of salt restriction[1368].

In the previously mentioned cohort study, NHANES-I, a gradually increased risk of heart failure was noted with rising salt consumption among roughly 5000 overweight American men and women, but it was not seen among those with normal weight (BMI <25)[692]. After adjusting for known cardiovascular risk factors, the relative risk for heart failure was 1.43 (95% CI 1.07–1.91) with a sodium intake of >114 mmol/day, compared with <50 mmol/day (these two groups represented the highest and lowest quartile of the population with regard to salt intake). An additional finding was that a high energy intake was associated with an increased risk of heart failure.

Calorie restriction

Obesity increases the risk of heart failure through various mechanisms[1427], but there are no studies specifically designed to assess the effect of weight loss on future risk of heart failure. However, a few studies have found improved heart function in various physiological tests (relevant to heart failure) after weight loss[34,381,1149,1407]. Two independent echocardiographic studies of healthy obese subjects found markedly improved myocardial performance index after weight loss[381,1149]. In the Swedish Obese Subjects Study of 4047 extremely obese individuals, there were 2 incident cases of heart failure in the bariatric surgery group and 5 in the control group during 10 years of follow-up[1673]. The difference is far from statistically significant, and an enormous amount of participants (in such good health) would be needed to clarify the issue in a proper randomised controlled trial.

Other factors

L-Carnitine contributes to the transport and oxidation of fatty acids in the muscle cells. A lack of carnitine has been discussed as a contributing cause of reduced muscle function in the case of heart failure[212,1865]. Carnitine can be supplied either from meat and fish or synthesised from the essential amino acids methionine and lysine. Since cereals are low in both of these amino acids, an excessive intake of cereals may contribute to a lack of carnitine[329,1179].

Secondary prevention

Once heart failure is established, the situation is very different, and some evidence actually suggests that both salt restriction and weight loss may be hazardous. Hence, early prevention seems prudent.

Salt intake

The conventional wisdom that people with diagnosed heart failure should restrict sodium intake to less than 130 mmol/day (<3 g/day sodium or <7.5 g/day sodium chloride)[784,2001] has lately been called into question. The traditional advice has been based on observational studies and physiological principles, while controlled trials have been lacking. In 2007, a randomised controlled trial was published, possibly the first of its kind[1397]. The study compared a 'normal' (120 mmol Na) with a low sodium diet (80 mmol Na) in 232 Italian patients with heart failure (88 women, 144 men). All were prescribed a very high dose of diuretic (furosemide 250–500 mg twice a day) and were advised to drink 1000 mL daily. Despite the rather modest sodium restriction, readmission due to worsening condition was more common in the low sodium group ($P < 0.05$), and levels of brain natriuretic peptide, a marker of heart failure, were higher in that group (685 ± 255 pg/mL compared to 425 ± 125 pg/mL; $P < 0.0001$). As the authors state, further studies are required to determine if the effect was due to the combination of a high dose diuretic and a low sodium diet, or if a low sodium diet is harmful in itself.

Regardless of the previously mentioned study, sodium restriction in heart failure requires careful supervision, especially in patients undergoing pharmaceutical treatment (which is virtually always the case). A restricted salt intake should be implemented in consultation with a physician or heart failure specialist nurse. It is highly recommended that reductions in salt intake are brought about gradually over a 2-week period or more in order to avoid adverse effects of a sudden imbalance in the renin–angiotensin system.

Fluid restriction

Patients with confirmed heart failure frequently experience thirst, which they themselves often attribute to the diuretic treatment. However, the thirst may be caused by heart failure itself and can sometimes even develop in the case of a high fluid intake. The patient should be cautioned about a drinking too much water and other fluids in particular if serum sodium tends to be low. The objective is to keep the weight stable after fluid retention is under control. Guidelines generally recommend 1–1.5, sometimes 2, litres of fluid per day but the evidence is uncertain.

Weight control

As already stated, overweight and increased waistline are ideally addressed before the first sign of heart failure. Once heart failure is present, weight loss has been associated with increased mortality in several observational studies[1425]. Heart failure patients are often more or less undernourished[265], and loss of muscle mass (sarcopenia) may contribute to further development of the disease[1637]. Traditional weight loss often leads to a loss of muscle mass, rather than reduced fat[103,504]. In the case of more severe heart failure, malnutrition often develops with wasting and general weight loss (cachexia). If the patient concurrently develops fluid retention (oedema), as a consequence of the failing heart, their net weight does not necessarily change. Underweight and cachexia have been shown to be an independent risk factors for serious complications among patients with chronic heart failure, in addition to impaired oxygen absorption, low ejection fraction (a measure of the heart's pumping strength) and pronounced shortness of breath[55,1878].

It is therefore a balancing act between beneficial and detrimental weight loss. In evaluating dietary changes, it can be helpful to carry out a whole-body measurement with dual-energy X-ray absorptiometry (DXA) or at least a bioimpedance analysis (BIA) before and after the diet change.

Conclusion

An ancestral-like diet that is rich in protein and minerals and low in salt, and which is based on lean meat, fish, vegetables and fruits, is probably beneficial in the prevention of heart failure. In the case of definite heart failure, the situation is more uncertain. One reason for trying a protein-rich diet is that it apparently reduces high levels of serum urate[403], a strong prognostic indicator of increased mortality among heart failure patients[54]. Another, even more hypothetical, argument is that such a diet may reverse leptin resistance and thereby restore nitroso-redox balance[1576]. Such restoration is thought to explain the remarkable results of the A-HeFT drug trial, where a combination of isosorbide dinitrate and hydralazine reduced total mortality by 43%, as compared with placebo, in African Americans with heart failure[587].

4.10   Dementia

Adult-onset dementia is traditionally divided into Alzheimer's disease and dementia associated with atherosclerosis, so-called vascular dementia (there are also other, less common forms). However, it has been claimed that the two conditions actually overlap one another, and that the previous division may sometimes be artificial[384]. Traditional cardiovascular risk factors increase the risk for dementia, such as glucose intolerance[323,1458,1977,1992], hypertension[906,1130,1663] and overweight[631,918]. The process probably begins quietly, early in a person's life, with subtle cognitive changes already in their 20s that can be a potential measure of the risk of developing Alzheimer's disease[1692].

One of the characteristics of Alzheimer's disease is the build-up of a certain type of amyloid (substance with a particular microscopic appearance), which many believe to be the primary cause of Alzheimer's[667,1896]. There are indications that these amyloid deposits can be reduced with improved blood lipids or increased insulin sensitivity[346,1426].

Drug treatment of high blood pressure has been found to slightly improve cognitive performance and memory, but not to benefit learning capacity[170]. Whether blood pressure lowering with the use of lifestyle is more efficient can only be speculated upon. A similar uncertainty relates to dyslipidaemia: some evidence suggests that statins are beneficial for future dementia, but randomised controlled trials in demented patients have been negative and primary preventive trials are lacking[1223,1604]. The opposite, an increased risk with statin treatment, has been claimed as well[1519]. Hence, it seems more sensible to prevent dementia through lifestyle changes[104].

Prevalence studies

There are no systematic studies of the occurrence of dementia in non-urbanised populations. We saw no sign of adult-onset dementia on the Trobriand Islands[1041]. We did not perform a systematic screening using scientifically acceptable methods, but we actively asked the residents of Kitava and parts of the Kiriwina and Kaileuna islands, which included a total of at least 6000 persons. Loss of comprehension during old age was categorically denied. The residents understood what we meant because there were two people on Kitava who had impaired cognitive ability since childhood. We met both of these individuals, aged 20–30 years, and with evident learning disability. All ages, even those who did not sign up for testing, otherwise demonstrated well-maintained cognitive skills.

Dementia is not a discrete disease. When an older person starts to lose their communication skills, their closest relatives tend to notice, particularly in this type of society. If adult-onset dementia had been nearly as common as in the West, this phenomenon would have been well known to residents. Many examples were given of other diseases that were described clearly, carefully and identically in different villages. The descriptions of unusual deaths even four generations ago were largely consistent across the community.

Hugh Trowell has described how a British psychiatrist who worked for a long time in East Africa in the 1930s reported that 'senile dementia was a notable absentee'[1812]. Trowell was a painstakingly careful person, which is why this information has a certain amount of weight to it.

In the West, senile dementia is a very common reason why older people have to receive institutional care, perhaps even the most common reason[1161]. In Sweden, roughly 2% of retirees sought nursing care due to dementia[53]. Impaired cognitive functioning without dementia is even more common[1373].

Relevant dietary factors

There is very little research regarding the significance of specific dietary factors for adult-onset dementia. It would seem logical that vascular dementia can be prevented because of the relationship between diet and atherosclerosis, and the fact that type 2 diabetes, glucose intolerance, insulin resistance and hypertension are related to dementia[323,906,1130,1458,1663,1977,1992]. None of these risk factors have been addressed in dietary clinical trials. However, one randomised controlled trial found that daily supplementation with 800 µg of folic acid (corresponding to 400 g of spinach) improved performance on tests that measure information-processing speed and memory, domains that are known to decline with age, in older adults with raised total homocysteine concentrations[451]. This suggests that foods rich in folate, such as vegetables and liver, are beneficial. Studies of other vitamins or minerals have not shown convincing results[1914].

Two observational studies have found an increased risk for impaired cognitive functioning with a high total or saturated fat intake, as well as a reduced risk with a high intake of fatty fish[866,1244,1245]. One additional study from the USA and one from Finland confirmed these findings, but only among carriers of a genetic marker for Alzheimer's disease, namely an absence of apolipoprotein E epsilon4[972,1089]. Grant noted that the prevalence of Alzheimer's in 11 different countries was strongly and positively associated with total fat intake and, again, negatively with fish intake[612]. As usual with observational studies, there is a potential problem with confounders, and it is uncertain how large a role is played by fat or energy intake, since a high fat intake covaries with a low intake of fruits and vegetables (and other healthy lifestyle choices).

4.11   Cancer

Observational studies suggest that existing differences in dietary habits explain about 30% of the variation in risk of cancer in Western countries[899]. In addition, the incidence of some forms of cancer show such marked variation worldwide that the preventive potential is probably even larger[1391]. Furthermore, the most prevalent cancers show considerable covariation: in the years around 1980, two-thirds of the tenfold variation of prostate cancer incidence worldwide was explained by breast cancer incidence and 40% by colon cancer incidence[1084].

Prevalence studies

The occurrence of cancer and other malignant diseases among traditional people has only been studied sporadically. A low cancer incidence was reported among the hunter-gatherers in the Amazon[126], Malaysia[1430] and the Arctic[439,1588]. David Livingstone, who conducted research throughout large parts of Africa in the nineteenth century, felt that cancer was a 'disease of civilisation'[727]. This opinion was also shared by Trowell, who, after many years' work as a doctor in Uganda in the mid-1900s, carefully documented the occurrence of non-infectious diseases among the native population[1812].

The current incidence of cancer varies widely throughout developing and developed countries. The incidence of colorectal cancer (cancer of colon or rectum) varies up to 25-fold between countries with the highest rates (USA, Australia and New Zealand, and parts of Europe) and those with the lowest rates (Africa and Asia)[7]. Women who immigrate from countries with a low risk of breast cancer to countries with a high risk of the disease often increase their own risk after a period of time, and their daughters have an even higher risk level[7].

The residents of Kitava were not familiar with malignant cachexia, i.e. long-term emaciation that lasts months or years and ends in death. However, slow-growing, visible tumours could be described as an extremely rare occurrence. One older man passed away after having had a sore on his lower leg for several months that never healed. It probably involved tropical phagedenic ulcer, an infectious necrotizing ulcer of the skin and underlying tissues that is easily cured with penicillin, but otherwise becomes chronic and often develops into squamous cell carcinoma[1095,1219]. All middle-aged residents and senior citizens were familiar with the case, and it was described identically by respondents across the island[2007].

A 67-year-old man showed a hard, rough tumour on his mouth palate with the typical signs of oral cancer. Like the overwhelming majority of residents, he was a regular betel chewer but did not smoke. Oral cancer is a common form of cancer in this part of the world[89,712,1894]. It is well known that betel quid chewing is an important factor for oral cancer due to the strongly alkaline environment that develops in the mouth by adding slacked lime (from heated coral) to the betel quid[204,1107,1269,1309,1454,1636,1726,1746,1787]. In betel chewing, a common practice in large parts of Asia and Oceania, the areca nut (*Areca catechu*) is chewed together with leaves or seed mixture from the betel tree (*Piper chavica betel*) and a pinch of slaked lime.

A couple of people knew about an old woman a few generations back who had a tumour in the breast and passed away after a time. Jüptner observed a case of breast cancer in a pregnant woman on Kiriwina in the early 1960s (H. Jüptner, personal communication). Her relatives refused to let her be operated on, and she died less than 1 year after childbirth. Up until the 1980s, women regularly went topless, which provided good observation opportunities.

Jüptner was originally a gynaecologist and obstetrician. During his five years as a doctor on the Trobriand Islands with its 12 000 inhabitants (in 1990 there were roughly 25 000), he diagnosed 10–15 cases of ovarian cancer, which is a higher incidence than in the rest of Papua New Guinea ($P < 0.02$)[1231] or in the USA ($P < 0.008$)[709].

Jüptner found no cases of cervical cancer (the most common gynaecological cancer in Papua New Guinea[1231]) and no other malignancies, but he performed very few autopsies. He saw no cases of Burkitt's lymphoma, which is not uncommon in other coastal regions with widespread malaria[712].

Stanhope published an article in a journal with a summary of cancer deaths on Kiriwina based on the work of four different Australian doctors during the 1960s[1712]. Of the 139 deaths (10 470 person-years), three to six were determined to be caused by cancer: one tongue cancer, two unclear but histopathologically (microscopically) confirmed cases of cancer, one possible stomach cancer, one possible lung cancer and one possible thyroid cancer.

Even if the overall picture is somewhat unclear, it seems that the Trobriand Islanders have a low incidence of superficial malignancies (cancers of the skin/throat apart from the oral cavity, malignant lymphoma, superficial lymph node metastases, breast cancer), obstructive (constrictive) or otherwise expansive cancer in the abdomen/pelvis (cancer in the gastrointestinal tract, liver and uterus) and cancer in the urinary tract or prostate.

Prehistoric skeletal remains

In contrast to the diseases discussed in previous chapters, skeletal cancer is traceable in bone remains from our ancestors. However, estimates of the true occurrence of cancer among prehistoric hunter-gatherers on this basis are fraught with great inaccuracy. Uncertain diagnostic tools, unclear age estimates, lack of standardisation, too few individuals, non-representative selection, changes that occurred after death (diagenesis) as well as incomplete knowledge of the lifestyle of the population under examination are the greatest concerns[800,856,1732].

Nevertheless, it is possible to draw inferences. Within the field of palaeopathology (the study of prehistoric diseases) there is wide agreement that metastasising cancers are uncommon in the preagricultural skeletal remains[257,307,312,648,800,1512,1539,1910]. However, malignant tumours originating in the skeleton (e.g. myeloma and sarcoma), which are uncommon in all modern populations, were occasionally un-covered. As with modern Westerners, myeloma is the most common of these. Thus, in preagricultural humans, primary bone malignanices seem to have been more common than cancers metastasising to bone. In contrast, in the Western world, at least 98% of people with malignant bone tumours have metastatic cancer. This dis-similarity adds to the evidence that the most common cancers of modern societies are largely preventable.

Relevant dietary factors

There is currently broad consensus that diet affects the occurrence or growth of cancer, or both, but there is only fragmentary good knowledge regarding which specific foods increase or decrease the risk[7,899]. Many experts advocate a high intake of fruits and vegetables, although the results of epidemiological studies have been varied. For low-fat, high-fibre diets, there is less convincing evidence in cancer prevention. Vegetarianism does not seem to lower the risk of death from cancers[900], suggesting that meat is not a major culprit.

In 2007, the World Cancer Research Fund (WCRF) and the American Institute of Cancer Research (AICR) published a review by an international panel of experts on the connection between diet and cancer, including factors that are indirectly influenced by nutrition such as weight and stature[7]. Considerable emphasis was put on observational studies, while randomised controlled trials were sometimes neglected. In Table 4.16, which lists the diet-related factors for which the panel thought there was convincing evidence of a cancer connection, overweight emerges as a major culprit. However, although overweight increases the risk of several cancers, most cases are evidently not convincingly explained by this or other factors. Thus, most of the many-fold higher incidences of cancer in the Western world are not explained. All Westerners are high-risk individuals, and the additional risk from being overweight or obese instead of lean is typically rather small.

Breast cancer

Overweight and weight gain in adulthood has been found to increase the risk of postmenopausal breast cancer, the most common cancer in women in the Western world[7,23,479,658,677]. Nineteen out of 24 cohort studies have shown increased risk with increased body fatness, which was statistically significant in seven[7]. On aver-age, an estimated 3% (95% CI 1–4) increase in risk per two units increase in BMI was found. The associations with BMI and adult weight change seem to be stronger both for aggressive and for hormone receptor-positive cancers[23]. Available cohort studies also show increased risk of postmenopausal breast cancer with increased waist circumference, which was statistically significant in two out of eight studies[7]. Meta-analysis was possible on four studies, giving an estimated 5% increase in risk (95% CI 0–10) per 8 cm increase in waist circumference.

Table 4.16 Diet-related factors which, according to the World Cancer Research Fund and the American Institute for Cancer Research, are convincingly related to the risk of developing cancer[7].

Form of cancer	Decreases risk	Increases risk
Breast	Lactation	Alcoholic drinks
		Body fatness[a]
		Adult attained height[b]
Colon, rectum	Physical activity	Body fatness[a]
		Abdominal obesity
		Adult attained height
		Red meat[c]
		Processed meat[d]
		Alcoholic drinks
Pancreas	–	Body fatness[a]
Kidney	–	Body fatness[a]
Endometrium	–	Body fatness[a]
Oesophagus	–	Alcoholic drinks
		Body fatness[a]
Oral cavity, throat	–	Alcohol
Liver	–	Aflatoxins
Lung	–	Arsenic in drinking water
		β-carotene supplements[e]
Nasopharynx	–	–
Stomach	–	–
Gallbladder	–	–
Ovary	–	–
Cervix	–	–
Prostate	–	–
Bladder	–	–
Skin	–	–
Other	–	–

[a]No defined lower limit.
[b]Convincing for postmenopausal (and probable for premenopausal) breast cancer.
[c]The term 'red meat' refers to beef, pork, lamb and goat from domesticated animals.
[d]The term 'processed meat' refers to meats preserved by smoking, curing, or salting, or addition of chemical preservatives.
[e]The evidence is derived from studies using high-dose supplements (20 mg/day for β-carotene; 25 000 IU/day for retinol) in smokers.

The WCRF/AICR panel also found convincing evidence that breast cancer incidence is increased by factors that generate a rapid growth in height and increased stature[7]. Both of these are related to early puberty, which was also pointed out by the panel. One possible mechanism is excessive tissue growth due to hyperinsulinaemia or insulin resistance (see Section 4.6).

Although not mentioned by the panel, casein has been shown in rat experiments both to cause insulin resistance[377,993,1808] and to accelerate the growth of breast cancer compared with whey[644] or soya protein[683]. The results of epidemiological studies in humans have been contradictory with regard to dairy consumption[1237].

Total fat intake is strongly associated with breast cancer in worldwide comparisons[269], but within separate Western populations the association is small or non-existent[202,249,1651,1689], and an 8-year dietary intervention program including a low-fat diet (the Women's Health Initiative Dietary Modification Trial) did not significantly prevent breast cancer[1447]. The non-significant 9% decrease ($P = 0.07$) was more likely due to caloric restriction and increased intake of fruits and vegetables. Hence, it seems more important to focus on body fat than on dietary fat[1689].

Colorectal cancer

There is increasing evidence that points to a connection between insulin resistance and colorectal cancer (see Section 4.6)[313,630,1597,1805] and most cohort studies support a gradually increased risk with increasing BMI[7], and in particular with increasing waistline[362,626,840,1851].

The role of meat has been discussed for many years. Based on observational studies, the WCRF/AICR panel found convincing evidence that red meats (from domesticated animals) and processed meats are a cause of colorectal cancer. The proposed causative compounds are substances formed on cooking at high temperature (polycyclic aromatic hydrocarbons and heterocyclic amines), processing (nitrates and nitrites) or during intestinal metabolism (N-nitroso compounds)[7]. However, no adverse association has been found for poultry or fish[281,1090,1315], despite that these provide the same compounds[884,1675]. With regard to polycyclic aromatic hydrocarbons, the contribution from cereals is actually larger than from meat, although the levels are lower than in meat, in particular grilled meat[7]. As for nitrate, vegetables account for 70–97% of the intake in high-income countries[7]. All this may indicate the presence of confounders (e.g. health-conscious people tending to avoid foods conceived as harmful), or that other factors than red meat are more important at the population level. Between 1963 and 1998 in the UK, when the intake of red meat decreased by 25%, the incidence of colorectal cancer *increased* by 64%[729]. Furthermore, vegetarians do not have a lower risk of colorectal cancer death than omnivores[900].

There is no randomised controlled trial specifically addressing meat, but in the very large Women's Health Initiative Dietary Modification Trial, the intervention group decreased their intake of red meat by 10%, whereas the control group increased their intake by 10% (mean difference 20%; 95% CI 15–25). Despite this marked difference, there was no effect on colorectal adenomas or cancers during 8 years[153].

Contrary to common belief, and to the judgement of the WCRF/AICR panel, cereal fibre probably does not prevent colorectal cancer. Six randomised controlled trials[32,193,802,1106,1188,1590], the three largest ones published in 2000, and a meta-analysis of these studies[75] have now convincingly refuted this idea. All six trials evaluated the effect on the recurrence of colorectal adenomas, benign tumours from which most colorectal cancers arise, in people already diagnosed with adenoma. There was no overall effect of dietary fibre on incidence or recurrence of adenomas, although one study found an *adverse* effect on adenoma recurrence of soluble fibre (ispaghula husk)[193], and another one found a significant *increase* in the number of large adenomas after 4 years of wheat bran supplementation[802]. Even more worrying were the results from the two trials that were large enough to study true cancer incidence, which, as a matter of fact, was higher in the fibre supplemented group: 17 out of 1426 subjects were diagnosed with colorectal cancer in the fibre group as compared to 6 out of 1370 control subjects (relative risk 2.7; 95% CI 1.1–6.9; $P = 0.04$)[32,1590]. Observational studies do not support an important effect[7,1314,1851,1886], and the risk of confounding is considerable[1222,1388], partly because of the long-held notion that whole-grain foods are healthful[1936].

It is quite remarkable that none of the randomised controlled trials, which were published in the *New England Journal of Medicine* (two studies), the *Lancet* (one study) and other high-ranked journals, is cited in the WCRF/AICR report.

Prostate cancer

As discussed in Section 4.6, individuals with insulin resistance or the metabolic syndrome have an increased risk for prostate cancer[657] as well as a worse prognosis[656]. From an international perspective, the incidence of both prostate cancer and breast cancer varies many-fold and they covary by almost 20% ($R^2 = 0.18$; $P = 0.03$; adapted from [1392]). These two forms of cancer are also the ones that specifically affect the domestic dog, an animal which easily develops insulin resistance[309,907].

Among American physicians, high milk consumption is associated with increased risk of prostate cancer[280], and other cohort studies have generally found similar results[7]. In an international comparison of 65–74-year-old men in 41 countries, 73% of the mortality from prostate cancer was attributed to the non-fat portion of milk, i.e. milk proteins and lactose[610]. Similarly, the US Multi-ethnic Cohort study found low-/non-fat milk to be related to an increased risk and whole milk to a decreased risk of prostate cancer[1387]. Another American cohort study found that skim milk, but not other dairy foods, was associated with increased risk of advanced prostate cancer[1389].

Since 1996, there has been some hope that antioxidant supplementation with selenium and vitamins E and C could prevent prostate cancer, but recent large-scale randomised trials have put an end to this hope[564,575,1060]. Thus, lifestyle confounders probably explain the associations found in earlier cohort studies[564].

Diet in established cancer

Research about the optimal diet for people with cancer is scarce[7]. One study found that in patients with stage III *colon cancer* (spread to nearby lymph nodes but not to other parts of the body) treated with surgery and chemotherapy, a more 'Western' dietary pattern was associated with a higher risk of cancer recurrence and early death[1218]. However, there is no particular type of diet that can currently be recommended to hinder growth or metastasis of cancer[437]. On the other hand, there are also no known contraindications against a high intake of meat, fish, vegetables, fruits and nuts.

One study found that women with resected, early-stage *breast cancer* who were randomly assigned a very low-fat diet had a lower relapse rate during the first 7 years of follow-up[294]. They also lowered their energy intake more than the control group, and they lost 2.7 kg more than the control subjects ($P = 0.005$). However, only women with oestrogen receptor-negative cancers seemed to benefit.

Some people have the impression that it is not bad to be slightly overweight when affected by *any cancer*. This idea essentially lacks scientific support and is possibly based on the simple fact that people with advanced cancer often become wasted and emaciated. Although underweight may impose a risk, in particular in the case of malnutrition, overweight patients with recently diagnosed cancer do not have a better prognosis. Rather, much evidence indicates that being overweight increases the risk for recurrence and reduces the likelihood of survival[437]. Thus, among 14 709 French women with breast cancer, the risk of death increased by 32% among the overweight (95% CI 22–42) and by 53% among the obese (95% CI 37–72), compared to women with BMI below 25[1114]. In addition, obese patients had an increased risk of developing gynaecological or gastrointestinal cancer. An earlier meta-analysis found a mean 56% increase in mortality among obese women with breast cancer[1550]. Similarly, obese patients have poorer prognosis in prostate[545,656], colorectal[424] and renal cancer[49].

Soya products cannot be recommended, particularly not for women being treated for *breast cancer* with tamoxifen, since the tumour-inhibiting effect seems to be counteracted by genistein[447,846,852]. Genistein, the dominant phytoestrogen in soya bean, potentially stimulates the growth of oestrogen-dependent breast cancers by acting as a so-called promoter that accelerates the progress of existing breast cancer[42,321,1464,1622,1803]. The idea that soya consumption would explain the relatively low risk of breast cancer in women living in Japan is open for debate[730]. There are all sorts of reasons why breast cancer could have been less common in Japan than in Europe and North America. On these grounds, the former enthusiasm for soya has lately turned into caution[447,1445].

While irrelevant to most readers, the use of yam (*Dioscorea batatas*) as a staple food may also not be advisable for women with *ovarian cancer*. A high intake of yam could likely result in a high uptake of diosgenin, an endocrine disruptor with contraceptive properties[6,64,148,1976]. Speculatively, this could explain the seemingly high rate of ovarian cancer in the Trobriand Islands.

Future research

Even the most radical sceptic would have to agree that ancestral diets need to be tested in relevant animal cancer models. The foods that an animal eats in its natural environment should be studied to see if they have any effect on the occurrence and progression of cancer, as compared to the standard feeds given today. Any species-specific differences that may exist in terms of cancer should also be studied in this light.

The attention around diet and cancer has probably been too concentrated on substances that can initiate (start) cancer (e.g. mutagens from grilled foods and polycyclic aromatic hydrocarbons). Exposure to natural pesticides (chemical agents) has always been high among plant eaters. Indeed, the exposure to natural pesticides among modern humans is estimated to be several thousand times higher than exposure to synthetic pesticides. The total intake was even higher during the Palaeolithic era than it is today, but on the other hand, it was spread across a larger number of substances through a significantly wider selection of plant species and varieties. Besides being exposed to carcinogenic substances in the diet, humans have always been exposed to endogenous carcinogenic substances, i.e. those that are produced by the body, as well as by ionisation and ultraviolet radiation. 'Nature is not benign,' as Ames, the father of the commonly used Ames' test for carcinogenicity, stated[48].

Some of the focus should be shifted to the processes that are part of the body's defence system against premature cancer and metastasis[1189], systems that have been developed and refined over hundreds of millions of years in a finely tuned balance with the available foods. Cancer develops slowly before symptoms develop, and many of the steps along the way could be affected by diet.

4.12 Osteoporosis

The global burden of osteoporosis is heavy, and even more so in European countries[356,836]. The highest prevalence is seen in Scandinavian countries[356]. In her lifetime, every second Swedish woman will break one or more bones due to osteoporosis. This gigantic public health problem is not always described in a relevant or clear way, especially when it comes to the lifestyle changes involved. You sometimes get the impression that long daily walks and a high calcium intake will solve most of the problem, but this is not true. The effect of each of these interventions has been small in randomised controlled trials, and they are not expected to have a major impact on the average woman's fracture risk[888,1762,1957]. It seems obvious that other lifestyle factors are present. Again, an evolutionary perspective may be able to provide us with important insights.

Osteoporosis is characterised by bones with low density, disturbed microarchitecture and poor strength[1467]. Bone density, the percentage of bone tissue in relation to the surrounding tissue, can be measured with a bone densitometer (primarily DXA). The increased risk of fracture with low bone density is comparable to the increased risk for stroke in relation to blood pressure, but it is higher than the increased risk for myocardial infarction in relation to serum cholesterol[1150,1320] (see Table 4.17). Other validated modifiable risk factors are, according to a 2003 report from the Swedish Council on Technology Assessment in Health Care (a national body for evidence based medicine): physical inactivity, underweight, low sun exposure, propensity to fall, smoking, high alcohol consumption, impaired sight and long-term oral cortisone treatment (www.sbu.se: search osteoporosis). The

Table 4.17 Probability of 10-year risk of hip fracture according to bone density categories (*T* scores, assessed with dual-energy X-ray absorptiometry) in 70-year-old Australian women with or without prior fracture (not due to major trauma)[1295].

T scores	Prior fracture	No prior fracture
1	1.0	0.4
0	2.3	0.7
−1	5.3	1.7
−1.5	7.9	2.5
−2	11.8	3.8
−2.5	17.4	5.7
−3	25.2	8.6

Note: The *T* score is the number of standard deviations above or below the mean for a healthy young adult of the same sex and from the same population. A *T* score of −2.5 or less is classified as osteoporosis in case of prior fracture and as osteopenia in case of no prior fracture.

well-documented, non-modifiable risk factors are high age, earlier fracture, female sex, early menopause, genetics and ethnicity. Tall stature is included in the latter group, although it may to some extent be modifiable, as discussed in Section 4.6.

Skeletal strength can be good even in the event of low bone density[719]. As for any material, other qualities like elasticity can be crucial for optimal durability. The strength can only be measured by subjecting a section of the skeleton to various degrees of stress until it cracks, a procedure which is obviously difficult in living subjects. Therefore, osteoporosis is a rather elusive disorder, as shown in one study where 54% of women with hip fracture had not been osteoporotic at DXA screening 5 years earlier[1885].

Prevalence studies

There are very few studies of the occurrence of osteoporosis and bone fractures among aboriginal populations and none at all for hunter-gatherers. Despite an equally low or lower bone density and often a lower calcium intake than in the West, existing data suggest that hip fractures are uncommon among non-urbanised, ethnic populations[17,120,186,1446,1607,1697].

We have unpublished data indicating that osteoporotic fractures are rare or absent in the Trobriand Islands, Papua New Guinea, and that this cannot be explained by high bone density, as measured with DXA on the forearms (P. Johansson, O. Johnell, W. Schiefenhövel, C. Wong and S. Lindeberg, unpublished data). A review of 4310 diaries in a clinic in Losuia, Kiriwina from December 1995 to October 1999, showed that all fractures were attributable to a powerful force, such as a fall from a coconut tree, assault or similar incidents. Our findings are consistent with the records of Jüptner and Schiefenhövel (personal communications), medical doctors with extensive experience from the islands.

The entire population of Kitava above the age of 60 was filmed from the side while standing, where a lack of thoracic kyphosis (exaggerated forward bending of the upper thoracic spine) was noted (S. Lindeberg, unpublished data). This condition is very common among older Westerners[680]. Even if thoracic kyphosis may have other causes than osteoporosis[1755], these findings provide further evidence that osteoporotic fractures are uncommon on the Trobriand Islands.

Barss noted a strikingly low incidence of hip fractures in Milne Bay province, the district with 135 000 inhabitants which includes the Trobriand Islands[120]. During his four years of service, he diagnosed three hip fractures in persons of Australian descent but none in the domestic population, which made up the overwhelming majority of patients. He saw many older persons, but no hip fractures and just a few distal radius fractures. Other types of fractures associated with accidents were relatively common.

However, if traditional populations have been relatively free of low-trauma fractures, Eskimos apparently constitute an exception. X-rays and several studies measuring bone density show that Eskimos in northern Alaska and Canada (Inuit and Yupik) during the end of the 1960s and beginning of the 1970s often suffered from osteoporosis[671,1167,1168,1402]. The bone density was generally low compared with white populations. Compared with Westerners, age-related bone loss started earlier in life and was more pronounced. At this time in history, however, their lifestyle began to be affected by Western eating habits with sugar and grains, as well as the start of modern, Western diseases[439,1059,1136,1138,1520,1643].

Across developed and developing countries, a clear variation in the incidence of hip fractures has been noted. In one international comparison, the risk of hip fracture was roughly 28 times higher in Sweden than in Turkey[870]. The probability that a 50-year-old woman today will suffer from a hip fracture at least once in their life is 28.5% in Sweden versus 1% in Turkey. (For any fracture and all ages, the risk is 50% among Swedish women.) Countries can be divided into the categories of very high risk for hip fracture (Norway, Iceland, Sweden, Denmark, USA), high risk (Taiwan, Germany, Switzerland, Finland, Greece, Canada, Holland, Hungary, Singapore, Italy, Great Britain, Kuwait, Australia, Portugal), medium risk (Hong Kong, France, Japan, Spain, Argentina, China) and low risk (Turkey, Korea, Venezuela, Chile). Much of this worldwide variation of hip fracture rates is explained by latitude[835], underscoring the preventive effect of sunlight and vitamin D as discussed below.

The worldwide pattern of vertebral fractures is similar to that of hip fractures, but not identical[836]. For instance, Japanese women have, compared to American women, a higher risk of vertebral fractures and a more pronounced lack of trabecular bone, a loss that also starts earlier in life[807]. During the second half of the twentieth century, the incidence of vertebral fractures declined in Japan, while it increased in the West.

Prehistoric skeletal remains

Fractures

Despite a large number of documented fractures in fossilised bones from Palaeolithic hunter-gatherers, osteoporotic fractures are considered to be rare in prehistoric skeletons south of the Arctic circle[19,1512,1910]. This conclusion is based on the overall picture of the location and type of the fractures, robustness of the bone and the available knowledge of the lifestyle. For example, fractures of the hip and the distal forearm are virtually non-existent. However, due to uncertain age estimates of the skeletal specimens and a limited number of skeletons, proper comparisons with modern populations are impossible.

A well-healed compound fracture of the neck of the femur was noted in a pre-historic hunter-gatherer in Australia[1910]. The bone was strikingly robust and was considered to originate from a man. Mild trauma fracture was deemed improbable, rather it was more likely that he jumped or fell from a great height. A distal ulnar fracture resulting from fending off a blow from a stick, for example, is the single most common fracture[1288,1512,1910]. This type of fracture dominates those adults currently living on the Trobriand Islands, in particular women (P. Johansson, un-published data).

In skeletons from Eskimos, vertebral compression fractures seem to be overrepre-sented, which has been attributed to reckless rides on Komitaks, a type of flat sleigh without bumpers[1212]. Vertebral compression fractures were noted in 36 of 80 adult Eskimos in his material. In a study of the Aleuts, a population closely related to the Eskimos, the prevalence was 22%[1984]. This can be compared with a prevalence of 25.3% (95% CI 22.3–28.2) among current American women over the age of 50[326]. The incidence of clinically diagnosed vertebral fractures, as opposed to those found at radiological screening, among women in the same population was 5.3 per 1000 person-years.

Bone density

Determining the bone density in skeletons that have been buried in the ground for long periods of time is associated with serious methodological difficulties[1512,1544]. Some authorities consider it almost impossible to determine the porosity, density and mineralisation of prehistoric bones[811]. Others, however, feel that there is sup-port for the idea that Palaeolithic populations had more robust skeletons than early farmers, not just due to the higher bone density, but also because of a more favourable structure[19,462,1544]. The idea was that increased axial strength in the long bones was achieved with a more oval and less rounded cross section, and with the higher percentage of trabecular bone tissue at the expense of cortical bone.

One osteological study compared forearm bone density in two groups of prehis-toric North American hunter-gatherers, one of which supplemented hunting and gathering with farming[1412]. He determined that the age-related loss of trabecular bone was greater in the latter group and that the farming hunter-gatherers did not distinguish themselves from Westerners. However, such comparisons over time are not reliable because of diagenesis (effects of the soil on the skeleton).

Osteological studies of prehistoric Eskimos, with given reservations, provide a consistent picture of a higher occurrence of osteoporosis than in modern West-ern populations[991,1166,1506,1789]. The general impression is that peak bone mass is achieved at a young age, similar to Westerners, but that the loss of bone after the age of 50 is more pronounced. Harper found evidence of a geographic gradient, with thicker, more compact (the outer layer) long bones among the oldest aboriginal Eskimos around the Bering Sea[671]. The bone thickness declines, the further east and south-east one travels along Canada's north coast to Greenland.

Relevant dietary factors

The effect of a Palaeolithic diet on skeletal strength is an open question. Strictly speaking, the same is true for other dietary models, partly because of the low relative impact of known dietary factors[1077]. Bone fragility can increase through a variety of disturbances, as already mentioned, but many questions remain unanswered. The risk for osteoporotic fractures increases with underweight, low sun exposure, calcium deficiency, physical inactivity, smoking and high alcohol consumption. Calcium deficiencies can develop from a low intake of calcium, low calcium bioavailability or elevated calcium excretion by the kidneys. If people of the Northern Hemisphere would remove dairy products from its position as the primary source of dietary calcium, many experts are concerned that osteoporotic fractures will increase even more than today. However, the risk may be lower than anticipated, as discussed below.

Vitamin D

Vitamin D facilitates calcium absorption in the intestines. It is not strictly a vitamin since all the required amount can be met by sunlight exposure which converts inactive precursors in the skin to the active form of vitamin D[1965]. However, modern humans spend much time indoors and roughly one quarter (25%) of the required amount of vitamin D is now supplied from food (mainly fish, meat and milk).

Much evidence indicates that vitamin D deficiency is common among Westerners, especially in elderly people, where the primary cause involves the long periods of time spent indoors[1080,1197,1199,1786,1853]. Vegans are also at risk, partly because vegetables do not contain vitamin D[984,1134,1215]. However, although it is widely accepted that vitamin D status is determined by the measurement of the circulating concentration of 25-hydroxyvitamin D, the cut-off value to define low vitamin D status remains controversial[379,1061,1965]. There is also a remarkable paradox in that extensive sun exposure in several studies does not suffice to raise serum 25-hydroxyvitamin D above the accepted cut-off levels[167,814,2000,2031]. Hence, other factors could hypothetically increase our need for vitamin D, possibly by way of vitamin D receptor resistance. Obese people are characterised by lower plasma levels of 25-hydroxyvitamin D[937,1691,1970], which is apparently not explained by reduced sun exposure[672]. In some, but not all studies, vitamin D status has improved after weight loss[1491]. These findings could imply that an unhealthy Western lifestyle increases vitamin D requirements.

During the Palaeolithic era, there was probably no need for dietary vitamin D due to the large amounts of time spent outdoors. However, north of the polar circle, the winter sun is so low in the horizon that the process of converting vitamin D may have been insufficient. This could partly explain the high prevalence of vertebral fractures among the Eskimos, as outlined above. Even today, people at northern latitudes, such as Scandinavians, have a markedly increased risk of hip fractures[835].

Unfortunately, vitamin D supplementation has a marginal effect, at least in elderly people. In a Cochrane review of randomised placebo-controlled trials in older people, vitamin D alone (without calcium or other additional supplements) showed no effect whatsoever on hip fracture (7 trials, 18 668 participants; relative risk 1.17; 95% CI 0.98–1.41) or vertebral fracture (4 trials, 5698 participants; relative risk 1.13; 95% CI 0.50–2.55)[94]. Another meta-analysis did not find vitamin D to add any benefit on top of calcium supplementation[1762]. However, in people with low vitamin D serum concentration (25-OH-vitamin D_3 <25 nmol/L), a tendency for greater risk reduction of fracture was seen (relative risk for fracture 0.86 vs 0.94; $P = 0.06$). In addition, the dose of vitamin D was low in most trials, and the preventive effect was better ($P = 0.03$) in the high-dose trials (at least 800 IU/day; relative risk 0.84; 95% CI 0.75–0.94) than in the low-dose trials (less than 400 IU/day; relative risk 0.87; 95% CI 0.71–1.05). Other studies also indicate that the dose of vitamin D should be at least 800 IU/day[171]. Another meta-analysis of randomised controlled trials came to a slightly different conclusion: combining vitamin D with calcium is more important than increasing the dose of vitamin D above 800 IU/day[199]. In that study, vitamin D reduced the risk of hip fractures only when calcium supplementation was added.

In summary, taking extra vitamin D late in life seems to have little effect on bone strength in most people, and the risk of side effects is not negligible, in particular hypercalcaemia[94]. Preferably, we should spend much time outdoors throughout life.

Calcium intake

In elderly Western women, calcium supplementation alone (i.e. without vitamin D) probably prevents fractures, in particular fractures of the hip and backbone. In contrast, fractures of the lower arm, the most common type of fracture, are apparently not prevented. In a meta-analysis of 17 placebo-controlled trials in men and women ($n = 52\,625$), calcium treatment alone was associated with a 10% risk reduction in fractures of all types combined (95% CI 0–20)[1762]. Some of the lack of effect appears to be caused by people not taking the prescribed calcium supplement. The treatment effect was also better with calcium doses of 1200 mg/day or more than with doses of less than 1200 mg/day (risk ratio 0.80 vs 0.94; $P = 0.006$). The average calcium intake in Sweden is 900 mg/day among women and 1000 mg/day among men (www.slv.se). Any positive effect on bone mass should be weighed against recent evidence that calcium supplementation may increase the risk of myocardial infarction, at least when it is given alone[191]. This evidence comes from a randomised placebo-controlled trial in 1471 postmenopausal women, half of whom were randomised to receive calcium supplementation. During 5 years of follow-up, there were 45 myocardial infarctions in the calcium group and 19 in the placebo group ($P = 0.01$). The combined incidence of myocardial infarction, stroke or sudden death was also higher, 101 events, compared to 54 in the placebo group ($P = 0.008$). A recent observational study found similar results[2032].

In children, the benefit of calcium is more uncertain, partly because exceptionally large and long-term trials would be needed to evaluate the effect on fracture incidence. One Cochrane meta-analysis of 19 randomised controlled trials in healthy children ($n = 2859$) found no clinically significant effect on bone density of calcium supplementation (including food sources)[1956,1957]. There was a small effect on forearm bone density (standardised mean difference 0.14 g/cm^2; 95% CI 0.04–0.24). This effect is expected at best to reduce absolute fracture risk in children by 0.1–0.2% per year. A later randomised controlled trial with a calcium-fortified fruit drink in 96 girls aged 12 showed a small increase of bone mineral density at all sites which rapidly vanished after supplements were no longer provided[977]. Possibly, dietary calcium has been overemphasised for the building of strong bone in children with crucial factors yet unexplored. A lifelong excess of calcium supplementation has even been suggested to increase the risk of fractures at old age[923]. In this context, it is noteworthy that recent calcium balance studies indicate that human calcium requirements are lower than previously thought[783].

Dairy products

The value of dairy products is also uncertain. Controlled trials of dairy foods for bone health in children have not been conclusive. Three trials included in a meta-analysis (which found no effect)[981] were excluded in the Cochrane review of calcium supplementation mentioned above[1956,1957], as they were not placebo-controlled[250,278] or did not have adequate randomisation[1158]. Instead, four other placebo-controlled trials using milk extract supplementation were included in the Cochrane review[197,291,342,810]. The overall effect, with or without the first three trials, was a slight positive effect of uncertain clinical importance in children. In adults, several studies do not indicate an important effect of dairy foods, with the possible exception of females younger than 30 years[1921]. A cross-over trial in postmenopausal women found metabolic effects of expected benefit for bone strength[196].

In contrast to many of the intervention trials, observational studies of increased fracture rates[606,865] and lower bone density[1160,1518] in young milk abstainers are slightly worrying, although it may be the substitutes, such as soft drinks, that are harmful rather than the displacement of milk in itself[1029]. One study found 50 children in the ages of 3–13 who did not drink milk, usually due to lactose intolerance or because they didn't like the taste, to have lower bone density than controls[606]. As many as 16 of the 50 children had suffered a fracture (expected number was 6; $P < 0.001$). More research is clearly warranted as to the role of milk and its bioactive constituents[234,1832], in particular among children who stick to other parts of a Western diet.

Calcium absorption

The absorption of calcium in the intestines (i.e. its bioavailability) is affected by certain dietary factors, of which the most quantitatively important one is probably phytic acid in cereals and beans. Through the process of chelate bonding, phytic acid forms insoluble salts, phytates, with calcium, iron, zinc and magnesium, which effectively prevent their absorption[259,542,668,1243,1535,1571,1572,1703]. There is no evidence of long-term adaptation to compensate for this reduced uptake. Phytate is therefore a common cause of mineral deficiencies in vegetarians[488,590,669] (see Section 4.13 for further discussion of phytic acid).

The idea that phytic acid in cereals may contribute to osteoporosis would possibly explain why the disease is common among domestic pigs, in particular breastfeeding sows[410]. The recommended calcium intake widely exceeds what is possible for wild pigs to obtain, which indicates an abnormally high amount of calcium needed for grain-fed pigs. Broiler chickens that are raised on certain grain-based, concentrated feeds in order to grow quickly often develop a very obvious brittle skeleton (Einarsson, L., personal communication). Even among laying hens, osteoporotic fractures are common during incubation, but breeding helps promote hens that are more resistant to life on the egg farm[1931].

Salt intake

A potentially important cause of osteoporosis as a result of negative calcium balance is the normal level of salt consumption in Western countries[261,732,1155,1318]. More than 15 short-term studies in humans have clearly shown that urinary calcium excretions are positively correlated to sodium intake[501,809,1155,1159,1648]. The reabsorption of sodium and calcium in the kidneys is positively correlated to each other. Increased sodium intake leads to increased sodium excretions via the kidneys, which increases the calcium excretion level.

With a typical Western salt intake (100–250 mmol/day), the lowest 'obligatory' calcium excretion is 100 mg/day, the level below which calcium excretions will not drop any further with a reduced calcium intake. The excretion level is commonly called 'obligatory', but this is misleading because the threshold drops with reduced salt consumption[1319]. Available evidence indicates that compensatory mechanisms, such as increased calcium absorption in the gut, do not fully offset the negative effect on bone calcium[700,1155]. In particular, older women may not be able to compensate for the increased calcium losses caused by dietary sodium.

In experiments on rats, a high salt intake (at a realistic level) has resulted in accelerated bone loss[277,604,605,976,1216,1577]. In humans, a 2-year observational study found a gradual increase in bone loss with increasing salt intake among older women[405]. We did not see any effect of salt restriction on bone loss in an unpublished randomised controlled trial of 60 to 69-year-old women ($n = 90$) (S. Lindeberg, B. Forsberg, S. Elmståhl and O. Johnell, unpublished data). Bone density was measured with DXA prior to the experiment, as well as 6 and 12 months afterwards. Salt intake was calculated from the daily level of urinary sodium excretions. Thirty women were randomised to sodium restriction, but only 22 of them completed the study and only 6 subjects reached the goal of <50 mmol Na/day. In addition, the study's population had a relatively low sodium intake at baseline (113 ± 43 mmol Na/day).

Some studies suggest that reducing the salt intake from 150 to 100 mmol Na/day (corresponding to 9 and 6 g NaCl, respectively) has a marginal effect on bone loss[310]. Therefore, a decrease to ancestral levels (<50 mmol/day) may be advisable in order to achieve the desired effect.

Potassium intake

Alkaline salts of potassium, such as potassium bicarbonate and potassium citrate (which occur in particularly high amounts in vegetables and fruits) help prevent calcium loss via the kidneys in both young men and pre- and postmenopausal women[143,1013,1014,1611], even with a high salt intake[1246]. Potassium supplementation is particularly efficient in subjects with large urinary excretion of calcium[540]. In a study of 60 postmenopausal women, the effect of common salt on renal calcium excretion was completely reversed with potassium citrate supplements[1618]. After moderate salt restriction (87 mmol Na/day) for 3 weeks, the women were randomly assigned a high salt intake using sodium tablets (225 mmol Na/day) plus potassium citrate (90 mmol/day) or a high salt intake plus a placebo. During the 4 weeks with a high salt intake plus placebo, calcium excretion increased by 42 ± 12 mg/day without, but fell by 8 ± 14 mg/day with potassium citrate supplements ($P = 0.008$). Biochemical markers for bone destruction were only affected in the high salt intake plus placebo group.

Two non-controlled trials found increased bone mass of the backbone[1370] and forearm[1864] after long-term treatment with potassium citrate among patients with recurrent kidney stones. Furthermore, in an observational study of 994 women between the ages of 45 and 49, bone density showed a gradual positive correlation with potassium intake[1291]. Similar findings have been noted in older men and women[1822] and children[845].

Acid-base balance

There is growing evidence that acid-producing foods can adversely affect bone mass through low-grade metabolic acidosis which enhances calcium losses from the skeleton[37,233,247,449,515,1012,1103,1163,1292,1495,1611,1618,1822,1879,1924]. Foods which provide acid precursors in excess of base precursors yield a net endogenous acid production (NEAP), and this leads to greater urinary excretion of calcium, magnesium and nitrogen, and probably bone loss. Bone tissue is our main buffer against systemic acidosis why this aspect of diet may have been seriously underestimated.

Foods that are alkalising are typically rich in potassium and it is sometimes hard to separate these two beneficial factors. However, one randomised, controlled, double-blind trial in 161 postmenopausal women found that potassium citrate, which is alkalising, enhanced vertebral bone mass while potassium chloride, which is acidifying, caused significant bone loss[819].

Acid-producing foods include cereal grains, dairy products (particularly cheese), meat, fish, nuts, eggs and beans. Furthermore, dietary salt has an acidifying effect due to the chloride ion. All non-grain plant foods, such as fruits, root vegetables (including potatoes) and leafy vegetables, provide alkali excess and may thus protect the bone[36,541,1494,1610]. Due to the low proportion of such foods, most Western diets result in a net acid load. Among northern European children and adolescents, it has been estimated that grains, dairy products and meat+fish+eggs each contribute with about one-third of the daily acid load[36]. The particularly high acidity of cheese[36,1494] could possibly explain why cheese, compared to milk, may have less beneficial effects on bone[1921].

Most ancestral diets, even high meat variants, are apparently on the right side of the acid–base balance. One study found a NEAP of -88 ± 82 mEq/day (mean $\pm$ SD) for 159 different hypothetical preagricultural diets, compared to +48 for the average US diet (a positive value corresponds to a net acid load)[1610]. However, the Eskimos' exceptionally protein-rich diet based on meat and fish is an exception.

Protein intake

There is a long held debate as to whether, and under what circumstances, dietary protein has an anabolic (constructive) or catabolic (destructive) effect on bone[194,1371,1609]. Several studies from recent years suggest that many Westerners may have a protein intake that is too low to maintain optimal bone density[195,699,701,790,894,1455].

Three randomised controlled trials have found reduced bone loss of protein supplementation among elderly women with a previous hip fracture[1601,1775,1798]. However, in all these studies the supplements also contained vitamins and minerals which may have been responsible for the beneficial effect.

A large observational study showed a gradual preventive effect of increased protein intake among 55–69-year-old women[661]. Women in the lowest quartile of protein intake had a threefold higher risk of hip fracture than women in the highest quartile. A majority of observational studies have shown a gradual increase in bone mass with increasing protein intake[37,406].

However, the effect of dietary protein on bone is not straightforward. At an optimal protein intake, the provided amino acids can be used for building bone, but when the intake exceeds requirements, a further increase of dietary protein may contribute to bone loss[127,1609]. The window of optimal protein intake apparently varies, depending on the net acid load of the diet[127,1609].

A disputed issue is the extent to which protein from meat, fish, milk and vegetables have different effects on bone health and calcium losses. Available studies have provided varying results and do not support the preference of one kind of protein for the other[1154,1156,1257,1619,1915], and vegetarians do not have higher bone density than meat eaters[119,1290]. Soya protein has been suggested to prevent osteoporosis, but in the studies in question, often experiments on rats, the control group received casein[69,674,1355,1436,1988]. It is therefore unclear whether casein may have an unfavourable effect, or if soya protein may actually be favourable for the skeleton. One study noted reduced bone density and strongly elevated parathyroid hormone levels in pigs that were fed soya protein compared with another group that received fish meal[1036]. Increased levels of parathyroid hormone is a marker of bone loss.

The cardiovascular connection

Cardiovascular disease and osteoporosis are both common in Western countries. Furthermore, individuals with one of the two conditions are at increased risk for the other. In one study, 25% of women with hip fracture had known ischaemic heart disease, compared with 12% among age-matched control subjects[1621]. It has also been found that people with osteoporosis generally have more advanced atherosclerosis[787,1562]. The underlying mechanisms are not known but various suggestions have been made, such as insulin resistance (see below), leptin resistance[877], hypercholesterolaemia and oxidised LDL[1380], Wnt signalling and PPAR-γ antagonism[627] and transfer of calcium from the skeleton to the arterial wall[739].

Among breeding mice with an increased susceptibility for atherosclerosis, the same fat-rich chow that causes atherosclerosis also reduces bone mineral content[1382,1949].

Insulin resistance and diabetes

Many studies have analysed the complex relationship between insulin metabolism and bone strength[1796]. Much evidence indicates that insulin enhances bone formation through inhibition of osteoclast activity[555,1785]. Osteoporosis is characterised by an increased amount of glycosylated proteins, which may also be relevant[708]. Middle-aged and elderly people who have diabetes and marked insulin deficiency, in particular people with type 1 diabetes, have lower bone density and increased risk of fractures[740]. In contrast, conditions with hyperinsulinaemia, such as increased waistline, impaired glucose tolerance and early stages of diabetes type 2, are generally associated with high bone mass despite decreased or normal bone strength[911,1796]. One study of more than 300 000 Canadians found a reduced rate of osteoporotic fractures in individuals with newly diagnosed diabetes, and an increased rate with longer duration of diabetes, compared with non-diabetic people[1018]. Similarly, a recent Japanese study found an increased risk of vertebral fractures in type 2 diabetes that was not associated with lower bone mass[1978].

Diet-induced insulin resistance in rats causes brittle bones without reducing the bone density[1557,2002]. These findings again bring up the fact that skeletal strength is not determined simply by bone density[1892]. The hypothesis that insulin resistance is associated with excess fat outside the fat tissues is also potentially relevant for osteoporosis[593,627]. One study in white US women found a strong inverse correlation between bone mineral density, as measured by DXA, and the amount of fat in the bone marrow, which explained 55% of the variation in bone mineral density[1642].

To further complicate the issue, the glitazones (thiazolidenediones), a new type of drug for type 2 diabetes, lead to increased insulin sensitivity, lower bone density and increased fracture risk[1078].

Underweight

Bone density is lower and the risk of fractures is higher among very underweight (skinny) Westerners, in particular among those with a BMI below 18[385]. In Western populations, such a low BMI often indicates general malnutrition in the elderly and anorexia in young women. In contrast, morbid obesity (BMI ≥35) is associated with a slightly decreased risk of fractures in elderly individuals (15% risk reduction in one meta-analysis[385]), while no such benefit is apparent at young age: In fact, in one study of late adolescent females, excess weight in the form of fat mass was associated with a slightly reduced bone mass[1429]. Thus, bone growth during adolescence appears not to be enhanced by overweight or obesity.

After age 20–30, there is on average a gradual decline of bone mass with increasing age[767]. Among elderly people, this decline is more pronounced in people who lose weight[926]. However, in one study of elderly Australian women, bone loss was associated with weight loss only after age 70 and not in women who were physically active[1296]. Nevertheless, intentional weight loss may be a risk factor for low bone density, as seen in a 2-year controlled lifestyle intervention trial among premenopausal women aged 44–50 years[1384]. After an initial BMI of 25, women in the intervention group lost 0.4 kg, whereas control women gained 2.6 kg ($p = 0.011$). The intervention group experienced significantly greater hip bone loss (–0.20%/year) than the control group (–0.03%/year). Other similar studies of shorter duration have shown variable results[1384,1635,1867]. For the sake of bone strength, weight loss programmes should include physical activity.

Unfortunately, ancestral diets have not been studied in controlled trials with regard to bone health. A Danish study found that a high protein intake protected against bone loss during weight loss, and that bone loss correlated with reduced body fat, but not with reduced muscle mass[1680].

Alcohol

Heavy drinkers of alcohol are at increased risk for hip fracture, while a moderate intake appears to have no or little effect (in any direction)[741,1255,1563].

Summary

Abstaining from dairy products may not be as risky as we used to think for people switching to a salt-free, Palaeolithic diet with lots of green vegetables and fruits. Children and young people who reduce their milk consumption without improving their diet in other respects, however, may be at increased risk for bone fragility in later life, even if they are physically active. In troublesome cases, supplementary calcium and possibly vitamin D should be considered. More dietary studies are urgently needed.

4.13 Rickets

Rickets involves a softening of the skeleton due to deficiencies in two important food ingredients: calcium and phosphorus[921,1555]. Severe childhood cases can result in bent long bones, a crooked spine, muscle weakness and in the worst cases, death. In adults, the disease often results in a deformed pelvis, which can prevent women from delivering children. In many countries it was commonly called 'the English disease', a name which originates from the disease's epidemic spread in England during the beginning of urbanisation and industrialisation. Just 100 years ago, the majority of children in northern Europe were afflicted with the disease.

Rickets in osteological material

Rickets causes a number of permanent changes to the skeleton, such as bowing deformities of long bones, thickening of the growth zones and many other deformities. Most of these are specific to rickets, which is why they can be relatively easily identified by osteologists[1739]. Therefore, it is possible to draw certain conclusions from the disease's dramatic variation during prehistoric and historic times.

Skeletal changes due to rickets are seldom seen in prehistoric hunter-gatherers, and may be absent altogether[1739]. However, they certainly began to appear at the time of agriculture, and thereafter they showed a low prevalence for several thousand years, until they gradually increased throughout Europe during the Middle Ages, at least in the cities[1739]. There were no cases of rickets in any of the skeletal material from the mediaeval Swedish city of Lund ($n = 3305$) (C. Ahlström, personal communication). The dietary habits of the examined population are considered to have been quite good, similar to many other population groups during the Middle Ages[68]. The intake of meat and vegetables was high, among other things.

For obvious reasons, relatively few osteological studies have been done on skeletal populations from the past three centuries, but skeletal changes indicative of rickets have been seen in 25% of the skeletal populations from the eighteenth- and nineteenth-century Norwich[1739].

Rickets in medical literature

The first physician to describe a widespread public disease that corresponds with rickets is the Roman Soranus (98–138) from Ephesus[1739]. He noted a high incidence in the area around Rome, but no cases in Greece, or in Alexandria.

The disease does not turn up in the literature again until 1500 years later, when it is mentioned in the London death records of 1634[178,1337]. Of the 10 900 deaths that year, 14 were attributed to 'rickets'. By comparison, 13 people were executed,

32 drowned, 3 hanged themselves, 6 were murdered, 143 died of puerperal fever (child-bed fever) and 1279 from other feverish diseases. Only 1 person died of the plague that year, compared with 25% of London's population in 1625 and close to 10% in 1636.

Shortly before 1645, Francis Glisson (1597–1677) reported a new disease to The College of Physicians in London[178]. Glisson was born in the town of Rampisham in Dorset, and grew up in the county. In 1650, after more than five years of discussions with the college faculty, he wrote a thesis entitled 'De Richitide sive Morbo Peurili qui Vulgo The Rickets' [About rickets or a childhood disease that common people call the Rickets])[720]. One year later, Glisson wrote the following together with two co-authors: 'This disease became first known as near as we could gather from the relation of others, after sedulous enquiry, about thirty years since, in the counties of Dorset and Somerset . . . since which time the observation of it hath been derived unto all the southern and western parts of the Kingdom'[589].

Around the same time, and possibly without knowledge of the discussions described above, clergyman Thomas Fuller (1608–1661) from Exeter in Devonshire county, which borders Dorset and Somerset, wrote: 'There is a disease of infants . . . having scarcely as yet gotten a proper name in Latin, called The Rickets; wherein the head waxeth to great, whilst the legs and lower parts wane too little'[589].

It appears that primarily children in the upper and middle classes were affected by the disease in the seventeeth century[589]. During the eighteenth and nineteenth centuries, when, according to several sources, the disease reached epidemic levels in the industrial cities of Western Europe, it seems that the lower class suffered to a greater degree[1739]. The disease became so common that it partially paved the way for the new medical discipline of orthopaedics, which literally means 'the art of straightening out children' (the term was coined in France in 1741). It was also partly responsible for the development and spread of caesarean sections starting in England. The prevalence of the disease was high among children in rural Sweden in the nineteenth century[711]. Some sources suggest that more than 80% of children in the cities of Western Europe and North America suffered from the disease at the beginning of the twentieth century[589,720,743,1739].

Relevant dietary factors

Vitamin D

Vitamin D is the most important hormone for regulating calcium metabolism and preventing calcium deficiency through effects on the intestines, kidneys, parathyroid glands and the skeleton. Rickets includes a spectrum of diseases from a simple lack of vitamin D to a dietary lack of calcium even with an adequate intake of vitamin D[1016,1417].

The current explanation that rickets became widespread in English cities due to their dark living quarters and cramped alleyways has been rather widely accepted, especially in the light of the connection between skin and vitamin D. However, there has been a certain amount of scepticism because of the short amount of time outdoors that is needed to achieve conversion of active vitamin D in the skin (see Section 4.12). Additional reasons for scepticism come from the case descriptions of rickets among children in the Swedish countryside at the beginning of the last century[1326]. Attempts have been made to explain a certain percentage of these cases by the custom of wrapping small infants in cloth and keeping them indoors, but this information is difficult to assess. The markedly high occurrence of the disease in the Middle East, North Africa and India in recent years does not seem to be fully explained by a lack of sunlight[164,398,476,1093,1329,1522].

The fact that the disease responds well to vitamin D supplementation is, of course, not necessarily proof that a lack of the vitamin is the main cause. It is well known that the need for vitamin D is affected by other factors.

Cereals

A potential contributing factor that has received remarkably little attention is a high intake of grain products. Roughly 10 000 years ago, humans started to base much of their diet on grains. During the Middle Ages and the beginning of the Modern Age, cereals gradually made up a larger portion of the diet in Europe (M. Morell, personal communication).

Besides the fact that cereals are relatively low in calcium (calculated per unit of energy), they also contain phytate, which inhibits the absorption of calcium[542,1572]. Ethnic populations with an exclusive grain-based diet have an increased risk for rickets, even in sunny countries. Among Asian Indians, it has been shown that a high intake of chapati (flat cakes of unleavened bread) increases the incidence of rickets, and that excluding chapatis from the diet can alleviate the disease[531]. Not even rats seem to be genetically fully adapted to a grain-based diet in this respect[506], although their high intestinal phytase activity indicates a certain amount of adaptation[797].

The discovery that oats can cause rickets was made by Mellanby in the 1930s, when he found that puppies raised on oats suffered from rickets[1200]. He became aware of the calcium-binding effect of phytic acid[227], and showed this was the factor that caused rickets[673]. McCance and Widdowson later demonstrated the negative effects of highly refined flour (which has a higher phytic acid content) on the mineral balance of humans[1171], as well as the ability to improve calcium absorption by destroying phytates[1170]. These findings were later confirmed in numerous studies[542,668,1243,1535,1571,1572,1703].

Since phytic acid is mainly found in the germ part of the seed, whole grain flour is more unhealthy than refined flour in this respect. However, the seed also contains phytases that can break down the phytic acid under beneficial circumstances[259,985,1278,1570,1749]. In the best case, if the seeds are tossed in the right way, soaked and allowed to sit at proper temperature and pH for a sufficient number of hours (or days), the phytic acid can almost be eliminated. Sourdough fermentation (using the proper, old-fashion method) and other fermentation processes are example of these types of methods.

It is well known that self-supporting farming communities used fermentation[254], but whether the purpose was to break down phytic acid is unknown. Moisture and heat treatment were probably also common[563]. Grain eaters from northern latitudes seem to have fermented their grain more often than other ethnic groups (M. Sherwood, personal communication). These types of methods have been largely lost with the development of large-scale, grain-based food production during the agricultural revolution that preceded the industrialisation of Europe. The various types of grains distinguish themselves in that out of our four most popular cereals, it is most difficult to reduce phytic acid in oats. Hence, it is interesting to note that rye and barley, whose phytate levels are the easiest to reduce, were the dominant types of grains in the eighteenth-century northern Europe, and oats were probably more common among certain coastal populations in Scandinavia.

In terms of Dorset and Somerset, which were the first areas in England to be affected by rickets, it is tempting to speculate about the potential significance of brewer's yeast, which allowed bread to rise more quickly than using the sourdough method. Brewer's yeast is made from the yeast fungus, *Saccharomyces cerevisiae*, of which two types are used in breweries, top yeast and bottom yeast. In order for the yeast to be used in bread baking, top yeast is required. This is the original type of yeast that was replaced in most countries by a type of bottom yeast that was developed in Germany, which enabled beer to be preserved for significantly longer periods of time. As late as the early twentieth century, top yeast was still used in England, but almost nowhere else in Europe. Brewer's yeast arrived in England from France, but the exact trail is unknown. A glance at a map does not leave a lot to the imagination. It is not far from England to Normandy, whose northern tip points directly toward Dorset county, and the then-capital Dorchester, which was famous for its breweries. Is it possible that the new method for baking bread with brewer's yeast came from France (compare French bread) to England via Normandy and Dorset? The fact that baking bread with quick-rising yeast spread to the cities before the countryside, and the fact that it was popular among the well-to-do before the poorer folk is consistent with the spread of rickets in England. However, this hypothesis suffers from a serious problem: It cannot easily be tested. It appears very difficult to determine the intricate details of bread baking and beer brewing at that time. Another interesting aspect is that grain prices, which historically reflected consumption[1239], rose sharply in England during the early seventeenth century, after having remained stable for many years[1782].

Other factors

Several of the dietary factors that were discussed in terms of osteoporosis are also probably relevant for rickets. One of them is common salt, which was consumed in increasing amounts in Europe during and after the Middle Ages, due to the growth of food preservation techniques (being able to stretch out food supplies for a short period of time during the year by preserving and storing it).

4.14   Iron deficiency

The most common cause of anaemia in Sweden is a lack of iron, and the second most common cause is a lack of vitamin B_{12}. Both deficiencies can be prevented by a diet based on meat, fish, fruits and vegetables, without cereals and beans. For iron, this occurs primarily through better absorption of iron in the intestinal tract. Our clinical experience has shown that a Palaeolithic diet is effective for many fertile women with a tendency for anaemia, when other causes have been excluded.

Prevalence studies

The occurrence of iron deficiency in hunter-gatherers has not been sufficiently studied, but available data indicate that dietary iron deficiency is an uncommon cause of anaemia, and that average haemoglobin levels are generally satisfactory[312]. The prevalence of anaemia is relatively low in the majority of hunter-gatherer populations, and is usually caused by intestinal parasites. When the Bushmen of South Africa switched to a Western lifestyle, their haemoglobin levels dropped[308].

Today, iron deficiency is one of the most common deficiency diseases around the globe[1469,1987]. In developing countries, it is a large public health problem and the most important reason why close to half of all children and fertile women have anaemia. Chronic minor intestinal bleeding due to hookworm infection, a high intake of grains, and low intakes of vitamin C and meat, are the dominant causes in these countries.

A Swedish study showed that every second girl in the ninth grade had iron deficiency[646]. Among the 9% who were vegetarians, a full 80% had iron deficiency. Many women need iron supplementation during pregnancy, which suggests that large groups of women suffer from an inadequate diet. The prevalence of iron deficiency in Sweden from 1994–2000 increased from 40 to 49%. Prior to that, from 1944 to 1994, Swedish flour was enriched with iron, but nevertheless four out of ten girls still suffered from iron deficiency. One reason for the halted iron enrichment was the risks of elevated iron levels in the body for people with haemochromatosis. However, since enriched iron has a low bioavailability, it only makes up about 4–8% of the iron that can be absorbed by the body. Therefore, reintroducing the process of enriching flour with iron would only change the situation to a limited extent.

Incidentally, humans are the only known species to display lower blood counts in females than males[1546]. The sexes of other species do not vary in this respect, not even among apes with menstrual bleeding.

Prehistoric

Some prehistoric and historic skeletons show thickening and increased porosity of parts of the skull, sometimes with small holes on the surface. The condition is called porotic hyperostosis and there is a certain amount of support that it is specific to chronic anaemia[1538,1561,1599,1738,1835]. In the case of anaemia, the activity in the bone marrow increases, which then increases in volume as a way to compensate. In medicine, we rather refer to a process called 'bossing of the bones', in particular the condition 'erythroid hyperplasia', i.e. excessive growth in the blood-forming bone marrow. In osteology, when porotic hyperostosis occurs on the roof of the eye sockets it is denoted '*cribra orbitalia*'.

Certainly, anaemia in prehistoric hunter-gatherers, just like today, had many different causes. Two of the most common were probably iron deficiency anaemia and haemolytic anaemia. Some skeletal material, which is limited in terms of geography or time, displays a high frequency of porotic hyperostosis. Osteologists often consider iron deficiency and haemolytic anaemia to be the dominant causes. Several researchers, however, have asserted that iron deficiency alone is such a dominant significant causal factor that its occurrence can be determined by the frequency of these skeletal changes. However, in current populations, it is doubtful whether chronic iron deficiency gives rise to porotic hyperostosis, which is not a typical trait at all. It is theoretically possible that the bone marrow expands as long as there is iron available, but not after the iron deposits are empty. Iron deficiency, therefore may have been more common than what the fossil record suggests.

An increase in the frequency of porotic hyperostosis has been noted in the skull remains of humans after the emergence of agriculture, which supports the idea of a higher incidence of chronic anaemia in this group than among earlier hunter-gatherers[312,744,983]. There are two factors that are the dominant plausible causes for this increase, namely, iron deficiency and infections. Infectious diseases became a greater problem with increased population density and poor sanitary conditions, which developed when humans began to remain in fixed settlements[468,1105].

Relevant dietary factors

An increased prevalence of iron deficiency after the development of agriculture would actually be expected due to a reduced intake of meat, fish and vegetables, as well as an increased intake of cereals and beans. The iron level is only affected to a minor extent by the amount of iron in the food, while its absorption is of greater significance[200].

Meat and fish contain haem iron, which is absorbed to a greater extent than iron from vegetables[647]. In addition, there is an unidentified factor in meat that increases the iron's absorption[1536]. Iron deficiency in Western children is effectively prevented by the early introduction of meat[495,1498,1985].

Fruits and vegetables are probably another explanation for the beneficial effect of a Palaeolithic diet on iron levels, primarily through improved iron absorption of vitamin C.

Low phytate intake. Cereals and beans impair iron absorption because the iron is bound with phytates to a great degree[1088,1535]. There is no evidence of long-term adaptation to the effects of phytates[228].

As mentioned earlier, one of the more obvious problems with a vegetarian diet is the development of iron deficiency, which often affects vegetarians, in particular vegans. A high intake of grains and beans contribute to this condition to a considerable degree[488,590,669]. Soya beans also contain other substances that impede iron absorption besides phytates[1099]. Drinking tea during mealtime impairs iron absorption even further[647].

4.15   Autoimmune diseases

A wide range of diseases are caused by autoimmune reactions, where the immune system attacks the body's own cells and tissues. Roughly 5% of the population in the West is estimated to have some type of autoimmune disease[373].

There are many thoughts around the development of autoimmunity, which are mainly based on molecular biological studies[373,963]. A few of the mechanisms that appear to be relevant are presented here in terms of an evolutionary nutritional perspective. The concept that returning to more traditional eating habits can more or less prevent some autoimmune diseases is largely based on compilations by Loren Cordain[339] and David Freed[543,544].

Relevant mechanisms

For millions of years, our ancestors' ability to defend against infection from bacteria and viruses was based on identifying the outer surfaces of harmful proteins and learning to recognise them when they reappear. An immunity develops as a result, and in the case of a new infection, this defence mechanism could strike back quickly and effectively.

In the case of autoimmunity, the immune system somehow loses the basic ability to distinguish between the body's own proteins and foreign proteins. We are forced to eat, but we then risk ingesting proteins or peptides that can activate the immune system if they work their way through the intestinal wall and into the body[339].

Increased amount of potential antigens in the intestines. Three factors in agrarian-based food increase the concentration of potential antigens in the intestines: (1) Consumption of 'foreign' proteins from staple foods like milk, cereals and beans, (2) Reduced breakdown of dietary proteins due to trypsin and chymotrypsin inhibitors (a type of enzyme inhibitor) in cereals and beans,[436,1034,1404,1405,1989,1997] and (3) Disrupted balance of bacteria in the gut due to plant lectins, with overgrowth of antigen-producing bacteria[110] (see Table 4.18).

Increased intestinal permeability. In order to prevent undigested proteins and peptides from entering the body, the epithelial cells of the intestines are tightly glued to each other by means of so-called tight junctions (*zonulae occludentes*)[854]. Lectins in beans and grains open these tight junctions and thereby increase intestinal permeability to allow undesired molecules to pass through[616,1033,1460,1671]. Gliadin, the glycosylated gluten protein in wheat, has also been shown to activate zonulin

Table 4.18 Effects of plant lectins on gastrointestinal and immunological functions.

Effect	References
Promotes growth of Q(K/R) RAA-bearing intestinal bacteria such as *Escherichia coli* and *Lactococcus lactis*	110, 1033, 1460
Binds to polysaccharides and epithelial cells of the intestines, irritates tight junctions, increases endocytosis, shortens microvilli	1033, 1671a, 1460
Increases intestinal permeability	616, 1033, 1671
Strengthens HLA class II expression in the intestines	1927a
Stimulates T-cell proliferation	302a, 1831a
Stimulates gamma-interferon (IFN-γ)	1420a, 1086a
Results in abnormal ICAM expression in T-cells	933a, 1645a
Stimulates cytokine production (IL-1, TNF-α)	521a, 1850a

Note: ICAM, intercellular cell adhesion molecule; IL-1, interleukin 1; TNF-α, tumour necrosis factor α.
Source: Adapted from Reference 339.

signaling, apparently leading to increased intestinal permeability[438,978]. Another relevant barrier is the glycocalyx covering each cell surface facing the gut lumen[533], but this has barely been studied in this aspect. When bacteria in the intestines produce lectins, this can have a dramatic effect on the clinical picture of the host through the increased intestinal permeability[990]. Even glycoalkaloids in potatoes have been shown to increase intestinal permeability[1395].

Increased vascular permeability. Other barriers that are part of the protection against autoimmunity include the blood–brain barrier and the blood–testicle barrier. These involve the body's own antigen-protection for the cells and proteins of the immune system. The ability of foreign proteins to permeate the blood–brain barrier has been shown to increase with the consumption of wheat lectin[106,1148,1869].

Molecular mimicry. One mechanism that is often suggested to be behind autoimmunity is the cross-reaction that develops when one of the body's own proteins is deceptively similar to an outside protein (obtained from food or a microorganism)[1548]. In a misguided attack against the foreign protein, autoimmunity may develop and eventually destroy the body's own tissues. The risk of molecular mimicry is expected to increase with the consumption of proteins that are new for humans as a species.

Gluten intolerance may have possibly developed in this way[1276,1999]. Possibly, molecular mimicry is also a basis for allergies[1511,1548]. The global spread of allergies corresponds with the spread of the autoimmune diseases[179], and hay fever is a relatively new disease that arrived with the agrarian revolution 200 years ago[492].

Genetic factors. Each human inherits a specific HLA genotype (human leukocyte antigen), i.e. the proteins that cause rejection reactions to transplanted organs. The HLA genotype is strongly related to the risk for certain autoimmune diseases. In several cases, patients with autoimmune diseases have shown structural similarities between HLA and bacterial antigens. Therefore, heredity should be regarded in this and many other cases as providing an increased tendency to react to adverse environmental factors.

Polyclonal stimulation of lymphocytes. It is not just substances from bacteria that can activate lymphocytes polyclonally, i.e. regardless of what their antibodies or T-cells can bind to. Wheat lectin can do it as well[615].

Relevant diseases

Gluten intolerance

In the case of coeliac disease, the intestinal mucosal membrane is destroyed, which is caused by the consumption of gluten from grains, especially wheat and rye. The disease has a strong genetic component but is only expressed by eating cereals. By eliminating grains from the diet, the disease is completely cured, and the intestinal lining redevelops a normal appearance and function. Since many studies indicate that gluten intolerance arises from autoimmunity, this would suggest that a Palae-olithic diet could prevent and perhaps even remedy other autoimmune diseases. This type of statement will presumably not be met with as much scepticism to-day as it was when the Dutch physician Dicke suggested in the 1950s that wheat caused coeliac disease[1847]. Today, we realise that humans are not seed eaters by nature.

Coeliac disease is not the only manifestation of gluten intolerance. It is well known that dermatitis herpetiformis, an autoimmune skin disease, is also caused by gluten, but the problem with gluten is probably larger than that. In a study of 53 patients with unclear neurological symptoms which could not be assigned a specific diagnosis, antibodies against gluten (gliadin antibodies) appeared in 30 patients – more than half[635]. An additional 121 similar patients were then identified, the majority of which had ataxia (motion coordination disorder) or peripheral neuropathy (disease of the peripheral nervous system)[636]. In another study of 35 patients with peripheral neuropathy and gliadin antibodies, who were offered a gluten-free diet, 25 accepted and 10 refused the diet[638]. There was significant neurophysiological and clinical improvement in the gluten-free group, as opposed to worsening in the comparison group. The disease is now termed gluten ataxia.

The same research group also completed a report on ten patients with recurring headaches and gliadin anti-bodies, as well as unhealthy changes in the brain based on MRI tests [637]. All had episodic headaches, six had dizziness and four had ataxia. After a gluten-free diet, nine out of ten patients improved.

Rheumatoid arthritis

There are several reasons for testing a Palaeolithic diet on rheumatoid arthritis, a disease where autoimmunity is at least equally as probable as it is for coeliac disease. Many patients, especially those with presence of the so-called rheumatoid factor in the blood, display antibodies against wheat or milk proteins, or both[1336]. Fasting has long had a clear effect with clinical improvement and decreasing inflammation parameters[1678], which could be due to the elimination of antigenic dietary proteins. There is extensive support in the case of rheumatoid arthritis alone that show the role of these proteins in combination with a lectin-rich Western diet[339]. In dietary experiments on rabbits, joint inflammation similar to rheumatoid arthritis was caused by feeding them cow's milk[659,1925].

A Palaeolithic diet has a lot in common with the diets in the successful clinical intervention studies, such as gluten-free vegan diet and Mediterranean-like diet[640,920,1676,1677]. Similar to a Palaeolithic diet, both of these types of diets are rich in fruits and vegetables, low in fat, with a low omega-6/omega-3 ratio and contain no or little dairy products.

Three- to four-week intervention studies, with elemental diets where dietary proteins have been broken down into amino acids and oligopeptides, have not produced conclusive results[681,750,882]. Due to the relatively short study periods, and the possibility that oligopeptides can be perceived as antigens, these findings do not justify dismissing the above hypothesis regarding the importance of dietary proteins.

The hypothesis that meat contributes to rheumatoid arthritis has less support and is not substantiated by intervention studies[642]. In contrast, a relationship between rheumatoid arthritis and the intake of meat products has been observed in an epidemiological cohort study[1400] and an ecological study[611]. Countries with high meat consumption also have a high prevalence of HLA genotypes with a tendency for rheumatoid arthritis. However, an observation that is inconsistent with meat being a cause of rheumatoid arthritis is that the disease has become considerably more common among modern Eskimos, despite a markedly lower meat intake than in the past[1413,1588]. Therefore, confounding and other aspects of a healthy lifestyle may explain the association in observational studies.

A widely discussed question is whether rheumatoid arthritis is a new disease or whether it existed among prehistoric hunter-gatherers[1003]. It is difficult to distinguish between different types of joint inflammations and osteoarthritis (degeneration of joint cartilage and the underlying bone) in the available osteological material. Infectious arthritis was probably a common occurrence among Palaeolithic hunter-gatherers[856]. Therefore, the question must remain open. Rheumatoid arthritis is very common among the Pima Indians today, while other individual populations that were studied previously displayed a remarkably low prevalence[396].

Type 1 diabetes

It is well documented that type 1 diabetes develops as a result of an autoimmune reaction that destroys the insulin-producing cells in the pancreas[28,1821]. Therefore, it is worrisome that the geographical distribution of type 1 diabetes is strongly related to the consumption of dairy products. This relationship can be seen both on a global level[361,1258] and in individual regions such as Scandinavia[1793] or Italy[510]. One study attributed milk consumption to a total of 94% of the international variation in type 1 diabetes, with countries such as Finland and Sweden at the top and Japan at the bottom of the scale[361]. Similarly, in a comparison of nine regions in Italy, 70% of the diabetes variation was attributed to milk consumption[510]. The fact that these are not attributable solely to genetics is supported by the fact that type 1 diabetes is more common among the French descendants of Canada than among Frenchmen in France[361]. In the same way, the disease is more common among Japanese who immigrated to USA than those who remained in Japan. Prior to 1960, diabetes was a rarity in Japan[603].

Again, it might be the foreign proteins in the food, in this case from cow's milk, that are confused with similar proteins in the pancreatic cells through molecular mimicry[1906]. Suspicion has been particularly centred around one variant of casein, β-casein A1, whose consumption is strongly associated with the incidence of type 1 diabetes internationally ($R^2 = 0.96$), although such ecological associations need to be interpreted with some caution[486]. The slightly lower percentage of β-casein A1 in Icelandic milk may partly explain the low incidence of type 1 diabetes in Iceland[169]. However, the issue is debatable, partly because other milk proteins may trigger relevant immune reactions[676].

Further, milk proteins alone are probably not enough to trigger the autoimmune response, and additional environmental factors are apparently needed. In studies of rats and mice with a tendency for autoimmune type 1 diabetes (BBdp, diabetes prone BioBreeding mice, and NOD, non-obese diabetic mice) both wheat and soya protein have shown greater effects than casein on the development of diabetes[1603,1873]. In this rodent model, the strongest diabetes-promoting effect has been seen for wheat gluten[1603] and, in particular, a protein in wheat gluten named Glb1[1104]. Antibodies to this gluten fraction were present in 19 of 23 children with diabetes, and only 3 of 23 control children ($P = 0.03$)[1104]. Many researchers believe that increased intestinal permeability plays a key role for type 1 diabetes[1658,1844,2033], and both gluten-derived peptides and wheat lectin should be considered in this respect[112,339]. It may be relevant in this context to speculate on the several-fold increase of type 1 diabetes in New York between 1866 and 1922[493]. Unfortunately, the changes in food habits during this period have not been adequately characterised.

Multiple sclerosis

Multiple sclerosis (MS) is an autoimmune disease in the brain and spinal cord that leads to the selective destruction of the myelin sheath, the sheath around the nerve fibre, and the nerve fibre itself[318]. Only accidents are a more common cause of disability among young and middle-aged Westerners[682]. If one of two monozygotic (identical) twins develops the disease, the risk for the other twin is 30%, not 100%, which indicates that a certain environmental influence is needed.

The geographic distribution of MS is almost identical to that of type 1 diabetes, and as a result, the correlation with milk consumption is strong for MS as well[248,988,1128,1129]. Immunity against cow milk proteins via T-cells is very common among MS patients[625,1233,1954]. Antibodies against wheat gluten have also been found to be increased among MS patients[1490].

A pathologically increased permeability in the blood–brain barrier may be required to trigger an autoimmune attack against the central nervous system. One proven substance with this type of capability is wheat lectin[107].

Atherosclerosis

Atherosclerosis (see Section 4.3) is a disease characterised by inflammation and and the basic mechanism may be autoimmunity[551,1508]. The early atherosclerotic lesions consist of macrophages and T-cells, and more advanced lesions are filled with immune cells that can set up inflammatory responses[595,663,1028,1096,1938]. This knowledge lends further support to the idea that atherosclerosis can be prevented by a Palaeolithic diet.

Palaeolithic elimination diet

The evidence is accumulating that common proteins in our food can cause autoimmune reactions. It is time to discuss a Palaeolithic diet as a realistic alternative for preventing and treating autoimmune diseases. If one or several of them can be healed or alleviated through the elimination of dairy products, grains or beans, this would be quite a sensational breakthrough. There is a lot of evidence to indicate that motivated patients should try this approach.

In the case of ongoing autoimmune diseases, it is probably important to reduce the amount of circulating peptides and proteins that may be facilitating the autoimmune process. Therefore, consumption of antigenic proteins from dairy products, cereals and beans should be kept as low as possible. Enzymatic digestion of the same proteins in the gut should also be supported through a low intake of protease inhibitors from cereals and beans, including soya products. Finally, the intake of plant lectins from grains and beans should be minimised in an attempt to limit the permeability of the intestines and the blood–brain barrier, and prevent potentially damaging proteins and peptides (food-derived or coming from other sources) from entering the body.

5 Risks with the Palaeolithic diet

There are very few obvious risks with a Palaeolithic diet. For most people, the advantages seem to considerably outweigh the disadvantages. There are no nutrients in grains or milk, required by humans, that are not provided by a mixture of meat, fish, shellfish, vegetables, fruits, nuts and eggs. The effect of a high-protein intake on kidney function is dealt with in Section 4.4. The risk of osteoporosis with a low-calcium intake or weight loss is discussed in Section 4.12. A few additional risks have been addressed here.

5.1 Haemochromatosis

Genetic haemochromatosis is a hereditary disease that results in increased iron absorption. Around middle age, this leads to abnormal iron storage in the liver and other organs. Among northern Europeans, approximately 0.5% are homozygous carriers and approximately 10% may be heterozygotes[1301,1353].

The mutation behind haemochromatosis is considered to have originated among the Celts roughly 60 generations ago, i.e. approximately 1200 years ago[236]. A more recent estimate suggests that the mutation occurred in mainland Europe at least 6000 years ago[426]. The explanation for the rapid spread of the gene may be that it protected against severe iron deficiency caused by a grain-based diet[347]. In addition, a low intake of vegetables rich in vitamin C and the increased spread and higher virulence of intestinal parasites under high-density living conditions could have been contributing factors. Since heterozygotes also have increased iron absorption[236], there may have been a strong selective pressure in favour of the haemochromatosis gene.

Although humans are well adapted for meat-based ancestral diets, they are not necessarily appropriate for patients with genetic haemochromatosis. Heterozygous carriers can eat this type of foods, but they should check their iron status regularly after middle age. Measuring the serum ferritin is a simple and inexpensive way to check for haemochromatosis.

Some researchers feel that a high-iron intake can contribute to cardiovascular disease both in the carrier of the gene for haemochromatosis[1825] as well as those who are not carriers[1826]. Most evidence now suggests no increased risk for ischaemic heart disease (see Section 4.1) but possibly for stroke[482].

5.2   Iodine deficiency

One of the most intriguing essential nutrients in terms of evolutionary adaptations to past diets is iodine, a trace element which is required for thyroid hormone synthesis. The thyroid hormones are necessary for growth and development, particularly for the brain, and for metabolism. Severe iodine deficiency in infancy causes cretinism, which is considered to be the most common preventable cause of mental retardation worldwide[725]. In addition to mental retardation, cretinism is characterised by dwarfism and physical malformations including skull deformities and increased lordosis of the lumbar spine. Dobson has suggested that some of the upper Palaeolithic Venus figurines from mountainous parts of Europe and Asia may represent cretins among iodine-deficient terrestrial hunter-gatherers[428].

Today, milder forms of iodine deficiency with goitre (enlargement of the thyroid gland), but without mental retardation, are common in many regions of the Western world[397,1473]. The risk is greatest in areas where the soil has been depleted of iodine (mountainous regions or areas that are often flooded), but it is also prevalent in other parts of the world, including many European countries. Of 2855 Belgian children aged 6–12 years, 5.7% had goitre in 1998 (the frequency varied between 3.9 and 7.7% in the ten provinces of the country), and 3 years earlier, prior to national campaigns for iodine supplements, the percentage was 11%[397]. In most European countries, iodine deficiencies were common as late as 1992. The exceptions included Sweden, Norway, Finland, Austria and Switzerland, where iodine supplementation was introduced early, typically through table salt.

Without iodine enrichment of foods, few people reach the recommended iodine intake, 150 µg/day for adults and higher amounts during pregnancy and breastfeeding. Vegans run an increased risk of iodine deficiency[1037]. As people in developed countries consume less seafood, iodised salt and dairy products, they are expected to increase their risk of iodine deficiency. The recommended iodine density to be used for planning diets for groups of people is set at 18 µg/MJ. In order to prevent goitre, a daily dose of 50–75 µg or 1 µg/kg of body weight is considered sufficient for most people.

Shellfish and fish, especially seafood, and thyroid glands from various animals are exceptionally good sources of iodine (see Table 3.3). In contrast, nuts, meat (wild or domestic), organ meats (other than thyroids), fruits, and many roots and leafy vegetables are poor sources. Although preagricultural hunter-gatherers living off shore sometimes may have had access to high-iodine vegetables, a fish intake of less than 20% of total food intake (by weight) may not have been enough to meet the above recommendation for dietary iodine. Accordingly, at first glance it would seem that preagricultural humans were dependent on regular access to shellfish, or a very high intake of fish, preferably marine fish. Alternatively, they would need to be aware of the necessity that all family members regularly consume small amounts of thyroid glands from terrestrial mammals. In addition, a sufficient intake during pregnancy and long-term breastfeeding would be crucial for the developing infant brain. On the whole, this would seem to support the notion that humans are strictly dependent on marine food sources[357]. However, exploitation of the marine environment is first documented in the archaeologic record during the Middle Palaeolithic period (approximately 110 000 years BP), long after the emergence of fully modern humans, and stable isotope data suggest that inland aquatic foods were not utilised by hominins living in Europe until the mid-Upper Palaeolithic period (approximately 28 000–20 000 years BP)[1504].

In the light of the uncertainty that hominins evolved at fresh- and saltwater shorelines and became physiologically dependent on seafood[613], it is important to consider the role of goitrogenic substances in plant foods, substances which increase the requirement of iodine and may cause enlargement of the thyroid gland despite an adequate intake of iodine[560]. One group of such substances are flavonoids in beans that are able to suppress the synthesis of thyroid hormones by inhibiting the enzyme thyroxine peroxidase[431,649]. Another kind of goitrogens are cyanogenic glycosides which are produced by more than 2500 plant species. Their production and conversion to cyanide constitutes a well-studied defence mechanism against herbivory[596]. Cyanide can be acutely toxic when consumed in high amounts, but more relevant in this context is when it is ingested regularly in low concentrations. Cyanide is then converted to thiocyanate, a potentially goitrogenic substance which can increase the need for dietary iodine and may cause goitre, even when iodine intake is sufficient[431,560].

These are well-documented consequences of certain staple foods in the developing world. In particular, many staple foods that were domesticated in recent millenia (millet, maize, soya, cassava, sweet potatoes, lima beans, turnips, cabbage, cauliflower, rapeseed, mustard, onion, garlic, bamboo shoots and palm tree fruit) contain a variety of such goitrogens[431,560]. Kopp has suggested that a high-carbohydrate intake, for which humans would not be physiologically prepared, increases iodine requirements[939]. His argument is largely based on the notion that thyroid hormone levels are higher after consumption of high-carbohydrate diets, but these studies have not adjusted for potential goitrogens.

Thus, the reasons why large parts of the European population seem to need supplemental iodine are complex. Further studies are needed. There is insufficient data to suggest that humans, by way of natural selection, would have become totally dependent on marine food sources. Therefore, it is highly possible that human requirements for iodine are currently increased by some dietary factors. Further support for this line of thinking is the observation that iodine-depleted soils often did not coincide historically with endemic goitre[715]. The advantage of eating iodised salt to avoid goitre does not seem to outweigh the increased risk for stroke, cardiac failure, stomach cancer, osteoporosis and kidney stones.

5.3 Exaggerated drug effects

Pharmaceutical drugs are used and evaluated in Western humans (with Western dietary habits). The extent to which they would have a beneficial net effect on humans with Palaeolithic dietary habits has not been studied. In some cases, drastic changes in diet can lead to the effects of the medicine becoming stronger than desired. The positive side of this is that the need for the medicine may eventually be eliminated (in consultation with the treating physician).

Hypotension (abnormally low blood pressure)

Patients being treated with angiotensin-converting enzyme inhibitors, angiotensin receptor blockers or diuretics should be carefully monitored when switching to a salt-free Palaeolithic diet in order to avoid a sharp drop in blood pressure[1225]. It is best to make dietary changes in stages, e.g. by repeatedly cutting the salt intake in half, with a 1–2-week interval, and checking blood pressure after each reduction. In the case of gastroenteritis (stomach illness) and frequent diarrhoea, great caution is called for in the case of treatment with angiotensin-converting enzyme inhibitors.

Low blood sugar

Patients with type 2 diabetes who are on sulphonylurea preparations (glipizide, glibenklamide, glimepiride) are at risk for low blood sugar when making the radical switch to a Palaeolithic diet. If declining blood sugar level is suspected, the medicine should not be taken until consulted with a physician. This advice possibly also applies to newer insulin-releasing medicines such as repaglinide and nateglinide.

Warfarin-induced bleeding

Many of the foods that are part of a Palaeolithic diet are rich in vitamin K. Vitamin K is especially rich in vegetables (e.g. broccoli, spinach, brussels sprouts) as well as liver and kidney. Egg yolks contain smaller amounts.

The problem with vitamin K is that a sudden change in intake alters the effect of warfarin, so that it becomes more difficult to set the correct dose. If you suddenly eat large amounts of vitamin K, the need for warfarin also increases, which can result in blood thinning if the dose is not changed. On the other hand, if you are used to eating a lot of food that is rich in vitamin K and then you suddenly stop, there is a risk that the dose will become too high, which in the worst case can lead to internal bleeding.

Switching to a Palaeolithic diet during ongoing warfarin treatment should be done in consultation with a physician or nurse. In most cases, it is probably best to make the dietary changes gradually over a long period of time. If the warfarin treatment is planned to occur only for a few months, it is probably better to wait until after the exposure.

The most common cause for a disturbed balance is probably that the person is not eating at all, e.g. in conjunction with temporary illness. Dietary changes within the framework of normal Western dietary habits are not usually considered to be of great significance.

6 Viewpoint summary

This approach to diet and health is based on two well-documented principles of evolutionary biology. One is that humans, as is the case with other animal species, are genetically best suited to the types of food that were available in the ecological niche where they developed. The foodstuffs in our case were mainly meat, fish, shellfish, vegetables, fruits, nuts, insects and roots, in highly variable proportions and with great variety of plant foods. Conversely, the intake of dairy products, grains, rice, edible fats and refined sugar was negligible, even though these foods now make up the majority of the calories in a typical Western diet. Choosing foods in the first category appears to be the biologically correct way to maintain good health.

The other principle is that all species, even the plants and animals we consider food, have developed efficient systems to support the spread of their genes over the course of evolution. This includes toxins and other bioactive substances which are part of a plant's defence systems. Animals that we want to eat have been able to flee or counter-attack, and therefore they do not have the same need to poison their attackers as plants do. The seeds in fruits, on the other hand, increase their chances of germinating if the fruit is eaten; however, this assumes that the seed passes intact through the intestines. In order to reduce the intake of phytochemicals, our staple foods should preferably not be seeds, grains and beans, and should vary between different types of vegetables and root vegetables.

6.1 Evolutionary medicine instead of vegetarianism?

Traditional studies on the health effects of a person's lifestyle suffer from serious problems and can only provide limited information regarding the significance of individual lifestyle factors. The connections found between lifestyle and health are sometimes illusory, while the molecular biological models are severely oversimplified. It is also impossible to conduct double-blind studies of lifestyle changes.

In order to put any new knowledge about food into a comprehensible context, we all need analogies and models of the real world. One such common model has been vegetarianism, whose scientific support, however, is surprisingly weak. An alternative model is evolutionary medicine, which does not explain the development of the disease from a molecular biological perspective, although it fits well into such models. Instead, it explains the process in terms of evolutionary biology; those who were best suited to the available food were the ones who had the greatest chance of surviving into old age.

6.2   Traditional populations are spared from overweight and cardiovascular disease

Aboriginal populations, who do not consume foods that humans are not adapted for, have a disease panorama that is quite different from people in the Western world. Yet, this is not due to a lack of older persons. Myocardial infarctions, sudden cardiac death stroke and heart failure are uncommon or missing altogether in aboriginal peoples. The risk factor levels are also very beneficial. Blood pressure is low and does not increase with age as it does for us. Being overweight is not common, and everyone is very thin. Type 2 diabetes and insulin resistance do not seem to be present either.

The concept of normality is turned on its head with these types of comparisons. A normal, middle-aged European, with average levels of body weight, blood pressure and blood sugar has an average risk of dying of a heart attack. While this is 'normal' in Europe, we did not find any such cases in our Papua New Guinea study and no one died of a heart attack. We believe that this is due in large part to dietary habits, although the role of other lifestyle factors need to be addressed as well.

When traditional ethnic groups switch to a Western lifestyle, they suffer from exactly the same ills as we do, including abdominal obesity, hypertension, diabetes and cardiovascular disease. The spread of stroke after urbanisation in Africa and Papua New Guinea is only one of several noticeable examples.

6.3   Insulin resistance is more than abdominal obesity and diabetes

Our diet begins to make its marks on us early in life. Today's young people are becoming unnaturally tall and most girls are having their first menstruation before they are mentally mature enough to become mothers. Nearsightedness and acne are common occurrences. There is a lot to suggest that these health problems, similar to the most common forms of cancer in the West, are related to our current dietary habits. The mechanisms seem to be closely related to insulin resistance, a disorder that supposedly develops very early in the lives of Westerners.

Atherosclerosis is a disease that affects almost all Westerners. Animal experiments show that it is strongly dependent on the foods we eat. All types of fat have a negative impact, with the possible exception of omega-3 fat. Moreover, the types of protein in the diet are also significant factors. The milk protein casein has been shown to accelerate this process in many animal experiments, while protein from meat provides a preventive effect. The effect of 'foreign' proteins fits with the picture of atherosclerosis as an inflammatory or autoimmune disease. If grains also contribute to the disease, as has been suggested, it is plausible that plant lectins in seeds also have a negative impact.

6.4   Non-Europeans are affected the hardest

By all appearances, non-European ethnic groups have an especially low resistance to unhealthy food. Therefore, they often develop type 2 diabetes in adolescence and are 2–3 times more likely to develop nearsightedness than Scandinavians are. This indicates that the foods that have been eaten regularly by European populations since they became settled in the area are a contributing factor to insulin resistance, diabetes and myopia. Over time, descendants with the least resistance were eliminated according to the usual principles of natural selection. What remains today are northern Europeans who develop diabetes, but at a relatively older age.

It has been suggested that cow's milk contributes to type 2 diabetes, which would explain why this disease is less common after urbanisation in ethnic groups that have consumed milk for a long time. The hypothesis is supported by the fact that milk contributes to insulin resistance among beef calves and rats – effects that perhaps are not primarily dependent on milk fat.

6.5   'Foreign' proteins in the food

Proteins in meat, fish and shellfish are probably expected to be healthier than those in dairy products or beans. This is because the latter kinds of proteins seem to yield biologically active peptides with potential ability to disrupt various physiological processes. The most well-known example is gluten intolerance. The disease likely develops because a segment of gliadin in wheat is identical to a cellular protein in the gut. In the end, this can lead to the intestinal villi being broken down by an autoimmune process that cannot distinguish between the two proteins. When gliadin is excluded from the diet, the disease is alleviated, and the intestinal membrane completely recovers in terms of its appearance and function.

Other autoimmune diseases that potentially develop in the same way include type 1 diabetes, multiple sclerosis and rheumatoid arthritis. Among the biggest suspects in terms of type 1 diabetes are dairy products and wheat. Consuming grains or beans probably increases the amount of proteins that are not completely broken down before being absorbed into the body. This may also be significant in terms of the development of allergies, a group of diseases that are closely associated with autoimmunity.

6.6   Effects of an ancestral diet

Ancestral diets are characterised by a low content of salt, a high amount of minerals and vitamins, as well as a high percentage of omega-3 fatty acids. An important characteristic is that the diet can curb hunger with a moderate amount of calories and thereby counteract overeating. This essentially helps support a form of calorie restriction, which is a desirable approach for most middle-aged and older Swedes.

Available studies support the idea that this type of diet prevents cardiovascular diseases and type 2 diabetes, as well as improves blood pressure and blood lipids. One of several plausible mechanisms is improved insulin sensitivity. It may also be possible to prevent osteoporosis and various cancers such as breast, prostate and colorectal cancer, but more research is needed.

Therefore, humans are genetically suited to lean meat, fish, vegetables and fruits. These foods, preferably generated in a more organic manner than is currently the case, can be recommended as a staple diet, while the rest can be seen as compromises. Identifying and addressing the risks of common foods for common health problems should have a high priority in medical research.

6.7   The ancestral diet: a new concept

The optimal human diet is more than just the diet of our ancestors; it appears to have the potential to prevent many of the common public health problems of the West. Established experts in nutrition seem to be in agreement that this diet is very healthy. Some of them have certain reservations, however. In particular, it is feared that the calcium intake may sometimes become too low, and some feel that the protein intake is a little excessive – two problems that are discussed primarily in Sections 4.12 and 4.4. Others feel that the importance of fat and fibre has been overlooked.

The most common objections, however, do not apply to the use of lean meat, fish, fruits and green vegetables; rather, they apply more to the supposed absence of grains and low-fat dairy products. There is no doubt that a lot remains to be proven in terms of the theories and warnings that are proposed in this book. But it is important to point out that there are no nutrients in whole-grain bread and skim milk that cannot be just as easily obtained from an ancestral diet.

Another objection, and a highly relevant one, relates to sustainability. If the majority of humans on this planet shall avoid grains and increase their meat intake, then we clearly have a problem (although cutting dairy products is helpful). With or without such dietary changes, we will have to eat more locally produced foods, more starchy root vegetables and less ruminant meat, and we need to travel less. In our clinical experience, an ancestral-like dietary model does not require a higher meat intake than the present average (100 and 130 g/day for Swedish men and women, respectively).

7 Healthy eating

Non-recommended foods may be the ones that were rarely or never staple foods during human evolution. If diseases like overweight, type 2 diabetes and cardiovascular disease are partly caused by such foods, moderation of these foods is expected to be beneficial, while more severe restriction could be even more favourable. For diseases like autoimmune diseases, more strict avoidance of the specific culprits, whichever they are, may be necessary.

Grains

Humans can support themselves on a staple diet of various root vegetables supplemented with leafy vegetables and small amounts of fish, as they do in some parts of the Pacific. They can also support themselves on an extreme meat-based diet, as they used to do in the Arctic. However, neither humans nor other animals can live exclusively on grains without the risk of pellagra and beriberi. Even with a diet that is only half-based on cereals, there is still a risk of developing marginal deficiencies for certain nutrients. Not even specialised seed-eating mammals should be solely fed seeds in the long run.

Even if cereals, in particular whole grains, are more nutritious than some other Western foods, they still appear to be capable of damaging our health in several respects. I shall not repeat all the possible effects that have been discussed throughout this book. Some of the health risks are specific for certain types of seeds, but other risks apply to seeds in general.

Cereals have a low water content and are therefore rich in energy, which potentially explains why they seem to contribute to overfeeding of mammals, birds and even humans. We also suspect other components of grains to directly interfere with satiety mechanisms by way of endocrine disruption. The phytic acid in grains inhibits the absorption of iron, calcium, zinc and magnesium. Grains have a disadvantageous omega-6/omega-3 ratio and are low in many vitamins. They can theoretically contribute to autoimmunity and allergies due to their protein composition and their lectins.

Oats may possibly reduce a few of the problems that are associated with an exclusive wheat diet. Oats include soluble fibre, which are more healthy than fibre from wheat. However, oats still share many of the potential nutritional problems with different seed types. The problem with phytic acid is particularly pronounced in oats. Pasta often has a low glycaemic index, but otherwise it has no known advantages over other cereals. There is no convincing support that rice is more healthy than other cereals.

Dairy products

No free-ranging mammals drink milk as an adult apart from modern humans. Although human milk is good for babies and cow's milk is good for calves, a lifelong daily consumption of dairy products, or even human milk, may pose considerable risk for humans. There are indications from animal experiments and some human observational studies that milk products, even low-fat varieties, are a cause of atherosclerosis and hence myocardial infarction, and some forms of stroke, heart failure and dementia. They may also be possible causes of insulin resistance and autoimmunity. Their effect on bone density is not clear, as discussed in Section 4.12. Although the isolated exclusion of milk from an otherwise unhealthy Western diet may hypothetically carry some health risks, possibly including decreased bone strength, its incorporation into an ancestral diet is probably of no use. The mixture of wheat and milk as staple foods is common in many populations with Western disease, but not in any population where Western disease appears to be absent.

Refined fats

Margarines and oils supply empty calories with very little or no nutrients, thereby contributing to excess caloric intake and weight gain. Rapeseed oil, olive oil and linseed oil may be slightly better than other fats.

Sugar

Refined sugar, sweets and soft drinks only supply calories without minerals, vitamins or other nutrients, and probably increase the risk for overweight, insulin resistance, type 2 diabetes and the metabolic syndrome.

Beans

Beans probably were not eaten in large quantities during primate evolution. The risks associated with beans include their high levels of phytic acid, lectins, protease inhibitors, alkylresorcinols and phytoestrogens. Rats who are fed soya beans after weaning have limited growth, partly due to the effect of lectins.

These apprehensions certainly apply to soya beans. Two experts on health effects of soya beans at the US Food and Drug Administration (FDA), Doerge and Sheehan, the former chief of the Oestrogen Base Program, wrote in 1999 a public letter in protest of the FDA's approval of health claims for soya products (http://www.dcnutrition.com/news/Detail.CFM?RecordNumber=546). The researchers were concerned about the results of animal experiments where flavonoids in soya (genistein and daidzein) were found to have toxic effects on oestrogen-sensitive tissues and on the pancreas[431]. Particular caution is needed for children and adolescents children, but this has not prevented the large-scale development and marketing of soya-based infant formulas. Consumption of soya products during pregnancy has been suggested to increase the risk of abnormal development in the nerve system and reproductive organs of the offspring. It has been shown that realistic doses of genistein cause atrophy of the thymus in mice[1983]. Ishizuki et al. reported goitre and elevated individual thyroid-stimulating hormone levels, although still within the normal range, in 37 healthy iodine-sufficient adults without known thyroid disease, who were fed 30 g of pickled soya beans per day for as little as 1 month[431]. One study found genistein to disrupt female reproductive function in mice, but the effect in humans has not been examined[27].

On the other hand, it has also been suggested that flavonoids in soya beans have beneficial effects, including inhibiting the growth of cancer, but none of these effects have been proven convincingly[629]. With regard to breast cancer prevention, soya can no longer be recommended, as discussed in Section 4.11.

In old Chinese cuisine, soya products were eaten with caution, and the intake of genistein, e.g., is thought to have been well below the intake of 'health conscious' Westerners[369].

7.2 Recommended foods

Recommended foods are the ones that correspond to what was eaten during human evolution. Possibly, they play no important role in themselves for most Westerners, except replacing unhealthy staple foods. If the majority of modern humans consume enough calories and essential nutrients, as much evidence suggests, then the most efficient way to improve diet would be to avoid harmful dietary items, including the ones that may lead to overconsumption of food.

Lean meat

A reasonably high intake of lean meat, preferably from free-ranging animals without fortified feeds, ensures a high intake of high-quality proteins. Lean meat is satiating and combats obesity and thereby, likely, insulin resistance and the metabolic syndrome. Hypothetically, the risk for stroke and other cardiovascular diseases is reduced. The risk that undigested peptides could potentially be absorbed from meat and start an autoimmune or allergic reaction is probably quite low. Apart from protein, meat also supplies a high degree of iron, vitamin B_{12} and zinc.

Fish

Fish has the same advantages as lean meat and also contains omega-3 fatty acids, which have a number of more or less proven health effects. Fatty fish is particularly rich in these fatty acids.

Vegetables

A high intake of vegetables probably reduces the risk for many diseases. Compared with most other foods, vegetables are rich in a long list of nutrients with potential significance for reducing cardiovascular disease, dementia, cancer and osteoporosis.

Fruit

Fresh fruit is almost as beneficial as vegetables with the same type of nutritional benefits. The nutrient density (amount per unit of energy) of fruit is generally higher than in cereals but lower than in vegetables. Fructose poses no real threat since you need to consume huge amounts in order to exceed the safe limits.

Root vegetables

Humans are apparently well adapted for starchy root vegetables, which can be recommended as a staple food. Nevertheless, a certain amount of caution is advisable. They can sometimes contain more antinutritional substances than vegetables and fruits, although some of these are deactivated during boiling. Potatoes easily yield a high glycaemic load, which can be problematic for people with diabetes, at least in the short run, which is why some caution may be necessary. Varying the intake of different root vegetables and green vegetables as much as possible is recommended. Root vegetables are best cooked in a pressure cooker to deactivate the lectins and other bioactive proteins.

Tap water

The best drink at mealtime is tap water. Drinking water instead of juice, pop or beer helps to maintain a trim figure and combat insulin resistance. When you get used to it, tap water is an excellent mealtime drink. Mineral water provides too much unnecessary salt.

Nuts

Nuts are almost as beneficial a treat as fruit, but they should not be eaten in excess. Peanuts are not strictly nuts in a botanical sense and should be avoided. Even raisins and dried fruits are acceptable, but due to their low water content, just like nuts, they can provide an unnecessarily high-energy intake if you are not careful. Nuts also have the disadvantage of being a source of phytic acid and omega-6 fat.

7.3 Variation

One important issue is to increase the variation of plant foods in the diet, i.e. to spread the risks from biologically active substances as much as possible. When each of them is eaten in low amounts, they may be safe, whereas daily consumption of large amounts could pose a risk. Particular care needs to be taken with seeds and beans, and to a lesser extent with root vegetables.

In this context, the relationships between plant species may be critically important. For example, peanuts and soya beans belong to the same family (Fabaceae), which is why their lectins have a preference for similar hormone receptors[1848]. Hence, it is more important for people who are allergic to peanuts to be aware of this relationship than to reflect over what is meant by the word 'nuts'. Similarly, if a protein or a bioactive substance in potato turns out to be a health hazard, then other foods from the same nightshade family (Solanaceae), such as tomatoes, should be carefully considered. This kind of reasoning lay behind the scholarly warnings of potato and tomato when they were introduced into Europe in the eighteenth century: Was consumption of close relatives of the deadly nightshade really advisable?

Another aspect is the individual variation between human beings, families and even ethnic groups with regard to the upper safety level of a particular food. If you suffer from an illness, e.g. an autoimmune disease, you may wish to exclude your former staple foods because you suspect one of them to be the culprit. The obvious illustration is coeliac disease: If you exclude seeds containing gliadin and gliadin-like proteins from the diet, you are cured. In other cases, where the connection is less obvious, the ideal would be to test each person and each food for compatibility. In the future, this will perhaps be possible by means of genomics, proteomics, nutrigenomics and nutriproteomics.

7.4 Compromises

Very few people are able to follow this kind of dietary advice without compromises (I cannot manage this, for example). However, the greater the portion of our diet that is made up of ancestral-like foods, the better. For the majority of people, most of the suspected harmful dietary factors are, in all likelihood, benign in low doses. The problem is that no one knows what they are or what a safe limit is. No one knows which of our fears will turn out to be baseless. Much of this uncertainty will last for many years in the future.

A good start is to switch to an ancestral diet for everyday meals, with one or two compromises per week in the form of some favourite old food. The greater your illness (previous myocardial infarction, type 2 diabetes, autoimmunity, serious bowel disorder, etc.), the more important it is to be strict, particularly with the most suspicious food substances.

One way of making hot dishes more tasty, especially shortly after salt restriction, is to allow for limited amounts of sweet and hot sauces, pickled beets and the like. Although they contain some salt, the overall intake can be kept at reasonable levels if we do not overindulge, and if food is prepared without added salt. Oven baking, e.g. in earthenware dishes, can reduce the number of fried meals.

Glossary

Abdominal obesity Obesity concentrated around the abdomen that is associated with insulin resistance and increased risk for high blood pressure, cardiovascular disease and diabetes.

Academic medicine Scientifically based medicine that is taught at universities and colleges.

ACE inhibitors Drugs that inhibit angiotensin-converting enzyme (ACE), thereby countering arterial constriction, high blood pressure and its complications, including heart failure.

Acne Inflammation of the sebaceous glands in the skin, typically seen as red pimples in the face, and particularly prevalent among teenagers.

Adaptation A change by which an organism or species becomes better suited for its environment. Adaptation in an individual organism is typically caused by reversible physiological changes, while (genetic) adaptation in a species is by way of natural selection.

Adhesion The sticking together of cells or particles.

Agonist (Foreign) substance that triggers activity in a specific receptor.

Agglutination Lumping together, usually cells.

Alkaloids A class of substances containing nitrogen that are found in certain plants, especially in the plant families of buttercup, poppies and potatoes. They have pronounced physiological actions on humans.

All-cause death Death from any cause; total mortality.

Dietary advice by the American Heart Association Dietary standards according to the American Heart Association; total fat intake ≤30 E%, saturated fat 8–10 E%, dietary cholesterol <300 mg/day, polyunsaturated fat up to 10 E%.

Amylase An enzyme in saliva and pancreatic fluid that breaks down starch into glucose.

Amyloid Substance that is stored in different organs in the body and shares common histologic features in terms of colour and appearance, but can consist of various proteins or peptides.

Anabolic Relating to anabolism, the building of complex molecules from simple nutrients in the cells.

Anaemia 'Blood loss', low blood count, or percentage of haemoglobin (Hb) in the blood (a protein that transports oxygen throughout the body) that is too low.

Angina pectoris Chest pain caused by ischaemic heart disease.

Angiography Contrast X-ray of a blood vessel, carried out after introduction of a radiopaque substance.

Angiotensin II A protein whose presence in the blood promotes aldosterone production and tends to raise blood pressure.

Animal protein Dietary protein from the animal kingdom, including proteins from meat, fish, shellfish and dairy products. In my opinion, this is an inappropriate term, since milk proteins are relatively new for us as a species and have completely different effects than muscle proteins.

Antigen A substance that is foreign to the body and stimulates the creation of antibodies. The foreign substance is recognised by the organism via specific receptors on the surface of certain lymphocytes. During a reaction between the antigen and the receptors, either an antigen immunity or its opposite response, antigen tolerance, is generated. In the case of immunity, the immune system partly produces an increased number of lymphocytes that can combat the antigen in question, and also produces antibodies against the same antigen.

Apolipoproteins Proteins that are part of the blood's lipoproteins and are divided into four main groups, A, B, C and E, as well as other subgroups. The apolipoproteins are important for transporting lipoproteins through the cell membrane in connection with cell secretion or cell absorption. In addition, they control the activity in the enzymes that affect the fats in the lipoprotein particles.

Apoplexy A former name of (severe) stroke.

Arboreal Living in trees.

Arrhythmia A disorder with irregular or otherwise abnormal rhythm of the heart.

Ataxia Inability to coordinate muscle movement caused by disease in the cerebellum or by disturbed sense of touch.

Atherosclerosis An arterial disease, where fatty material is deposited in the inner layer of the vessel wall, which progressively becomes enlarged. It affects primarily large and average-sized arteries, e.g. aorta, coronary arteries and the large arteries in the legs and neck. It is the most common underlying cause of myocardial infarction, heart failure, stroke, non-Alzheimer dementia and many cases of renal failure.

Atherosclerotic Suffering from atherosclerosis.

Atrial fibrillation Continuous, exceedingly rapid contractions (fibrillation) of the musculature of the two upper cavities (atria) of the heart; a common disorder in Western populations.

Atrophy Thinning, degeneration of organs or tissue.

Autoimmune reaction Misdirected immune response where the immune system attacks the body's own structures, which can lead to autoimmune disease. Examples of such diseases include gluten intolerance, rheumatoid arthritis, type 1 diabetes and multiple sclerosis.

Baseline A minimum or starting point used for comparisons.

BBdp Diabetes prone BioBreeding mouse, a mouse with a high incidence of type 1 diabetes.

Benign Well intentioned.

Betel Mild, commonly occurring drug in Asia and Oceania. Areca nuts (*Areca catechu*) chewed together with leaves or seed mixture from betel tree (*Piper chavica betel*) and a pinch of slaked lime (calcium hydroxide) from, e.g., burnt coral. Areca nuts contain arecoline, a fluid oil with parasympathomimetic effects.

Bias A false interpretation of a statistical result due to a factor which correlates with the culprit factor and which is not properly allowed for in the analysis.

Bioactive substances Chemical substances that are synthesised by plants or animals and have a biological effect on the animals that consume them.

Bipedal Using only two legs for walking.

BMI See Body mass index.

Body mass index BMI, body weight in kg divided by the square of the body height expressed in meters (kg/m^2). One person who weighs 73 kg and is 1.70 m tall has a BMI of $73/(1.7)^2 = 25.3$.

Bovine Relating to cattle (family Bovidae).

Bypass operation Aorto-coronary bypass operation, coronary artery operation; an operation method in the event of constricted hardening of the coronary artery, where oxygenated blood from the aorta is routed past the blocked or constricted sites by means of a vascular transplant, commonly surface veins taken from the patient's legs, or arteries from the inside of the rib cage or from the arm.

Cachexia Severe emaciation as a result of significant, long-term malnutrition. In the West, the most common causes are cancer and other wasting diseases and conditions, where the general effect is the inability to eat sufficiently to compensate for the loss of energy, e.g. severe heart failure.

Calcium density See Nutritient density.

Cardiac Of or relating to the heart.

Cardiac arrest Heart stops due to sudden arrhythmia. Sometimes the arrest is temporary, and sometimes it leads to sudden death.

Cardiovascular diseases Diseases associated with the heart and blood vessels. Generally refers to diseases related to the hardening of the arteries in the heart and blood vessels.

Casein The dominant protein in milk.

Case–control study Retrospective study where patients who have fallen ill (cases) are compared with healthy control persons in terms of a particular variable, e.g. something in their lifestyle, which is suspected of causing the disease in question. A plausible source of errors is that awareness of the suspected lifestyle factor can influence the recollections of those who have fallen ill more than the control subjects.

Cereals Generic name for different types of seeds or grains (wheat, rye, corn, oats, rice, etc.).

CI See Confidence interval.

Coagulation (of blood) Clotting.

Cochrane Collaboration The Cochrane Collaboration is an international not-for-profit organisation, providing high-quality information about the effects of health care in accordance with the principles of evidence-based medicine (see this word). In the Cochrane Library, the collaboration regularly publishes systematic reviews, which are often referred to as 'Cochrane reviews' or 'Cochrane meta-analyses'.

Coenzyme Molecule needed in certain cases for the enzyme to be able to catalyse a chemical reaction.

Cognitive Having to do with cognition, i.e. knowledge or understanding.

Cohort A group of people; in epidemiological studies one that is followed over a period time (prospectively). Hence, cohort studies are prospective epidemiological studies analysing associations between exposure and outcome within separate populations.

Comparative studies Interdisciplinary studies of disease among different animal species.

Confidence interval The numeric range in which the true value for the population lies with a given probability; 95% confidence interval = 1–10 means that the true value has a 95% probability of being between these two limits.

Confounder Confounding factor, a factor (e.g. yellow fingers), which shows a statistical connection with a disease (lung cancer) and which covaries with the actual cause (smoking) without actually contributing to the development of the disease. Often the term 'residual confounding' is used, indicating the presence of unknown or unmeasured associated variables, after adjustment for the known ones.

Consecutive Following each other in time.

Controlled study Comparative study where a new treatment is given to one group of people (intervention group); this is compared with the best treatment thus far, which is given to another group (control group).

Coronary arteries The medium-sized blood vessels at the surface of the heart, supplying its musculature with nutrients and oxygen.

Coronary angiography X-ray of coronary artery using a contrasting agent that is injected into the coronary artery; can highlight atherosclerosis which constricts the blood flow.

Coronary heart disease Ischaemic heart disease, coronary disease; the most common type of cardiovascular disease and includes vascular spasms (angina pectoris) and heart attacks (myocardial infarctions). The main cause is hardening (atherosclerosis) in the coronary arteries of the heart.

Correlation Common variation between two variables (quantities) x and y, e.g. age (x) and blood pressure (y). This example shows a positive correlation, i.e. the blood pressure rises with age. In the case of a negative correlation, y drops while x rises. The degree of explanation, i.e. the size of the variation in y that can be explained by x is indicated in the correlation coefficient r or the determination coefficient R^2. The former can vary between -1 and $+1$, and the latter is the square of the former. Where $r = 0$, the two variables are not correlated. If $r = -1$ or $+1$, then x and y are in a straight line. If $r = 0.5$, then $R^2 = 0.25$. The latter can be expressed so that 25% of the variation in y can be explained by the variation in x.

Cortical bone The compact outer layer of the bone tissue.

Cross-sectional survey Epidemiological study at a specific point in time, in contrast to a prospective study that runs over a longer period of time.

Density Tightness, mass per volume.

Determination coefficient See Correlation.

DHA Docosahexaenoic acid; 22:6 omega-3; one of the two dominant omega-3 fatty acids in fatty fish.

Diagenesis Changes to the skeleton while it is interred in the ground through the effects of animals, roots, the earth's pressure, chemical reactions or temperature variations.

Diastolic blood pressure The lower value of the two values in a blood pressure reading, e.g. 140/90 mm Hg.

Digest To dissolve (food); chemically break down larger molecules into smaller ones.

Disease incidence See Incidence.

Domesticate Gradually taming wild animals. The process, which historically has continued for many generations, involves controlling plant propagation by gradually selecting the desired hereditary characteristics.

Double-blind study Study where the patients are randomly assigned into either a treatment group, which receives active treatment (often a drug) or a control group, which receives inactive substances that have the same look and taste of the active substance, i.e. a placebo. Both the patient and the examiner are 'blind', since the group to which each patient belongs is not revealed until the measurements are completed and the protocol can be broken. This technique spreads the effects of psychological anticipation equally across the treatment and the control groups, which helps when interpreting the results.

Dyslipidaemia Bad levels of blood lipids, i.e. high total cholesterol, high LDL cholesterol or low-HDL cholesterol.

DXA Dual-energy X-ray absorptiometry: a method for measuring bone density.

ECG Electrocardiography; recording of the electrical activity of the heart.

Ecological study An epidemiological study which compares populations, typically in different countries, with regard to associations between an exposure or a risk factor and an outcome variable, such as death or disease. One famous ecological study is the Seven Countries Study.

EGF Epidermal growth factor, a mammalian protein acting in the regulation of cell growth, proliferation and differentiation, among other things. Like several other endogenous and exogenous ligands, including milk-derived β-cellulin, it binds to and activates the EGF receptor, a tyrosine kinase receptor.

Ejection fraction A measurement within cardiology to measure how much of the blood in the heart's left ventricle is pumped out during the ventricular contraction (systole).

Elimination diet Diet where a person consciously avoids one or several foodstuffs for diagnostic purposes in order to clarify which foods are causing allergic reactions, or for treatment purposes, in order to avoid allergic or autoimmune reactions.

Endocytosis Absorption in a cell of bacteria, dead tissue or foreign particles.

Endometrium The mucus membrane lining the inside of the uterus.

Endothelial function Function of the endothelial cells in the blood vessel, i.e. the cells that cover the inside of the vessel against the blood stream. In addition to regulating vascular tone by releasing nitrous oxide, the endothelium has a number of other functions, which include, e.g., forming a barrier between the blood stream and the tissues, participating in the process of coagulation and fibrinolysis (processes that affect blood clot formation), as well as remaining metabolically active in the conversion of triglycerides to free fatty acids and glycerol via the enzyme lipoprotein lipase.

Endothelial dysfunction Reduced endothelial functioning (see Endothelium); considered an early sign of atherosclerosis, possibly because the reduced amount of nitrous oxide has a negative effect on macrophages and smooth musculature. Further evidence of the significance of endothelial dysfunction is its association with various risk factors for ischaemic heart disease, such as smoking, hypertension, type 2 diabetes and dyslipidaemia.

Endothelium Interconnected layer of cells that coat the inside of blood vessels, the lymph system and the inside of the heart. (In this book, it only refers to the cellular layer in the blood vessel.)

Energy-dense foods Foods with a high calorie content per unit of weight. Typically, the term refers to processed foods that are high in sugar, starch or fat and low in micronutrients.

Energy percent (E%), percentage of the total dietary energy consumption.

Epidemiology The study of the incidence (occurrence) and prevalence (distribution) of diseases in the population in relation to measurable factors such as blood pressure or dietary habits. Epidemiological studies are most often observational studies, i.e. the surrounding environment is studied as it is, without intervening in it.

Epithelial cell cancer Cancer radiating from the epithelial cells, a large group of cancers that most often cover the surfaces of glands or build up on the surface of them; the most common forms of epithelial cell cancer include breast cancer, prostate cancer and colorectal cancer.

Essential amino acids Amino acids that are necessary for normal life functions but cannot be formed by an organism. The term generally applies to animals since bacteria and plants, in most cases, can form all 20 amino acids that are included in proteins. The essential amino acids for humans include arginine, phenylalanine, histidine, isoleucine, lysine, methionine, threonine, tryptophan and valine.

Evidence-based medicine EBM, trend in academic medicine without connections to the industry (1) based on clinical and patient-related issues and not just those that research by chance becomes interested in, (2) places easily accessible and continuously updated knowledge bases at the disposal of the clinic and (3) in cases where systematic compilations are absent, they provide the tools needed for each doctor to gain an acceptable understanding of answer to his or her clinical question. Some of the founders of the movement have defined EBM as, 'the conscientious, explicit, and judicious use of current best evidence in making decisions about the care of individual patients'[1551].

Excretion The elimination or expelling of waste matter. Undigested food residues are excreted in faeces, while the waste products of metabolism are excreted by the liver and kidneys.

Explanatory variables In medical statistics, the factor(s) that explain the variation in sickness in a population. For example, blood pressure is one of the explanatory factors behind stroke, i.e. blood pressure and the risk of stroke covary.

Extinct Having no living members.

Fasting insulin The amount of serum insulin in a fasting person.

Fatty liver Liver steatosis, fatty degeneration in the liver; abnormal accumulation of fat in the liver cells (hepatocytes). Most often caused by lipotoxicity/insulin resistance. Can also be caused by overconsumption of alcohol.

Ferritin A protein that absorbs and stores iron.

Fibrinolysis Enzymatic dissolution of blood clots; a process in the body that combats blood coagulation.

Fibrosis Increased storage of connective tissue.

Fitness An organism's ability to survive and reproduce in a particular environment.

Folate The salt of folic acid, a vitamin.

Follicle Smaller, bag-shaped hole, e.g. hair follicle or ovarian follicle.

Follicular Referring to the follicle.

Forage To obtain food, to search (widely) for food.

Founder population A small parent population with distinctive genetic feature(s), emerging from a larger population.

Frequency formula Food frequency questionnaire, questionnaire to be completed indicating how often and how much a person eats of a certain food.

Funnel plot A scatter graph showing the relationship, in a meta-analysis of randomised controlled trials, between treatment effect and some measure of trial weight, such as sample size or standard error.

Gastrointestinal tract Relating to the stomach and intestines (gut).

GI See Glycaemic index.

Glitazones Thiazolidenediones; a group of drugs that intensify the effects of insulin and improve the use of glucose in the musculature, while halting the creation of new glucose in the liver; used primarily for type 2 diabetes.

Glucose A simple sugar that is an important energy source for living organisms; a component of starch and other carbohydrates.

Glucose tolerance The body's capacity to metabolise (dietary) glucose. Impaired glucose tolerance, or glucose intolerance, leads to high levels of blood sugar after a carbohydrate-rich meal. Most often, insulin resistance is present (see this term). Approximately one-third of people with glucose intolerance later develop diabetes, one-third become normalised, while the remainder continue to have impaired glucose tolerance. Glucose intolerance, which is a risk factor for cardiovascular disease, is present in most patients with ischaemic heart disease and stroke.

Glucose tolerance test Laboratory test to determine the body's glucose tolerance (see this term). The blood sugar on an empty stomach is measured, and then a 75-g glucose solution is ingested, usually per-orally (through the mouth, i.e. drunk). The blood sugar is checked one or several times thereafter for up to 2 hours. In the intravenous glucose tolerance test, glucose is injected instead of drunk.

Gluten A mixture of two proteins in some cereal grains, one of which causes gluten intolerance. In wheat, the responsible protein is gliadin while in rye and barley they are, respectively, secalin and hordein. The other protein is glutenin, which is important for baking properties of leavened bread.

Glycaemic index GI, indicates how quickly and how high the blood sugar rises after consuming carbohydrate foods. The blood sugar is measured repeatedly after a person has ingested a quantity that is estimated to contain 50 g of digestible carbohydrates. The area between the starting value and the final blood glucose curve is an expression of the GI, which is expressed numerically in relation to a corresponding area after consuming 50 g of pure glucose which is set to $GI = 100$ (sometimes white bread makes up the reference level).

Glycaemic load Glycaemic index (see this term) multiplied by the total amount of carbohydrates in the meal. If high glycaemic index foods are rich in water and fibre, they may exert a rather low glycaemic load.

Glycation The attachment of sugar residues on proteins; a proposed cause of various inflammatory and toxic conditions.

Glycoalkaloids A group of alkaloids that are found in potatoes and tomatoes in the form of α-chaconine and α-solanine (these are also called solanidine glycosides).

HbA1c Glycated haemoglobin; provides diabetics with a picture of their average blood sugar over the past few weeks.

HDL High-density lipoprotein; particles in the blood that transport blood lipids, primarily cholesterol. The risk of cardiovascular disease drops with rising concentration of HDL cholesterol, and hence the name 'good' cholesterol.

Haemochromatosis Unhealthy storage of iron in various organs of the body.

Herbivore An animal that feeds on plants.

Heterocyclic amines The substances that are formed during frying or grilling food and which have been shown to produce cancer in animal experiments.

Heterozygote In terms of a particular hereditary trait (e.g. eye colour or carrier of haemochromatosis), a heterozygote is the individual who carries different genes in the chromosomal pair in question. This differs from homozygotes who have double sets of the gene. Heterozygote carriers often have no or mild symptoms of the disease.

Histochemistry Science that combines biochemical and histological methods to identify, localise and, if possible, determine the amount of various substances in the microscopic building blocks of the tissues, particularly in the cells.

Histology The study of tissue; study of the microscopic structure of normal tissues (cell types, interstitial material and fibrous structures, architecture, as well as the structural and functional coordination of the cells). The term is often used synonymously with microscopic anatomy (in reality, the microscopic structure of the organ) and also includes cytology in this case (study of cells).

Histopathology The study of unhealthy changes in the tissues of the body. The term is now used only in a limited sense to indicate the method of diagnosing disease from microscopic slices of tissue either during an autopsy or in samples from living persons (biopsy).

HLA Human leucocyte antigen; a system of hereditary, tissue-bound structures that can constitute an antigen for the recipient during transplantation. The HLA genotype also affects the risk for autoimmune reactions.

Hominin Hominid, a primate of the family of humans and their bipedal ancestors, including various species of Homo, Australopithecus and Ardipithecus. The term is increasingly replacing the older word 'hominid', which often includes chimps and gorillas. Unfortunately, some researchers refer to these as hominins. Thus, at present, both terms are not precisely defined. Gräslund has employed the family name *Prehomo* for all early human ancestors living between 6 and 2 million years ago (until the emergence of *Homo*).

Hunter-gatherer lifestyle The traditional prehistoric human lifestyle, where meat, fish, fruits, vegetables, nuts, leaves and shellfish, in varying proportions, were staple foods.

Hyaline Structureless, transparent substance without inflammatory cells that are formed by breaking down body tissue.

Hyaline sclerosis Hyaline storage and necrosis in small arteries and arterioles, very common in the heart musculature of dogs. In humans, a form of hyaline sclerosis develops in the smaller blood vessels of the kidneys in patients with diabetes or hypertension.

Hydrolysis Chemical breakdown of a substance through reaction with water.

Hyperinsulinaemia Elevated concentration of insulin in plasma, often secondary to insulin resistance; risk factor for type 2 diabetes and cardiovascular disease.

Hyperplasia Enlargement of the organs through increased number of (normal-sized) cells in a tissue (cf. hypertrophy). Unhealthy hyperplasia can contribute to the development of tumours.

Hypertrophy Organ enlargement through increased cell size, without the addition of new cells (cf. hyperplasia). The increase in the size of individual cells is connected to the new production of cell components and is not solely the result of cellular swelling (absorption of fluids). Sometimes hypertrophy is a physiological response to increased performance requirements, e.g. increase in the muscle mass during training.

Hypertension High blood pressure.

IGF-1 Insulin-like growth factor-1, somatomedin C; the body's own hormone with effects similar to growth hormone and insulin.

In vitro Indicates that experiment or observation is made in a reaction vessel, test tube, petri dish, etc., and not in a living body (in vivo).

Impaired fasting glucose Slightly increased blood/plasma/serum glucose when 2-hour glucose is normal at the oral glucose tolerance test; fasting plasma glucose 6.1–6.9 mmol/L and 2-hour plasma glucose <7.8 mmol/L.

Incidence A measure used in epidemiology for the occurrence of a disease within a population; the incidence indicates how many new cases occur during a certain period of time within a specific population group. See Prevalence.

Induce Call forth, cause, start.

Intestinal permeability Ability of large molecules that have not been broken down to pass through the intestinal mucous membrane.

Intravenous treatment Injection of medicine directly into the blood veins.

Initiation First state in the development of cancer caused by a carcinogenic substance; includes pre-neoplastic changes in the cell's genetic material.

Insulin An anabolic (body-building) hormone that facilitates the storage of glucose, fat and protein in certain tissues. It is formed in β-cells in the Langerhans' islet cells of the pancreas.

Insulin sensitivity See Insulin resistance.

Insulin resistance Reduced sensitivity to insulin in the receiving tissues, which can lead to the so-called metabolic syndrome with abdominal obesity, hypertension, dyslipidaemia, reduced glucose tolerance and type 2 diabetes. It can also contribute to excessive tissue growth and abnormal height, early puberty, myopia, acne, infertility, prostate enlargementand certain common forms of cancer (see Section 4.6).

Intervention Treatment or similar action to produce a given effect, such as reduced risk of becoming sick (see Randomisation).

Ischaemic heart disease Heart disease caused by atherosclerosis of the coronary vessels of the heart; includes myocardial infarction, angina pectoris and silent myocardial ischaemia, i.e. insufficient blood supply to heart musculature without chest pain.

L Litre

Lactase Enzyme found in the mucous membrane of the small intestines that breaks down lactose in the food.

Lactose Milk sugar, a disaccharide made from galactose and glucose.

LDL Low-density lipoprotein, particles in the blood that transport blood lipids, especially cholesterol. The risk of cardiovascular disease increases with rising concentration of LDL cholesterol, hence the name 'bad' cholesterol.

LDL/HDL ratio The ratio between the concentration of LDL and HDL cholesterol in the blood; the higher the ratio, the lower the risk for cardiovascular disease.

LDL oxidation Oxidation of LDL molecules in the blood vessel wall that is then thought to gradually cause hardening of the arteries.

Lectin See Plant lectin.

Left ventricular hypertrophy Enlargement of the heart's left chamber.

Lipoprotein Particles in the blood which transport fats and lipids.

Lymphocyte A type of white blood cell that is part of the body's immune response.

Lymphoma Generic term for malignant tumours originating from the lymphocytes in the lymphatic tissue; often originates in the throat.

Macronutrient Energy-providing nutrient: protein, fat or carbohydrate (alcohol is usually not included although it also provides energy). Macronutrient composition refers to the proportion of fat, carbohydrate and protein in a food (alcohol is usually not included).

Malignant Dangerous, deadly; used primarily for cancer.

Median The value that divides a set of ordinal data into two equal parts, i.e. there are the same number of values above the median as below it. See Quartile.

Menarche Age of first menstruation.

Menopause The ceasing of menstruation; the period in a woman's life when this occurs (typically between 45 and 50 years of age).

Meta-analysis A combined analysis of all published studies that compare a certain treatment, often after excluding those studies that do not meet certain scientific requirements. The strength of the analysis is that the number of trial subjects increases, which reduces the number of random factors. The weakness is the effect of error sources (see Section 3.2), which can be intensified if they recur in multiple studies. For example, health-conscious Westerners in different countries can have the same misunderstanding of what should be eaten, which can intensify the effect of confounders.

Metabolism Conversion of substances in the body; all biological reactions that take place in living organisms.

Metabolite A substance formed by metabolism of another, primary substance.

Metformin A drug against type 2 diabetes.

Microvilli Fibrous growths of the membrane on certain cells of the surface of the mucous membrane, which gives it the appearance of a tightly clipped brush. This greatly increases the surface of the cell, which is significant in terms of exchanging substances between the cell's insides and the surrounding area, e.g. in the intestines.

Mineral density See Nutritient density.

Mitogenic Causing cell division (mitosis).

Mitosis The most common form of cell division.

mmol Millimole, thousandth mol; SI unit for amount of a substance.

Monosaccharide The basic sugar unit of disaccharides and complex carbohydrates; consists of glucose, fructose, galactose and maltose.

Monounsaturated fat Unsaturated fatty acid with a double bond; the most commonly occurring fatty acid in nature, which is the dominant fatty acid in olive oil.

Mortality Death rate.

MRI Magnetic resonance tomography; radiological diagnostic method that is primarily used to diagnose diseases in the brain, spinal marrow, as well as slipped discs and tumours in the skeleton and musculature.

n Abbreviation of number, such as number of subjects in a study in humans.

Negative correlation The more of one thing, the less of the other (see Correlation).

Nested case–control study An observational study where cases and controls are taken from within a cohort study.

NOD Non-obese diabetic mouse, a mouse with a high incidence of type 1 diabetes.

Normal distribution Distribution of large group of randomly selected measurements, which in a biological context, are regularly distributed in such a way that the graphic image forms bell-shaped mathematical curve, the so-called Gauss curve. Body height, e.g., has a perfectly normal distribution, while body weight and many other biological variables must be put through logarithms before they display a normal distribution.

Nutrient density Concentration of nutrients calculated per unit of energy (kcal, MH) instead of per unit of weight.

Nutrients The substances that are part of food and are needed for the body's normal metabolism. They can be divided into those that primarily provide energy (energy-producing nutrients) and those that are needed to cover the body's energy needs. There are also those that are needed for growth (growth and maintenance) of tissues, and which cannot be formed in the body (essential nutrients), e.g. proteins and certain fatty acids, vitamins and minerals. Nutrients are often divided into macronutrients, i.e. those that occur in large amounts (e.g. proteins, fats, carbohydrates, calcium) and micronutrients, which are only needed in very small amounts, e.g. trace elements and vitamins. The energy-producing nutrients include carbohydrates, fats and proteins, and even alcohol.

Nut (1) Type of plant fruit, characterised by being dry and usually having a single seed. It does not open when it ripens; rather the entire fruit is spread around and opens when the seed starts to germinate. Sometimes the nuts have wings (as with birch trees) or brush-like structures (as with dandelions), which allows them to be spread by wind. Some nuts have spurs, which makes them stick to animal fur. Some fruits that are commonly called nuts, e.g. coconut and walnuts, are not nuts in the botanical sense.

Nut (2) Fruit, which when ripe, consists of an (often brown) hard, dry shell and an (often) edible fat core with a mild taste and which falls from trees or bushes unopened.

Observation study See Epidemiology.

Odds ratio The odds of an event occurring in one group divided by the odds in a reference group. An approximate estimate of relative risk in case–control studies (of rare events).

Omega-3 fatty acids The type of polyunsaturated fatty acids that are typical for fish and that are thought to protect against cardiovascular disease.

Oligopeptide Peptide which is made up of 10–20 amino acids. The limit up towards polypeptides is therefore fluid.

Oral glucose tolerance test See Glucose tolerance test.

Optimal Best or most favourable.

Osteoclast Cells that help break down bone tissue, which is a condition for normal metabolism and creation of new bone tissue. Osteoclast activity is stimulated by several factors, especially PTH and vitamin D.

Osteology The study of the vertebrate skeleton. Comparative osteology has a close connection to Palaeontology. Functional osteology deals with the shape of the skeleton in terms of function. Osteology is also used to determine the species from animal remains, e.g., in archaeological excavations (historical osteology) from the dung of wild animals, and crime scene investigations. Human osteology, i.e. the study of the human skeleton, is very important in the field of archaeological research.

Osteoporosis A disease with brittle bone; the most common cause of low-trauma fractures in elderly Westerners.

Lacto-ovo-vegetarian Person who does not eat meat or fish, but eats eggs and dairy products.

P Probability; a number between 0 and 1 that indicates the different outcomes of a random trial. If $P = 0.09$, there are 9 chances in 100 that the findings were the result of chance. The limit for statistical significance is often set to $P < 0.05$, where the chance is less than 1 in 100 that the findings were random.

p **for trend** The probability that there is a continuous and graded relationship between an explanatory variable, e.g. nut intake, and outcome, e.g. risk, for myocardial infarction.

PAI-1 Plasminogen activator inhibitor 1, a substance that contributes to clot formation and increases with metabolic syndrome.

Palaeolithic Old Stone Age; archaeological period covering the time between when humans started making tools, approximately 2.3 million years ago and the end of the last Ice Age, approximately 10 000 years ago.

Pancreas Organ that produces enzymes to break down the fat in various foods (lipase), starch (amylase), sugar (maltase) and protein (trypsinogen), as well as hormones such as insulin and glucagon, which are secreted in the blood and regulate blood sugar level.

Parathyroid glands (*Glandulae parathyreoideae*), pea-sized glands on the back side of the thyroid that produce parathyroid hormones (PTH). Internal secretion of PTH increases with falling calcium concentrations and vice versa. PTH increases the amount of calcium in the blood by increasing the absorption of calcium from the skeleton and intestines in conjunction with vitamin D, and reduces the amount of phosphate in the blood by increasing the urinary secretions.

Parathyroid hormone See Parathyroid glands.

Pathogenesis How a disease develops and grows.

PCO See Polycystic ovaries.

Peptide Chemical compound that consists of two or more amino acids, united through peptide bonds. Many peptides are created due to incomplete breakdown of proteins.

Peripheral arterial disease Disease of the large arteries in the legs or, more rarely, the arms; involves primarily reduced circulation due to atherosclerosis.

Permeability Ability to penetrate something.

Personal communication Piece of information given informally or at a conference, as opposed to published, peer-reviewed data.

Person-years Measure of incidence; indicates the number of persons per year. Often the number of people suffering from a disease is given per 100 000 person-years, i.e. per 100 000 persons per year.

Pesticides Chemical agents commonly used to protect plants against pests, similar to herbicides, fungicides and insecticides.

Phytate See Phytic acid.

Phytic acid Hexaphosphoric acid ester of meso-inositol; occurs in nature as calcium and magnesium salts; phytates. These appear to a large extent in plant seeds, where they probably constitute a way of storing phosphorus, which is released by the effect of the enzyme phytase when the seed germinates. A large amount of phytates in the food can inhibit the absorption of iron, calcium, zinc and magnesium from the digestive tract and thereby contribute to a lack of these minerals.

Phytochemicals Substances in (edible) plants which may be absorbed when ingested by humans and which are bioactive, i.e. have drug-like effects. In nutritional science they have generally been described as beneficial (or harmless), while plant ecologists often see them as part of the plant's defence system against herbivory.

Phytoestrogens Substances with oestrogenic or, in some cases, anti-oestrogenic effects that are formed by certain plants (phyto = plant); part of the larger group xenoestrogens (DDT metabolites, certain dioxins, etc.). The two main classes of phytoestrogens are the isoflavones (e.g. genistein and daidzein in soya) and the lignans.

Plant lectin Plant proteins that bind to certain type of sugar, and whose most important function is to protect against attack by plant-eating animals. The highest concentration is found in seeds, beans, potatoes and peanuts. Plant lectins are resistant to breakdown in the stomach/intestinal tract and can penetrate the mucous membrane of the intestines and become deposited in the internal organs, where they are thought to have a long list of significant, negative consequences including atherosclerosis, insulin resistance, cancer and autoimmune reactions.

Plant sterols Sterols formed by plants; includes phytoestrogens, campesterol, sitosterol, etc.

Plaque A small raised patch, such as one caused by atherosclerosis, i.e. an atherosclerotic plaque.

Plasma The pale, yellow or grey-yellow, fluid portion of blood, as distinguished from the serum obtained after coagulation. Blood includes plasma and blood cells.

Platelet A type of cell in the blood involved in clotting.

Polyclonal Having many different cell clones, 'cell families'. Contact with an antigen normally affects many different B and T lymphocytes, which then propagate and form a polyclonal immune response.

Polycystic ovary syndrome PCOS, disease with numerous small cysts in the ovaries. Hormone production in the ovaries is disturbed with increased secretion of male sex hormones as a result. Normal ovulation cannot take place and infertility is common. Missed or scant menstruations are also common, as well as increased hair growth and abdominal obesity.

Polycyclic aromatic hydrocarbons PAH, the substances that are formed during frying or grilling food and which has been shown to produce cancer in animal experiments.

Polysaccharide Large carbohydrate molecules consisting of a large number of monosaccharides; the most common ones are cellulose, starch and glycogen.

Porosity The characteristic of a material being porous, filled with holes; defined as the volume of the holes by volume of the entire material.

Positive correlation The more of one thing, the more of the other (see Correlation).

Post hoc analysis A statistical term for an analysis that was not pre-specified in the original design of the study.

Postmenopausal After menopause.

Potassium density See Nutrient density.

Prevalence Term in epidemiology for the percentage of the population that has a certain disease for a certain period of time (see Incidence).

Primary prevention Preventive measures designed to prevent the occurrence of disease in healthy people, as opposed to secondary prevention aiming at hindering further progression of manifest disease.

Prospective study An epidemiological study where a group (cohort) of individuals are followed prospectively, i.e. forwards in time. A common approach in observational studies (cf. Case–control study).

Prostatic hyperplasia Enlargement of the prostate; appears in benign (benign prostatic hyperplasia) and malignant form (prostate cancer).

Proteoglycan A compound consisting of a protein bound to large carbohydrates (polysaccharides).

PTCA Percutaneous transluminal coronary angiography (per = trough; cutis = skin; trans = across/through/beyond; lumen = central cavity, in this case the artery; coronary = one of the arteries that surround and supply the heart; angio- = relating to blood vessels; graphia = writing), X-ray of the blood vessels after injection of a radiopaque substance through a catheter introduced into the coronary arteries of the heart.

PTH Parathyroid hormone (see Parathyroid).

Publication bias Source of errors because published studies do not necessarily display the same results as those that are not published; the results from studies that do not support a researcher's results, e.g., may be published more seldom.

PubMed A free search engine for accessing the MEDLINE database of citations and abstracts of biomedical research articles.

Pulmonary Of or relating to the lungs (pulmones).

Quartile The value in statistical material that indicates the top or bottom 25% of values. The bottom quartile, the median and the top quartile divide the material into four equal parts. The first quartile constitutes the 25% with the lowest value, the second quartile are those with higher values up to the median, and so forth.

Quintile The value in statistical material that indicates the top or bottom 20% of values. The four quintiles divide the material into five equally large (fifths).

r, R^2 See Correlation.

Rickets Rachitis; older name was 'English disease', skeletal disease due to insufficient calcification of newly formed organic bone tissue.

Randomisation Random distribution of a material (e.g. trial subjects) in order to compare different forms of treatment.

Randomised controlled trial RCT, A random process determines who receives the new treatment (intervention group) and who receives an inactive treatment (placebo) or an older, established treatment (control group).

Receptor Either structure on/in cells or cell/cell systems designed to capture and transmit signals. Specific substances bind to the receptor which either activate (agonists) or block its effects (antagonists).

Regress Moving in reverse, in this sense, removing the formation of hardened arteries.

Renal Of or relating to the kidneys.

Relative risk The risk of a study group becoming ill divided by the risk of a control group. A relative risk of 1.0 means an equally high risk in both groups, and thereby no effect of the studied intervention or exposition, while a relative risk of 0.75 means 25% reduced risk. Relative risk is synonymous to risk ratio. In this textbook, the mean relative risk is generally presented in conjunction with its 95% confidence interval (see Confidence interval), i.e. relative risk 0.80 (0.64–0.97).

Replication Lat. *Replica'tio* 'repetition', 'circulation', 'circular motion', from *re'plico* meaning 'reproduce', 'unroll', 'unfold'. In the event of replication, the chemical bonds between both strands of the DNA coils are broken, and function as templates for the creation of new DNA by means of the enzyme DNA polymerase. The result is two identical DNA molecules with one old and one newly formed strand. Replication of the total genetic make-up of the cell is a preparatory stage for cell division, while smaller parts of the genetic material are replicated to repair incorrect or damaged DNA.

Residual confounding See Confounder.

Retinoids Natural and synthetic A-vitamin analogues which inhibit cell proliferation and facilitate apoptosis (programmed cell death).

Retinoid receptors Receptors in the cell nucleus that are divided into retinoic acid receptors (RAR) and retinoid X receptors (RXR). The body's natural retinoids (*trans*-retinol acid and 9-*cis*-retinol acid) work by binding to these two receptor families. Retinol receptors activate genetic transcription by bonding as RAR/RXR heterodimers or RXR homodimers to elements in the promoter region of the target genes, whose function is to limit the growth of certain types of cells.

Retrosternal Behind the breast bone (sternum).

Rheumatoid factor Antibodies against immunoglobulins; appear especially with rheumatoid arthritis.

Rheumatoid arthritis RA, chronic rheumatism of the joints, a joint disease with chronic inflammation in the joint capsule, leading to deterioration of adjacent articular cartilage and bone tissue.

Risk compensation Increased risk-taking behaviour among people randomised to a certain kind of lifestyle change, due to the feeling of belonging to the best of two or more comparable groups.

Rodent A gnawing mammal of an order that includes rats, mice, squirrels, hamsters, porcupines and their relatives, distinguished by their strong, constantly growing front teeth and no canine teeth.

Sarcopenia Loss of skeletal muscle mass, usually referring to age-related loss.

Satiation Satisfaction of appetite to the full; the process of bringing eating to an end. It mainly affects the amount of food eaten at that particular meal.

Satiety The feeling of fullness between meals. The higher satiety, the longer appetite is suppressed and the less likely a person is to eat between meals.

Saturated fat Fat with a high percentage of saturated fatty acids, i.e. those that are missing double bonds in their carbon chains. Saturated fat occurs foremost in dairy products and animal depot fat (lard).

Sclera The outer layer of the wall of the eyeball (apart from the front of the eyeball) consisting of strong connective tissue.

Secondary prevention Preventive treatment in the case of established diseases (e.g. myocardial infarction) in order to prevent becoming ill again (e.g. another heart attack).

Selection pressure Within the field of evolution, it means partly the impact that environmental factors have on a population which leads to natural selection, and partly the intensity of natural selection, measured, e.g., as the change in the frequency of a gene from one generation to another.

Serum Yellowish fluid that is extracted when blood is slowly compressed. Serum contains almost all the components of blood plasma except for fibrinogen. Most clinical-chemical laboratory tests are performed on serum, which is marked with S-, e.g. S-cholesterol.

Seven Countries Study A famous, international epidemiological, observation study, which was one of the first to study, on an international level, the possible relationships between eating habits and cardiovascular disease. The countries in the study included both Crete and Japan, which were found to have a particularly low risk of ischaemic heart disease.

Sickle cell anaemia Genetic lack of blood due to unusual haemoglobin structure. The disease is common in areas with widespread malaria. Heterozygous carriers have increased resistance to malaria, and have thereby had an survival advantage during evolution.

Significant A difference or a relationship is statistically significant if it is improbable that it is the result of chance (see P).

Single-blind study A comparative study where the test managers, but not the test subjects, know who receives which treatment. This is in contrast to double-blind study, where neither of the parties involved knows.

Squamous cell Flat cells in a single layer or multiple layers that line many of the body's surfaces, e.g. the skin.

Squamous cell carcinoma Cancer that originates from the squamous cell. The organs where squamous cell cancer most commonly develops include the skin, cervix, lungs, trachea and oesophagus.

SLU Statens Lantbruksuniversitet (Swedish University of Agricultural Sciences).

Spinal cord A long bundle of nerves inside the vertebral column. It is connected to the brain with which it forms the central nervous system.

Spontaneously hypertensive Becoming spontaneously hypertensive, i.e. developing hypertension (high blood pressure). Somewhat of a misleading term that often refers to a special breed of rats that always develops high blood pressure, without exception, when fed salty food.

STA Solanum tuberosum agglutinin, potato lectin.

Standard deviation Statistical measure of the distribution of data; the larger the distribution, the lower the certainty of group comparisons.

Standard error A measure of the statistical accuracy of an estimate, equal to the standard deviation of the theoretical distribution of a large population of such estimates.

Starch A type of carbohydrate consisting of long chains of glucose. There are two forms of starch: amylopectin and amylose. Amylopectin, which constitutes 75–80% of starch in most plants, has a high GI, while amylose has a low GI.

Statins A type of medicine used for dyslipidaemia, e.g. Zocord, Pravachol and Lipitor.

Statistically significant A difference or a relationship is statistically significant if it is improbable that it is the result of chance (see *P*).

Sterols A subgroup of steroids, defined on the basis of certain structural details. In humans, cholesterol is the quantitatively dominant sterol.

Streptozotocin diabetic rats Rats who are rendered diabetic by use of streptozotocin, a toxic substance which destroys the insulin-producing β-cells of the pancreas; an animal model of type 1 diabetes.

Systolic blood pressure The upper value of the two, in, e.g., 140/90 mm Hg.

T-cell T-lymphocytes; lymphocytes that are responsible for a specific immune response transmitted via the cells, in contrast to B-lymphocytes, which form circulating antibodies.

Taurine A sulfur-containing amino acid important in the metabolism of fats.

Thermodynamics The study of the conversion of energy into heat and different forms of work (essentially mechanical work and chemical reactions).

Thoracic kyphosis Exaggerated backward arching of the thoracic spine in the direction of a hunchback.

TIA Transient ischaemic attack; ministroke; a temporary blockage of the blood supply to the brain with symptoms lasting a maximum of 1 hour, usually less than 5 min.

Trabecular bone The same as porous or spongeous bone; the part of the skeleton that is inside the compact (cortical) bone. Vertebrae consist mostly of trabecular bone. The bone-generating effects of oestrogen are more pronounced on trabecular bone rather than cortical bone.

Trace elements Micromineral substances, i.e. mineral substances that the body only needs in very small amounts, with a daily requirement of 1–2 mg down to microgram amounts. Trace elements in humans and animals include fluoride, iodine, iron, copper, chromium, manganese, molybdenum, selenium and zinc.

Transcription The process where information in the DNA is transmitted to messenger-RNA; a stage in gene expression before, e.g., protein synthesis.

Triceps skinfold For example, triceps skinfold thickness; the thickness of the skin folds over the triceps muscle on the backside of the upper arm measured with a so-called calliper. A measure of the amount of a person's subcutaneous fat.

Triglycerides Esters formed from glycerol and three fatty acids; the most common form of stored fat in the body.

Thymus Organ inside the breast bone made of lymphatic tissue. Grows during childhood, and is largest during puberty when it gradually regresses. Important for the maturation of T-lymphocytes, and the immunity to infection connected with cells.

Type 1 diabetes Insulin-dependant diabetes; characterised by a lack of insulin, debuts most often before the age of 35.

Type 2 diabetes Non-insulin-dependent diabetes, age-related diabetes, generally debuts after the age of 30.

Ultrasonography A technique using ultrasound echoes to identify objects of distinct density in the body (tumours, fetuses, etc.).

Urate Salts from uric acid. Elevated amount of urate in the blood can cause gout and is a risk factor for cardiovascular disease (see also Section 4.6 under 'Gout').

Uric acid Organic acid containing nitrogen, which is formed when the purine bases adenine and guanine (which are part of DNA and RNA) are broken down. Uric acid in humans and primates, which primarily appears as urate, is not metabolised further; urate is primarily secreted in the kidneys. In mammals other than primates, uric acid is converted to a soluble compound (allantoine) before being excreted. In birds and certain reptiles, whose liver is unable to bind urine substances, uric acid is the most important end product of protein metabolism.

Vascular Referring to the blood vessel.

Ventricular fibrillation Flickering of the ventricle; cardiac dysrhythmia that is due to disorganised electrical activity in the ventricles of the heart. The electrical activation signals in the ventricular musculature are irregular and very rapid, with a frequency of approximately 300–500 per minute. The mechanical activation of the ventricles is uncoordinated and is no longer able to pump out blood. Ventricular fibrillation is characterised by the sudden loss of consciousness and arrested arterial pulse and breath. It is the most common cause for sudden, unexpected death and often occurs in the initial hours after a heart attack.

Vertebra Each of the small bones forming the backbone, or the spine.

Western diseases Diseases, such as cardiovascular disease, obesity and diabetes, that are prevalent in Western societies and are thought to be more or less caused by a Western lifestyle.

WGA Wheat germ agglutinin, wheat lectin.

References

1. Anon (1985) A pathological survey of atherosclerotic lesions of coronary artery and aorta in China. A coordination group in China. *Pathol Res Pract* **180**, 457–62.
2. Anon (1998) Blood pressure, cholesterol, and stroke in eastern Asia. Eastern Stroke and Coronary Heart Disease Collaborative Research Group. *Lancet* **352**, 1801–7.
3. Anon (2000) *Nationella riktlinjer för strokesjukvård.* Socialstyrelsen, Stockholm.
4. Anon (2001) *Hälso- och sjukvårdsrapport 2001.* Socialstyrelsen, Stockholm.
5. Anon (2002) MRC/BHF Heart Protection Study of antioxidant vitamin supplementation in 20,536 high-risk individuals: a randomised placebo-controlled trial. *Lancet* **360**, 23–33.
6. Anon (2004) Final report of the amended safety assessment of Dioscorea Villosa (Wild Yam) root extract. *Int J Toxicol* **23** (Suppl 2), 49–54.
7. Anon (2007) *Food, nutrition and the prevention of cancer: a global perspective.* World Cancer Research Fund in association with American Institute for Cancer Research, Washington, DC.
8. Anon (2007) Nutrition recommendations and interventions for diabetes: a position statement of the American Diabetes Association. *Diabetes Care* **30** (Suppl 1), S48–65.
9. Abate, N. & Chandalia, M. (2001) Ethnicity and type 2 diabetes: focus on Asian Indians. *J Diabetes Complications* **15**, 320–7.
10. Abbott, R.D., Wilson, P.W., Kannel, W.B. & Castelli, W.P. (1988) High density lipoprotein cholesterol, total cholesterol screening, and myocardial infarction. The Framingham Study. *Arteriosclerosis* **8**, 207–11.
11. Abel, E.D., Litwin, S.E. & Sweeney, G. (2008) Cardiac remodeling in obesity. *Physiol Rev* **88**, 389–419.
12. Abete, I., Parra, D. & Martinez, J.A. (2008) Energy-restricted diets based on a distinct food selection affecting the glycemic index induce different weight loss and oxidative response. *Clin Nutr* **27**, 545–51.
13. Adam-Perrot, A., Clifton, P. & Brouns, F. (2006) Low-carbohydrate diets: nutritional and physiological aspects. *Obes Rev* **7**, 49–58.
14. Adams, K.F., Schatzkin, A., Harris, T.B., *et al.* (2006) Overweight, obesity, and mortality in a large prospective cohort of persons 50 to 71 years old. *N Engl J Med* **355**, 763–78.
15. Adams, L.A. & Angulo, P. (2005) Recent concepts in non-alcoholic fatty liver disease. *Diabet Med* **22**, 1129–33.

16. Adams, M.R., Golden, D.L., Anthony, M.S., Register, T.C. & Williams, J.K. (2002) The inhibitory effect of soy protein isolate on atherosclerosis in mice does not require the presence of LDL receptors or alteration of plasma lipoproteins. *J Nutr* **132**, 43–9.

17. Adebajo, A.O., Cooper, C. & Evans, J.G. (1991) Fractures of the hip and distal forearm in West Africa and the United Kingdom. *Age Ageing* **20**, 435–8.

18. Adeli, K., Taghibiglou, C., Van Iderstine, S.C. & Lewis, G.F. (2001) Mechanisms of hepatic very low-density lipoprotein overproduction in insulin resistance. *Trends Cardiovasc Med* **11**, 170–6.

19. Agarwal, S.C. & Grynpas, M.D. (1996) Bone quantity and quality in past populations. *Anat Rec* **246**, 423–32.

20. Aguilera, C.M., Ramirez-Tortosa, M.C., Mesa, M.D., Ramirez-Tortosa, C.L. & Gil, A. (2002) Sunflower, virgin-olive and fish oils differentially affect the progression of aortic lesions in rabbits with experimental atherosclerosis. *Atherosclerosis* **162**, 335–44.

21. Ahima, R.S. & Osei, S.Y. (2004) Leptin signaling. *Physiol Behav* **81**, 223–41.

22. Ahmed, M.E. (1990) Blood pressure in a multiracial urban Sudanese community. *J Hum Hypertens* **4**, 621–4.

23. Ahn, J., Schatzkin, A., Lacey, J.V., Jr., *et al.* (2007) Adiposity, adult weight change, and postmenopausal breast cancer risk. *Arch Intern Med* **167**, 2091–102.

24. Aiken, G.H., Lytton, D.G. & Everingham, S. (1974) Atherosclerotic heart disease in urbanised Papua New Guineans. *P N G Med J* **17**, 248–50.

25. Aizawa, H. & Niimura, M. (1995) Elevated serum insulin-like growth factor-1 (IGF-1) levels in women with postadolescent acne. *J Dermatol* **22**, 249–52.

26. Aizawa, H. & Niimura, M. (1996) Mild insulin resistance during oral glucose tolerance test (OGTT) in women with acne. *J Dermatol* **23**, 526–9.

27. Akbas, G.E., Fei, X. & Taylor, H.S. (2007) Regulation of HOXA10 expression by phytoestrogens. *Am J Physiol Endocrinol Metab* **292**, E435–42.

28. Åkerblom, H.K., Vaarala, O., Hyoty, H., Ilonen, J. & Knip, M. (2002) Environmental factors in the etiology of type 1 diabetes. *Am J Med Genet* **115**, 18–29.

29. Al-Bander, S.Y., Nix, L., Katz, R., Korn, M. & Sebastian, A. (1988) Food chloride distribution in nature and its relation to sodium content. *J Am Diet Assoc* **88**, 472–5.

30. Al-Marzouki, S., Evans, S., Marshall, T. & Roberts, I. (2005) Are these data real? Statistical methods for the detection of data fabrication in clinical trials. *BMJ* **331**, 267–70.

31. Albert, C.M., Gaziano, J.M., Willett, W.C. & Manson, J.E. (2002) Nut consumption and decreased risk of sudden cardiac death in the physicians' health study. *Arch Intern Med* **162**, 1382–7.

32. Alberts, D.S., Martinez, M.E., Roe, D.J., *et al.* (2000) Lack of effect of a high-fiber cereal supplement on the recurrence of colorectal adenomas. Phoenix Colon Cancer Prevention Physicians' Network. *N Engl J Med* **342**, 1156–62.

33. Alderman, M.H. (2006) Evidence relating dietary sodium to cardiovascular disease. *J Am Coll Nutr* **25**, 256S–61S.

34. Alexander, J.K. (1985) The cardiomyopathy of obesity. *Prog Cardiovasc Dis* **27**, 325–34.

35. Alexander, J.K. (2001) Obesity and coronary heart disease. *Am J Med Sci* **321**, 215–24.

36. Alexy, U., Kersting, M. & Remer, T. (2007) Potential renal acid load in the diet of children and adolescents: impact of food groups, age and time trends. *Public Health Nutr*, 1–7.

37. Alexy, U., Remer, T., Manz, F., Neu, C.M. & Schoenau, E. (2005) Long-term protein intake and dietary potential renal acid load are associated with bone modeling and remodeling at the proximal radius in healthy children. *Am J Clin Nutr* **82**, 1107–14.

38. Allbaugh, L.G. (1953) *Crete: a case study of an undeveloped country.* Princeton University Press, Princeton.

39. Allen, J.S. & Cheer, S.M. (1996) The non-thrifty genotype. *Curr Anthropol* **37**, 831–42.

40. Allen, T.J., Waldron, M.J., Casley, D., Jerums, G. & Cooper, M.E. (1997) Salt restriction reduces hyperfiltration, renal enlargement, and albuminuria in experimental diabetes. *Diabetes* **46**, 19–24.

41. Allison, D.B., Zannolli, R., Faith, M.S., *et al.* (1999) Weight loss increases and fat loss decreases all-cause mortality rate: results from two independent cohort studies. *Int J Obes Relat Metab Disord* **23**, 603–11.

42. Allred, C.D., Allred, K.F., Ju, Y.H., Virant, S.M. & Helferich, W.G. (2001) Soy diets containing varying amounts of genistein stimulate growth of estrogen-dependent (MCF-7) tumors in a dose-dependent manner. *Cancer Res* **61**, 5045–50.

43. Allsop, K.A. & Miller, J.B. (1996) Honey revisited: a reappraisal of honey in pre-industrial diets. *Br J Nutr* **75**, 513–20.

44. Alpert, J.S., Goldberg, R., Ockene, I.S. & Taylor, P. (1991) Heart disease in native Americans. *Cardiology* **78**, 3–12.

45. Altman, D.G. (1991) *Practical statistics for medical research*. Chapman and Hall, London.

46. Amarenco, P., Bogousslavsky, J., Callahan, A., 3rd, *et al.* (2006) High-dose atorvastatin after stroke or transient ischemic attack. *N Engl J Med* **355**, 549–59.

47. Ambard, L. & Beaujard, E. (1904) Causes de l'hypertension arterielle. *Arch Gen Med* **1**, 520–33.

48. Ames, B.N., Magaw, R. & Gold, L.S. (1987) Ranking possible carcinogenic hazards. *Science* **236**, 271–80.

49. Amling, C.L. (2004) The association between obesity and the progression of prostate and renal cell carcinoma. *Urol Oncol* **22**, 478–84.

50. An, D. & Rodrigues, B. (2006) Role of changes in cardiac metabolism in development of diabetic cardiomyopathy. *Am J Physiol Heart Circ Physiol* **291**, H1489–506.

51. Anderson, J.W., Johnstone, B.M. & Cook-Newell, M.E. (1995) Meta-analysis of the effects of soy protein intake on serum lipids [see comments]. *N Engl J Med* **333**, 276–82.

52. Andersson, A., Tengblad, S., Karlstrom, B., *et al.* (2007) Whole-grain foods do not affect insulin sensitivity or markers of lipid peroxidation and inflammation in healthy, moderately overweight subjects. *J Nutr* **137**, 1401–7.

53. Andreasen, N., Blennow, K., Sjodin, C., Winblad, B. & Svardsudd, K. (1999) Prevalence and incidence of clinically diagnosed memory impairments in a geographically defined general population in Sweden. The Pitea Dementia Project. *Neuroepidemiology* **18**, 144–55.

54. Anker, S.D., Leyva, F., Poole-Wilson, P.A. & Coats, A.J.S. (1998) Uric acid independent predictor of impaired prognosis in patients with chronic heart failure. *J Am Coll Cardiol* **31**, 154A.

55. Anker, S.D., Ponikowski, P., Varney, S., *et al.* (1997) Wasting as independent risk factor for mortality in chronic heart failure. *Lancet* **349**, 1050–3.

56. Anthony, M.S., Clarkson, T.B., Bullock, B.C. & Wagner, J.D. (1997) Soy protein versus soy phytoestrogens in the prevention of diet-induced coronary artery atherosclerosis of male cynomolgus monkeys. *Arterioscler Thromb Vasc Biol* **17**, 2524–31.

57. Anthony, M.S., Clarkson, T.B. & Williams, J.K. (1998) Effects of soy isoflavones on atherosclerosis: potential mechanisms. *Am J Clin Nutr* **68**, 1390S–3S.

58. Appel, L.J., Brands, M.W., Daniels, S.R., *et al.* (2006) Dietary approaches to prevent and treat hypertension: a scientific statement from the American Heart Association. *Hypertension* **47**, 296–308.

59. Appel, L.J., Champagne, C.M., Harsha, D.W., *et al.* (2003) Effects of comprehensive lifestyle modification on blood pressure control: main results of the PREMIER clinical trial. *JAMA* **289**, 2083–93.

60. Appel, L.J., Espeland, M.A., Easter, L., *et al.* (2001) Effects of reduced sodium intake on hypertension control in older individuals: results from the Trial of Nonpharmacologic Interventions in the Elderly (TONE). *Arch Intern Med* **161**, 685–93.

61. Appel, L.J., Moore, T.J., Obarzanek, E., *et al.* (1997) A clinical trial of the effects of dietary patterns on blood pressure. DASH Collaborative Research Group. *N Engl J Med* **336**, 1117–24.

62. Appel, L.J., Sacks, F.M., Carey, V.J., *et al.* (2005) Effects of protein, monounsaturated fat, and carbohydrate intake on blood pressure and serum lipids: results of the OmniHeart randomized trial. *JAMA* **294**, 2455–64.

63. Appleby, P.N., Key, T.J., Thorogood, M., Burr, M.L. & Mann, J. (2002) Mortality in British vegetarians. *Public Health Nutr* **5**, 29–36.

64. Aradhana, Rao, A.R. & Kale, R.K. (1992) Diosgenin – a growth stimulator of mammary gland of ovariectomized mouse. *Indian J Exp Biol* **30**, 367–70.

65. Araneta, M.R., Wingard, D.L. & Barrett-Connor, E. (2002) Type 2 diabetes and metabolic syndrome in Filipina-American women: a high-risk nonobese population. *Diabetes Care* **25**, 494–9.

66. Araujo, E.P., De Souza, C.T., Gasparetti, A.L., *et al.* (2005) Short-term in vivo inhibition of insulin receptor substrate-1 expression leads to insulin resistance, hyperinsulinemia, and increased adiposity. *Endocrinology* **146**, 1428–37.

67. Arcaro, G., Cretti, A., Balzano, S., *et al.* (2002) Insulin causes endothelial dysfunction in humans: sites and mechanisms. *Circulation* **105**, 576–82.

68. Arcini, C. (1999) *Health and disease in early Lund: osteo-pathologic studies of 3,305 individuals buried in the first cemetery area of Lund 990–1536*. Ph.D., Lund, Lund.

69. Arjmandi, B.H., Getlinger, M.J., Goyal, N.V., *et al.* (1998) Role of soy protein with normal or reduced isoflavone content in reversing bone loss induced by ovarian hormone deficiency in rats. *Am J Clin Nutr* **68**, 1358S–63S.

70. Armour, J.C., Perea, R.L.C., Buchan, W.C. & Grant, G. (1998) Protease inhibitors and lectins in soya beans and effects of aqueous heat-treatment. *J Sci Food Agric* **78**, 225–31.

71. Armstrong, M.L. & Heistad, D.D. (1990) Animal models of atherosclerosis. *Atherosclerosis* **85**, 15–23.

72. Arnlov, J., Lind, L., Zethelius, B., *et al.* (2001) Several factors associated with the insulin resistance syndrome are predictors of left ventricular systolic dysfunction in a male population after 20 years of follow-up. *Am Heart J* **142**, 720–24.

73. Aro, A. (2001) Complexity of issue of dietary trans fatty acids. *Lancet* **357**, 732–3.

74. Aro, A., Antoine, J.M., Pizzoferrato, L., Reykdal, O. & van Poppel, G. (1998) Trans fatty acids in dairy and meat products from 14 European countries: the TRANSFAIR study. *J Food Compos Anal* **11**, 150–60.

75. Asano, T. & McLeod, R.S. (2002) Dietary fibre for the prevention of colorectal adenomas and carcinomas. *Cochrane Database Syst Rev*, CD003430.

76. Ascencio, C., Torres, N., Isoard-Acosta, F., *et al.* (2004) Soy protein affects serum insulin and hepatic SREBP-1 mRNA and reduces fatty liver in rats. *J Nutr* **134**, 522–9.

77. Ascherio, A., Rimm, E.B., Hernan, M.A., *et al.* (1998) Intake of potassium, magnesium, calcium, and fiber and risk of stroke among US men. *Circulation* **98**, 1198–204.

78. Ashrafian, H., Frenneaux, M.P. & Opie, L.H. (2007) Metabolic mechanisms in heart failure. *Circulation* **116**, 434–48.

79. Ashton, E. & Ball, M. (2000) Effects of soy as tofu vs meat on lipoprotein concentrations. *Eur J Clin Nutr* **54**, 14–19.

80. Asplund, K. (2002) Antioxidant vitamins in the prevention of cardiovascular disease: a systematic review. *J Intern Med* **251**, 372–92.

81. Assman, G., Schulte, H. & von Eckardstein, A. (1993) Hypertriglyceridemia/low high-density lipoprotein cholesterol syndrome. *Nutr Metab Cardiovasc Dis* **3**, 1–4.

82. Assmann, G., Cullen, P., Erbey, J., *et al.* (2006) Plasma sitosterol elevations are associated with an increased incidence of coronary events in men: results of a nested case-control analysis of the Prospective Cardiovascular Munster (PROCAM) study. *Nutr Metab Cardiovasc Dis* **16**, 13–21.

83. Aston, L.M., Stokes, C.S. & Jebb, S.A. (2008) No effect of a diet with a reduced glycaemic index on satiety, energy intake and body weight in overweight and obese women. *Int J Obes (Lond)* **32**, 160–65.

84. Astrup, A. (2006) Carbohydrates as macronutrients in relation to protein and fat for body weight control. *Int J Obes (Lond)* **30** (Suppl 3), S4–9.

85. Astrup, A., Grunwald, G.K., Melanson, E.L., Saris, W.H. & Hill, J.O. (2000) The role of low-fat diets in body weight control: a meta-analysis of ad libitum dietary intervention studies. *Int J Obes Relat Metab Disord* **24**, 1545–52.

86. Astrup, A., Meinert Larsen, T. & Harper, A. (2004) Atkins and other low-carbohydrate diets: hoax or an effective tool for weight loss? *Lancet* **364**, 897–9.

87. Atalan, G., Holt, P.E., Barr, F.J. & Brown, P.J. (1999) Ultrasonographic estimation of prostatic size in canine cadavers. *Res Vet Sci* **67**, 7–15.

88. Atkinson, F.S., Foster-Powell, K. & Brand-Miller, J.C. (2008) International tables of glycemic index and glycemic load values: 2008. *Diabetes Care* **31**, 2281–3.

89. Atkinson, L., Chester, I.C., Smyth, F.G. & ten Seldam, R.E.J. (1964) Oral cancer in New Guinea. A study in demography and etiology. *Cancer* **17**, 1289–98.

90. Attia, N., Tamborlane, W.V., Heptulla, R., *et al.* (1998) The metabolic syndrome and insulin-like growth factor I regulation in adolescent obesity. *J Clin Endocrinol Metab* **83**, 1467–71.

91. Au Eong, K.G., Tay, T.H. & Lim, M.K. (1993) Race, culture and Myopia in 110,236 young Singaporean males. *Singapore Med J* **34**, 29–32.

92. Austin, M.A. (2000) Triglyceride, small, dense low-density lipoprotein, and the atherogenic lipoprotein phenotype. *Curr Atheroscler Rep* **2**, 200–207.

93. Austin, M.A. & Hokanson, J.E. (1994) Epidemiology of triglycerides, small dense low-density lipoprotein, and lipoprotein(a) as risk factors for coronary heart disease. *Med Clin North Am* **78**, 99–115.

94. Avenell, A., Gillespie, W.J., Gillespie, L.D. & O'Connell, D.L. (2005) Vitamin D and vitamin D analogues for preventing fractures associated with involutional and post-menopausal osteoporosis. *Cochrane Database Syst Rev*, CD000227.

95. Axel, D.I., Frigge, A., Dittmann, J., *et al.* (2001) All-trans retinoic acid regulates proliferation, migration, differentiation, and extracellular matrix turnover of human arterial smooth muscle cells. *Cardiovasc Res* **49**, 851–62.

96. Azevedo, A., Bettencourt, P., Almeida, P.B., *et al.* (2007) Increasing number of components of the metabolic syndrome and cardiac structural and functional abnormalities – cross-sectional study of the general population. *BMC Cardiovasc Disord* **7**, 17.

97. Azevedo, A., Bettencourt, P., Dias, P., *et al.* (2006) Population based study on the prevalence of the stages of heart failure. *Heart* **92**, 1161–3.

98. Aziz, A. & Anderson, G.H. (2002) Exendin-4, a GLP-1 receptor agonist, modulates the effect of macronutrients on food intake by rats. *J Nutr* **132**, 990–95.

99. Backhouse, T.C. (1958) Melanesian natives and vascular disease: a note based on autopsy records, 1923–1934. *Med J Aust* **1**, 36–7.

100. Baker, J.F., Krishnan, E., Chen, L. & Schumacher, H.R. (2005) Serum uric acid and cardiovascular disease: recent developments, and where do they leave us? *Am J Med* **118**, 816–26.

101. Balanza Galindo, S. & Mestre Molto, F. (1995) [Cardiovascular risk factors in the fishing environment of Cartagena and Castellon]. *Rev Esp Salud Publica* **69**, 295–303.

102. Balen, A.H., Dresner, M., Scott, E.M. & Drife, J.O. (2006) Should obese women with polycystic ovary syndrome receive treatment for infertility? *BMJ* **332**, 434–5.

103. Bales, C.W. & Ritchie, C.S. (2002) Sarcopenia, weight loss, and nutritional frailty in the elderly. *Annu Rev Nutr* **22**, 309–23.

104. Ball, L.J. & Birge, S.J. (2002) Prevention of brain aging and dementia. *Clin Geriatr Med* **18**, 485–503.

105. Bang, H.O. & Dyerberg, J. (1972) Plasma lipids and lipoproteins in Greenlandic west coast Eskimos. *Acta Med Scand* **192**, 85–94.

106. Banks, W.A., Ibrahimi, F., Farr, S.A., Flood, J.F. & Morley, J.E. (1999) Effects of wheat-germ agglutinin and aging on the regional brain uptake of HIV-1GP120. *Life Sci* **65**, 81–9.

107. Banks, W.A. & Kastin, A.J. (1998) Characterization of lectin-mediated brain uptake of HIV-1 GP120. *J Neurosci Res* **54**, 522–9.

108. Bansal, S., Buring, J.E., Rifai, N., *et al.* (2007) Fasting compared with nonfasting triglycerides and risk of cardiovascular events in women. *JAMA* **298**, 309–16.

109. Banting, W. (1865) *Letter on corpulence, addressed to the public.* Mohun & Ebbs, New York.

110. Banwell, J.G., Howard, R., Kabir, I. & Costerton, J.W. (1988) Bacterial overgrowth by indigenous microflora in the phytohemagglutinin-fed rat. *Can J Microbiol* **34**, 1009–13.

111. Bao, D.Q., Mori, T.A., Burke, V., Puddey, I.B. & Beilin, L.J. (1998) Effects of dietary fish and weight reduction on ambulatory blood pressure in overweight hypertensives. *Hypertension* **32**, 710–17.

112. Barbeau, W.E., Bassaganya-Riera, J. & Hontecillas, R. (2007) Putting the pieces of the puzzle together – a series of hypotheses on the etiology and pathogenesis of type 1 diabetes. *Med Hypotheses* **68**, 607–19.

113. Barclay, A.W., Petocz, P., McMillan-Price, J., *et al.* (2008) Glycemic index, glycemic load, and chronic disease risk– a meta-analysis of observational studies. *Am J Clin Nutr* **87**, 627–37.

114. Bardiger, M. & Stock, A.L. (1972) The effects of sucrose-containing diets low in protein on ocular refraction in the rat. *Proc Nutr Soc* **31**, 4A–5A.

115. Barnard, R.J., Youngren, J.F. & Martin, D.A. (1995) Diet, not aging, causes skeletal muscle insulin resistance. *Gerontology* **41**, 205–11.

116. Barnes, D.J. (1990) Obstructive sleep apnoea: a new disease for Papua New Guinea? *P N G Med J* **33**, 225–7.

117. Barnes, R. (1961) Incidence of heart disease in a native hospital of Papua. *Med J Aust* **2**, 540–42.

118. Barnicot, N.A., Bennett, F.J., Woodburn, J.C., Pilkington, T.R. & Antonis, A. (1972) Blood pressure and serum cholesterol in the Hadza of Tanzania. *Hum Biol* **44**, 87–116.

119. Barr, S.I., Prior, J.C., Janelle, K.C. & Lentle, B.C. (1998) Spinal bone mineral density in premenopausal vegetarian and nonvegetarian women: cross-sectional and prospective comparisons. *J Am Diet Assoc* **98**, 760–5.

120. Barss, P. (1985) Fractured hips in rural Melanesians: a nonepidemic. *Trop Geogr Med* **37**, 156–9.

121. Barss, P.G. (1985) Prostatic disease in rural Melanesians. *Papua New Guinea Med J* **28**, 279–82.

122. Barth, C.A. & Pfeuffer, M. (1988) Dietary protein and atherogenesis. *Klin Wochenschr* **66**, 135–43.

123. Bartlett, C., Sterne, J. & Egger, M. (2002) What is newsworthy? Longitudinal study of the reporting of medical research in two British newspapers. *BMJ* **325**, 81–4.

124. Bartnik, M., Malmberg, K., Norhammar, A., *et al.* (2004) Newly detected abnormal glucose tolerance: an important predictor of long-term outcome after myocardial infarction. *Eur Heart J* **25**, 1990–97.

125. Bartnik, M., Ryden, L., Ferrari, R., *et al.* (2004) The prevalence of abnormal glucose regulation in patients with coronary artery disease across Europe. The Euro Heart Survey on diabetes and the heart. *Eur Heart J* **25**, 1880–90.

126. Baruzzi, R. & Franco, L. (1981) Amerindians of Brazil. In: *Western diseases: their emergence and prevention* (H.C. Trowell & D.P. Burkitt eds). Edward Arnold, London, pp. 138–53.

127. Barzel, U.S. & Massey, L.K. (1998) Excess dietary protein can adversely affect bone. *J Nutr* **128**, 1051–3.

128. Basabose, A.K. (2002) Diet composition of chimpanzees inhabiting the Montane forest of Kahuzi, Democratic Republic of Congo. *Am J Primatol* **58**, 1–21.
129. Bastian, S.E., Dunbar, A.J., Priebe, I.K., Owens, P.C. & Goddard, C. (2001) Measurement of betacellulin levels in bovine serum, colostrum and milk. *J Endocrinol* **168**, 203–12.
130. Bauer, J.E. & Covert, S.J. (1984) The influence of protein and carbohydrate type on serum and liver lipids and lipoprotein cholesterol in rabbits. *Lipids* **19**, 844–50.
131. Baur, J.A., Pearson, K.J., Price, N.L., *et al.* (2006) Resveratrol improves health and survival of mice on a high-calorie diet. *Nature* **444**, 337–42.
132. Bazzano, L.A., He, J., Ogden, L.G., *et al.* (2002) Fruit and vegetable intake and risk of cardiovascular disease in US adults: the first National Health and Nutrition Examination Survey Epidemiologic Follow-up Study. *Am J Clin Nutr* **76**, 93–9.
133. Beaglehole, R., Prior, I.A., Foulkes, M.A. & Eyles, E.F. (1980) Death in the South Pacific. *N Z Med J* **91**, 375–8.
134. Bechelli, L.M., Haddad, N., Pimenta, W.P., *et al.* (1981) Epidemiological survey of skin diseases in schoolchildren living in the Purus Valley (Acre State, Amazonia, Brazil). *Dermatologica* **163**, 78–93.
135. Becker, B.F., Reinholz, N., Leipert, B., *et al.* (1991) Role of uric acid as an endogenous radical scavenger and antioxidant. *Chest* **100**, 176S–81S.
136. Becker, W. (1982) *Svensk kost.* Statens Livsmedelsverk, Uppsala.
137. Becker, W. (1998) Transfettsyror. Nya data visar att innehållet i svensk kost är lågt. *Vår Föda* **5**, 20–23.
138. Becker, W. & Pearson, M. (2002) *Dietary habits and nutrient intake in Sweden 1997–98: The Second National Food Consumption Survey (in Swedish).* Swedish National Food Administration, Uppsala.
139. Becker, W. & Pearson, M. (2002) *Kostvanor och näringsintag i Sverige. Metod- och resultatanalys.* Livsmedelsverket, Uppsala.
140. Beilin, L.J., Burke, V., Puddey, I.B., Mori, T.A. & Hodgson, J.M. (2001) Recent developments concerning diet and hypertension. *Clin Exp Pharmacol Physiol* **28**, 1078–82.
141. Belderok, B. (2000) Developments in bread-making processes. *Plant Foods Hum Nutr* **55**, 1–86.
142. Belfiore, A. (2007) The role of insulin receptor isoforms and hybrid insulin/IGF-I receptors in human cancer. *Curr Pharm Des* **13**, 671–86.
143. Bell, R.R., Eldrid, M.M. & Watson, F.R. (1992) The influence of NaCl and KCl on urinary calcium excretion in healthy young women. *Nutr Res* **12**, 17–26.
144. Beltowski, J. (2006) Leptin and atherosclerosis. *Atherosclerosis* **189**, 47–60.
145. Bender, R., Jockel, K.H., Trautner, C., Spraul, M. & Berger, M. (1999) Effect of age on excess mortality in obesity. *JAMA* **281**, 1498–504.
146. Bender, R., Trautner, C., Spraul, M. & Berger, M. (1998) Assessment of excess mortality in obesity. *Am J Epidemiol* **147**, 42–8.
147. Bender, R., Zeeb, H., Schwarz, M., Jockel, K.H. & Berger, M. (2006) Causes of death in obesity: relevant increase in cardiovascular but not in all-cancer mortality. *J Clin Epidemiol* **59**, 1064–71.
148. Beneytout, J.L., Nappez, C., Leboutet, M.J. & Malinvaud, G. (1995) A plant steroid, diosgenin, a new megakaryocytic differentiation inducer of HEL cells. *Biochem Biophys Res Commun* **207**, 398–404.
149. Bengtsson, B. & Grodum, K. (1999) Refractive changes in the elderly. *Acta Ophthalmol Scand* **77**, 37–9.
150. Bennett, P.H. (1999) Type 2 diabetes among the Pima Indians of Arizona: an epidemic attributable to environmental change? *Nutr Rev* **57**, S51–4.
151. Benyshek, D.C. & Watson, J.T. (2006) Exploring the thrifty genotype's food-shortage assumptions: a cross-cultural comparison of ethnographic accounts of food security among foraging and agricultural societies. *Am J Phys Anthropol* **131**, 120–6.

152. Berenson, G.S., Srinivasan, S.R., Bao, W., *et al.* (1998) Association between multiple cardiovascular risk factors and atherosclerosis in children and young adults. The Bogalusa Heart Study. *N Engl J Med* **338**, 1650–6.

153. Beresford, S.A., Johnson, K.C., Ritenbaugh, C., *et al.* (2006) Low-fat dietary pattern and risk of colorectal cancer: the Women's Health Initiative Randomized Controlled Dietary Modification Trial. *JAMA* **295**, 643–54.

154. Berge, K.E., von Bergmann, K., Lutjohann, D., *et al.* (2002) Heritability of plasma noncholesterol sterols and relationship to DNA sequence polymorphism in ABCG5 and ABCG8. *J Lipid Res* **43**, 486–94.

155. Berger, J.D., Robertson, L.D. & Cocks, P.S. (2003) Agricultural potential of Mediterranean grain and forage legumes: anti-nutritional factor concentrations in the genus Vicia. *Genet Resourc Crop Evol* **50**, 201–12.

156. Bergeron, N. & Jacques, H. (1989) Influence of fish protein as compared to casein and soy protein on serum and liver lipids, and serum lipoprotein cholesterol levels in the rabbit. *Atherosclerosis* **78**, 113–21.

157. Bergstrom, A., Pisani, P., Tenet, V., Wolk, A. & Adami, H.O. (2001) Overweight as an avoidable cause of cancer in Europe. *Int J Cancer* **91**, 421–30.

158. Berner, Y.N. (2001) The contribution of obesity to dyspnoea in elderly people. *Age Ageing* **30**, 530.

159. Berry, E.M. (2001) Are diets high in omega-6 polyunsaturated fatty acids unhealthy? *Eur Heart J* (Suppl 3), D37–41.

160. Berry, S.J., Strandberg, J.D., Saunders, W.J. & Coffey, D.S. (1986) Development of canine benign prostatic hyperplasia with age. *Prostate* **9**, 363–73.

161. Bertomeu, A., Garcia-Vidal, O., Farre, X., *et al.* (2003) Preclinical coronary atherosclerosis in a population with low incidence of myocardial infarction: cross sectional autopsy study. *BMJ* **327**, 591–2.

162. Bessesen, D.H. (2001) The role of carbohydrates in insulin resistance. *J Nutr* **131**, 2782S–6S.

163. Betsholtz, C., Christmansson, L., Engstrom, U., *et al.* (1989) Sequence divergence in a specific region of islet amyloid polypeptide (IAPP) explains differences in islet amyloid formation between species. *FEBS Lett* **251**, 261–4.

164. Bhattacharyya, A.K. (1992) Nutritional rickets in the tropics. *World Rev Nutr Diet* **67**, 140–97.

165. Bigaard, J., Frederiksen, K., Tjonneland, A., *et al.* (2005) Waist circumference and body composition in relation to all-cause mortality in middle-aged men and women. *Int J Obes (Lond)* **29**, 778–84.

166. Billinghurst, J.R. (1970) The pattern of adult neurological admissions to Mulago hospital, Kampala. *East Afr Med J* **47**, 653–63.

167. Binkley, N., Novotny, R., Krueger, D., *et al.* (2007) Low vitamin D status despite abundant sun exposure. *J Clin Endocrinol Metab* **92**, 2130–5.

168. Biong, A.S., Veierod, M.B., Ringstad, J., Thelle, D.S. & Pedersen, J.I. (2006) Intake of milk fat, reflected in adipose tissue fatty acids and risk of myocardial infarction: a case-control study. *Eur J Clin Nutr* **60**, 236–44.

169. Birgisdottir, B.E., Hill, J.P., Thorsson, A.V. & Thorsdottir, I. (2006) Lower consumption of cow milk protein A1 beta-casein at 2 years of age, rather than consumption among 11- to 14-year-old adolescents, may explain the lower incidence of type 1 diabetes in Iceland than in Scandinavia. *Ann Nutr Metab* **50**, 177–83.

170. Birns, J., Morris, R., Donaldson, N. & Kalra, L. (2006) The effects of blood pressure reduction on cognitive function: a review of effects based on pooled data from clinical trials. *J Hypertens* **24**, 1907–14.

171. Bischoff-Ferrari, H.A. & Dawson-Hughes, B. (2007) Where do we stand on vitamin D? *Bone* **41**, S13–9.

172. Bissoli, L., Di Francesco, V., Ballarin, A., *et al.* (2002) Effect of vegetarian diet on homocysteine levels. *Ann Nutr Metab* **46**, 73–9.

173. Bitzer, M., Feldkaemper, M. & Schaeffel, F. (2000) Visually induced changes in components of the retinoic acid system in fundal layers of the chick. *Exp Eye Res* **70**, 97–106.

174. Bjelakovic, G., Nikolova, D., Gluud, L.L., Simonetti, R.G. & Gluud, C. (2007) Mortality in randomized trials of antioxidant supplements for primary and secondary prevention: systematic review and meta-analysis. *JAMA* **297**, 842–57.

175. Bjelakovic, G., Nikolova, D., Gluud, L.L., Simonetti, R.G. & Gluud, C. (2008) Antioxidant supplements for prevention of mortality in healthy participants and patients with various diseases. *Cochrane Database Syst Rev*, CD007176.

176. Bjerregaard, P., Jorgensen, M.E., Lumholt, P., Mosgaard, L. & Borch-Johnsen, K. (2002) Higher blood pressure among Inuit migrants in Denmark than among the Inuit in Greenland. *J Epidemiol Community Health* **56**, 279–84.

177. Bjerregaard, P., Young, T.K. & Hegele, R.A. (2003) Low incidence of cardiovascular disease among the Inuit – what is the evidence? *Atherosclerosis* **166**, 351–7.

178. Black, J. (1995) Rickets and the crippled child: an historical perspective [letter]. *J R Soc Med* **88**, 363–4.

179. Black, P. (2001) Why is the prevalence of allergy and autoimmunity increasing? *Trends Immunol* **22**, 354–5.

180. Black, R.E., Williams, S.M., Jones, I.E. & Goulding, A. (2002) Children who avoid drinking cow milk have low dietary calcium intakes and poor bone health. *Am J Clin Nutr* **76**, 675–80.

181. Black, R.N., Spence, M., McMahon, R.O., *et al.* (2006) Effect of eucaloric high- and low-sucrose diets with identical macronutrient profile on insulin resistance and vascular risk: a randomized controlled trial. *Diabetes* **55**, 3566–72.

182. Blake, J., Devereux, R.B., Borer, J.S., *et al.* (1990) Relation of obesity, high sodium intake, and eccentric left ventricular hypertrophy to left ventricular exercise dysfunction in essential hypertension. *Am J Med* **88**, 477–85.

183. Blankenhorn, D.H., Johnson, R.L., Mack, W.J., el, Z.H. & Vailas, L.I. (1990) The influence of diet on the appearance of new lesions in human coronary arteries. *JAMA* **263**, 1646–52.

184. Bleys, J., Miller, E.R., 3rd, Pastor-Barriuso, R., Appel, L.J. & Guallar, E. (2006) Vitamin-mineral supplementation and the progression of atherosclerosis: a meta-analysis of randomized controlled trials. *Am J Clin Nutr* **84**, 880–7; quiz 954–5.

185. Bloch, J.I. & Boyer, D.M. (2002) Grasping primate origins. *Science* **298**, 1606–10.

186. Bloom, R.A. & Pogrund, H. (1982) Humeral cortical thickness in female Bantu – its relationship to the incidence of femoral neck fracture. *Skeletal Radiol* **8**, 59–62.

187. Bobe, G., Young, J.W. & Beitz, D.C. (2004) Invited review: pathology, etiology, prevention, and treatment of fatty liver in dairy cows. *J Dairy Sci* **87**, 3105–24.

188. Boden-Albala, B., Sacco, R.L., Lee, H.S., *et al.* (2008) Metabolic syndrome and ischemic stroke risk: Northern Manhattan Study. *Stroke* **39**, 30–5.

189. Bodkin, N.L., Alexander, T.M., Ortmeyer, H.K., Johnson, E. & Hansen, B.C. (2003) Mortality and morbidity in laboratory-maintained Rhesus monkeys and effects of long-term dietary restriction. *J Gerontol A Biol Sci Med Sci* **58**, 212–19.

190. Bokemark, L., Wikstrand, J., Attvall, S., *et al.* (2001) Insulin resistance and intima-media thickness in the carotid and femoral arteries of clinically healthy 58-year-old men. The Atherosclerosis and Insulin Resistance Study (AIR). *J Intern Med* **249**, 59–67.

191. Bolland, M.J., Barber, P.A., Doughty, R.N., *et al.* (2008) Vascular events in healthy older women receiving calcium supplementation: randomised controlled trial. *BMJ* **336**, 262–6.

192. Bønaa, K.H., Njolstad, I., Ueland, P.M., *et al.* (2006) Homocysteine lowering and cardiovascular events after acute myocardial infarction. *N Engl J Med* **354**, 1578–88.

193. Bonithon-Kopp, C., Kronborg, O., Giacosa, A., Rath, U. & Faivre, J. (2000) Calcium and fibre supplementation in prevention of colorectal adenoma recurrence: a randomised intervention trial. European Cancer Prevention Organisation Study Group. *Lancet* **356**, 1300–6.

194. Bonjour, J.P. (2005) Dietary protein: an essential nutrient for bone health. *J Am Coll Nutr* **24**, 526S–36S.

195. Bonjour, J.P., Ammann, P., Chevalley, T. & Rizzoli, R. (2001) Protein intake and bone growth. *Can J Appl Physiol* **26**, S153–66.

196. Bonjour, J.P., Brandolini-Bunlon, M., Boirie, Y., *et al.* (2008) Inhibition of bone turnover by milk intake in postmenopausal women. *Br J Nutr* **100**, 866–74.

197. Bonjour, J.P., Carrie, A.L., Ferrari, S., *et al.* (1997) Calcium-enriched foods and bone mass growth in prepubertal girls: a randomized, double-blind, placebo-controlled trial. *J Clin Invest* **99**, 1287–94.

198. Bonnefille, R., Potts, R., Chalie, F., Jolly, D. & Peyron, O. (2004) High-resolution vegetation and climate change associated with Pliocene Australopithecus afarensis. *Proc Natl Acad Sci USA* **101**, 12125–9.

199. Boonen, S., Lips, P., Bouillon, R., *et al.* (2007) Need for additional calcium to reduce the risk of hip fracture with vitamin D supplementation: evidence from a comparative metaanalysis of randomized controlled trials. *J Clin Endocrinol Metab* **92**, 1415–23.

200. Bothwell, T.H. (1996) Iron balance and the capacity of regulatory systems to prevent the development of iron deficiency and overload. In: *Iron Nutrition in Health and Disease* (L. Hallberg & N.-G. Asp eds). John Libbey, London, pp. 3–16.

201. Bowen, J., Noakes, M., Trenerry, C. & Clifton, P.M. (2006) Energy intake, ghrelin, and cholecystokinin after different carbohydrate and protein preloads in overweight men. *J Clin Endocrinol Metab* **91**, 1477–83.

202. Boyd, N.F., Stone, J., Vogt, K.N., *et al.* (2003) Dietary fat and breast cancer risk revisited: a meta-analysis of the published literature. *Br J Cancer* **89**, 1672–85.

203. Boyd, R. & Silk, J.B. (2006) *How humans evolved*. Norton, New York.

204. Boyle, P., Macfarlane, G.J., Maisonneuve, P., *et al.* (1990) Epidemiology of mouth cancer in 1989: a review [see comments]. *J R Soc Med* **83**, 724–30.

205. Brancati, F.L., Kao, W.H., Folsom, A.R., Watson, R.L. & Szklo, M. (2000) Incident type 2 diabetes mellitus in African American and white adults: the Atherosclerosis Risk in Communities Study. *JAMA* **283**, 2253–9.

206. Brand Miller, J.C. & Colagiuri, S. (1994) The carnivore connection: dietary carbohydrate in the evolution of NIDDM. *Diabetologia* **37**, 1280–6.

207. Brand-Miller, J. (2005) Optimizing the cardiovascular outcomes of weight loss. *Am J Clin Nutr* **81**, 949–50.

208. Brand-Miller, J., Hayne, S., Petocz, P. & Colagiuri, S. (2003) Low-glycemic index diets in the management of diabetes: a meta-analysis of randomized controlled trials. *Diabetes Care* **26**, 2261–7.

209. Brand-Miller, J.C. & Colagiuri, S. (1999) Evolutionary aspects of diet and insulin resistance. *World Rev Nutr Diet* **84**, 74–105.

210. Brand-Miller, J.C., Colagiuri, S. & Gan, S.T. (2000) Insulin sensitivity predicts glycemia after a protein load. *Metabolism* **49**, 1–5.

211. Brand-Miller, J.C., Holt, S.H., Pawlak, D.B. & McMillan, J. (2002) Glycemic index and obesity. *Am J Clin Nutr* **76**, 281S–5S.

212. Brass, E.P. & Hiatt, W.R. (1998) The role of carnitine and carnitine supplementation during exercise in man and in individuals with special needs. *J Am Coll Nutr* **17**, 207–15.

213. Braudel, F. (1981) *The structures of everyday life: The limits of the possible*. Collins, London.

214. Bravata, D.M., Sanders, L., Huang, J., *et al.* (2003) Efficacy and safety of low-carbohydrate diets: a systematic review. *JAMA* **289**, 1837–50.

215. Breinl, A. (1915) On the occurrence and prevalence of diseases in British New Guinea. *Ann Trop Med Parasitol* **9**, 285–335.

216. Brendler, C.B., Berry, S.J., Ewing, L.L., *et al.* (1983) Spontaneous benign prostatic hyperplasia in the beagle. Age-associated changes in serum hormone levels, and the morphology and secretory function of the canine prostate. *J Clin Invest* **71**, 1114–23.

217. Bresson, J.L. (1998) Protein and energy requirements in healthy and ill paediatric patients. *Baillieres Clin Gastroenterol* **12**, 631–45.

218. Brett, M. & Barker, D.J. (1976) The world distribution of gallstones. *Int J Epidemiol* **5**, 335–41.

219. Briel, M., Ferreira-Gonzalez, I., You, J.J., *et al.* (2009) Association between change in high density lipoprotein cholesterol and cardiovascular disease morbidity and mortality: systematic review and meta-regression analysis. *BMJ* **338**, b92.

220. Briggs, R.D., Rubenberg, M.L., O'Neal, R., M., Thomas, W.A. & Hartroft, W.S. (1960) Myocardial infarction in patients treated with Sippy and other high-milk diets. *Circulation* **21**, 538–42.

221. Brighenti, F., Benini, L., Del Rio, D., *et al.* (2006) Colonic fermentation of indigestible carbohydrates contributes to the second-meal effect. *Am J Clin Nutr* **83**, 817–22.

222. Broekhuizen, L.N., Mooij, H.L., Kastelein, J.J., *et al.* (2009) Endothelial glycocalyx as potential diagnostic and therapeutic target in cardiovascular disease. *Curr Opin Lipidol* **20**, 57–62.

223. Bronte-Stewart, B., Keys, A. & Brock, J.E. (1955) Serum-cholesterol, diet and coronary heart disease: Inter-racial survey in Cape Peninsula. *Lancet* **2**, 1103.

224. Brouwer, I.A., Raitt, M.H., Dullemeijer, C., *et al.* (2009) Effect of fish oil on ventricular tachyarrhythmia in three studies in patients with implantable cardioverter defibrillators. *Eur Heart J* **30**, 820–6.

225. Brown, L., Rosner, B., Willett, W.W. & Sacks, F.M. (1999) Cholesterol-lowering effects of dietary fiber: a meta-analysis. *Am J Clin Nutr* **69**, 30–42.

226. Brownlee, M. (2005) The pathobiology of diabetic complications: a unifying mechanism. *Diabetes* **54**, 1615–25.

227. Bruce, H. & Callow, R. (1934) Cereals and rickets. The role of inositolhexaphosphoric acid. *Biochem J* **28**, 517–28.

228. Brune, M., Rossander, L. & Hallberg, L. (1989) Iron absorption: no intestinal adaptation to a high-phytate diet. *Am J Clin Nutr* **49**, 542–5.

229. Bruning, J.C., Michael, M.D., Winnay, J.N., *et al.* (1998) A muscle-specific insulin receptor knockout exhibits features of the metabolic syndrome of NIDDM without altering glucose tolerance. *Mol Cell* **2**, 559–69.

230. Brunner, E. (2006) Oily fish and omega 3 fat supplements. *BMJ* **332**, 739–40.

231. Brunner, E.J., Shipley, M.J., Witte, D.R., Fuller, J.H. & Marmot, M.G. (2006) Relation between blood glucose and coronary mortality over 33 years in the Whitehall Study. *Diabetes Care* **29**, 26–31.

232. Bruno, G., Biggeri, A., Merletti, F., *et al.* (2003) Low incidence of end-stage renal disease and chronic renal failure in type 2 diabetes: a 10-year prospective study. *Diabetes Care* **26**, 2353–8.

233. Buclin, T., Cosma, M., Appenzeller, M., *et al.* (2001) Diet acids and alkalis influence calcium retention in bone. *Osteoporos Int* **12**, 493–9.

234. Budek, A.Z., Hoppe, C., Michaelsen, K.F. & Molgaard, C. (2007) High intake of milk, but not meat, decreases bone turnover in prepubertal boys after 7 days. *Eur J Clin Nutr* **61**, 957–62.

235. Buettner, R., Scholmerich, J. & Bollheimer, L.C. (2007) High-fat diets: modeling the metabolic disorders of human obesity in rodents. *Obesity (Silver Spring)* **15**, 798–808.

236. Bulaj, Z.J., Griffen, L.M., Jorde, L.B., Edwards, C.Q. & Kushner, J.P. (1996) Clinical and biochemical abnormalities in people heterozygous for hemochromatosis [see comments]. *N Engl J Med* **335**, 1799–805.

237. Bunn, H.F. & Higgins, P.J. (1981) Reaction of monosaccharides with proteins: possible evolutionary significance. *Science* **213**, 222–4.

238. Burattini, R., Di Nardo, F., Casagrande, F., Boemi, M. & Morosini, P. (2009) Insulin action and secretion in hypertension in the absence of metabolic syndrome: model-based assessment from oral glucose tolerance test. *Metabolism* **58**, 80–92.

239. Burger, J., Kirchner, M., Bramanti, B., Haak, W. & Thomas, M.G. (2007) Absence of the lactase-persistence-associated allele in early Neolithic Europeans. *Proc Natl Acad Sci USA* **104**, 3736–41.

240. Burkitt, D.P., Walker, A.R. & Painter, N.S. (1974) Dietary fiber and disease. *JAMA* **229**, 1068–74.

241. Burr, M.L., Ashfield-Watt, P.A., Dunstan, F.D., *et al.* (2003) Lack of benefit of dietary advice to men with angina: results of a controlled trial. *Eur J Clin Nutr* **57**, 193–200.

242. Burr, M.L., Fehily, A.M., Gilbert, J.F., *et al.* (1989) Effects of changes in fat, fish, and fibre intakes on death and myocardial reinfarction: diet and reinfarction trial (DART) [see comments]. *Lancet* **2**, 757–61.

243. Burton-Freeman, B.M. & Keim, N.L. (2008) Glycemic index, cholecystokinin, satiety and disinhibition: is there an unappreciated paradox for overweight women? *Int J Obes (Lond)* **32**, 1647–54.

244. Buse, J.B., Ginsberg, H.N., Bakris, G.L., *et al.* (2007) Primary prevention of cardiovascular diseases in people with diabetes mellitus: a scientific statement from the American Heart Association and the American Diabetes Association. *Diabetes Care* **30**, 162–72.

245. Buse, J.B., Polonsky, K.S. & Burant, C.F. (2003) Type 2 diabetes mellitus. In: *Larsen: Williams textbook of endocrinology*, 10th ed. (P.R. Larsen, H.M. Kronenberg, M. S. & K.S. Polonsky eds). Saunders, Philadelphia, PA, pp. 1427–83.

246. Buse, M.G., Robinson, K.A., Marshall, B.A., Hresko, R.C. & Mueckler, M.M. (2002) Enhanced O-GlcNAc protein modification is associated with insulin resistance in GLUT1-overexpressing muscles. *Am J Physiol Endocrinol Metab* **283**, E241–50.

247. Bushinsky, D.A. (1998) Acid-base imbalance and the skeleton. In: *Nutritional aspects of osteoporosis*, Vol. 7 (P. Burckhardt, B. Dawson-Hughes & R.P. Heaney eds). Springer, New York, pp. 208–17.

248. Butcher, J. (1976) The distribution of multiple sclerosis in relation to the dairy industry and milk consumption. *N Z Med J* **83**, 427–30.

249. Byrne, C., Rockett, H. & Holmes, M.D. (2002) Dietary fat, fat subtypes, and breast cancer risk: lack of an association among postmenopausal women with no history of benign breast disease. *Cancer Epidemiol Biomarkers Prev* **11**, 261–5.

250. Cadogan, J., Eastell, R., Jones, N. & Barker, M.E. (1997) Milk intake and bone mineral acquisition in adolescent girls: randomised, controlled intervention trial. *BMJ* **315**, 1255–60.

251. Calhoun, D.A., Jones, D., Textor, S., *et al.* (2008) Resistant hypertension: diagnosis, evaluation, and treatment: a scientific statement from the American Heart Association Professional Education Committee of the Council for High Blood Pressure Research. *Circulation* **117**, e510–26.

252. Camacho-Hubner, C., Woods, K.A., Miraki-Moud, F., *et al.* (1999) Effects of recombinant human insulin-like growth factor I (IGF-I) therapy on the growth hormone-IGF system of a patient with a partial IGF-I gene deletion. *J Clin Endocrinol Metab* **84**, 1611–6.

253. Cambien, F., Warnet, J.M., Vernier, V., *et al.* (1988) An epidemiologic appraisal of the associations between the fatty acids esterifying serum cholesterol and some cardiovascular risk factors in middle-aged men. *Am J Epidemiol* **127**, 75–86.

254. Campbell, Å. (1950) *Det svenska brödet: en jämförande etnologisk-historisk undersökning*. Svensk bageritidskrift, Stockholm.

255. Campbell, C. & Arthur, R. (1964) A study of 2000 admissions to the medical ward of Port Moresby General Hospital. *Med J Aust* **1**, 989–992.

256. Cancello, R. & Clement, K. (2006) Is obesity an inflammatory illness? Role of low-grade inflammation and macrophage infiltration in human white adipose tissue. *BJOG* **113**, 1141–7.

257. Capasso, L.L. (2005) Antiquity of cancer. *Int J Cancer* **113**, 2–13.

258. Cappuccio, F.P., Markandu, N.D., Carney, C., Sagnella, G.A. & MacGregor, G.A. (1997) Double-blind randomised trial of modest salt restriction in older people. *Lancet* **350**, 850–4.

259. Caprez, A. & J., F.-T.S. (1982) The effect of heat treatment and particle size of bran on mineral absorption in rats. *Br J Nutr* **48**, 467–75.

260. Capuano, V., Lamaida, N., Fattore, L., D'Antonio, V. & Di Quacquaro, G.S. (1998) The increased frequency of hypercholesterolemia in southern Italy is induced only by changing diet quality? *Panminerva Med* **40**, 55–7.

261. Carbone, L.D., Barrow, K.D., Bush, A.J., *et al.* (2005) Effects of a low sodium diet on bone metabolism. *J Bone Miner Metab* **23**, 506–13.

262. Carey, V.J., Walters, E.E., Colditz, G.A., *et al.* (1997) Body fat distribution and risk of non-insulin-dependent diabetes mellitus in women. The Nurses'Health Study. *Am J Epidemiol* **145**, 614–9.

263. Carmel, R. (1997) Cobalamin, the stomach, and aging. *Am J Clin Nutr* **66**, 750–9.

264. Caron, M. & Seve, A.-P. (2000) *Lectins and Pathology*, Taylor & Francis, London.

265. Carr, J.G., Stevenson, L.W., Walden, J.A. & Heber, D. (1989) Prevalence and hemodynamic correlates of malnutrition in severe congestive heart failure secondary to ischemic or idiopathic dilated cardiomyopathy. *Am J Cardiol* **63**, 709–13.

266. Carretero, C., Trujillo, A.J., Mor-Mur, M., Pla, R. & Guamis, B. (1994) Electrophoretic study of casein breakdown during ripening of goat's milk cheese. *J Agric Food Chem* **42**, 1546–50.

267. Carroll, K.K. (1978) The role of dietary protein in hypercholesterolemia and atherosclerosis. *Lipids* **13**, 360–5.

268. Carroll, K.K. (1982) Hypercholesterolemia and atherosclerosis: effects of dietary protein. *Fed Proc* **41**, 2792–6.

269. Carroll, K.K. & Khor, H.T. (1975) Dietary fat in relation to tumorigenesis. *Prog Biochem Pharmacol* **10**, 308–53.

270. Carson, G. (1957) *Cornflake crusade*. Rinehart, New York.

271. Castell, C., Tresserras, R., Serra, J., *et al.* (1999) Prevalence of diabetes in Catalonia (Spain): an oral glucose tolerance test-based population study. *Diabetes Res Clin Pract* **43**, 33–40.

272. Catchpole, B., Ristic, J.M., Fleeman, L.M. & Davison, L.J. (2005) Canine diabetes mellitus: can old dogs teach us new tricks? *Diabetologia* **48**, 1948–56.

273. Cedergren, M.I. (2004) Maternal morbid obesity and the risk of adverse pregnancy outcome. *Obstet Gynecol* **103**, 219–24.

274. Cefalu, W.T., Wagner, J.D., Bell-Farrow, A.D., *et al.* (1999) Influence of caloric restriction on the development of atherosclerosis in nonhuman primates: progress to date. *Toxicol Sci* **52**, 49–55.

275. Ceschi, M., Gutzwiller, F., Moch, H., Eichholzer, M. & Probst-Hensch, N.M. (2007) Epidemiology and pathophysiology of obesity as cause of cancer. *Swiss Med Wkly* **137**, 50–6.

276. Chalkley, S.M., Hettiarachchi, M., Chisholm, D.J. & Kraegen, E.W. (2002) Long-term high-fat feeding leads to severe insulin resistance but not diabetes in Wistar rats. *Am J Physiol Endocrinol Metab* **282**, E1231–8.

277. Chan, A.Y., Poon, P., Chan, E.L., Fung, S.L. & Swaminathan, R. (1993) The effect of high sodium intake on bone mineral content in rats fed a normal calcium or a low calcium diet. *Osteoporos Int* **3**, 341–4.

278. Chan, G.M., Hoffman, K. & McMurry, M. (1995) Effects of dairy products on bone and body composition in pubertal girls. *J Pediatr* **126**, 551–6.

279. Chan, J.M., Rimm, E.B., Colditz, G.A., Stampfer, M.J. & Willett, W.C. (1994) Obesity, fat distribution, and weight gain as risk factors for clinical diabetes in men. *Diabetes Care* **17**, 961–9.

280. Chan, J.M., Stampfer, M.J., Ma, J., *et al.* (2001) Dairy products, calcium, and prostate cancer risk in the Physicians' Health Study. *Am J Clin Nutr* **74**, 549–54.

281. Chao, A., Thun, M.J., Connell, C.J., *et al.* (2005) Meat consumption and risk of colorectal cancer. *JAMA* **293**, 172–82.

282. Chardigny, J.M., Destaillats, F., Malpuech-Brugere, C., *et al.* (2008) Do trans fatty acids from industrially produced sources and from natural sources have the same effect on cardiovascular disease risk factors in healthy subjects? Results of the trans Fatty Acids Collaboration (TRANSFACT) study. *Am J Clin Nutr* **87**, 558–66.

283. Charles, D., Ness, A.R., Campbell, D., Davey Smith, G. & Hall, M.H. (2004) Taking folate in pregnancy and risk of maternal breast cancer. *BMJ* **329**, 1375–6.

284. Chen, C.Y., Scurrah, K.J., Stankovich, J., *et al.* (2007) Heritability and shared environment estimates for myopia and associated ocular biometric traits: the Genes in Myopia (GEM) family study. *Hum Genet* **121**, 511–20.

285. Chen, J., He, J., Wildman, R.P., *et al.* (2006) A randomized controlled trial of dietary fiber intake on serum lipids. *Eur J Clin Nutr* **60**, 62–8.

286. Chen, Z., Peto, R., Collins, R., *et al.* (1991) Serum cholesterol concentration and coronary heart disease in population with low cholesterol concentrations [see comments]. *BMJ* **303**, 276–82.

287. Cheng, T.O. (2000) Systolic and diastolic blood pressures and urinary sodium excretion in mainland China. *QJM* **93**, 557–8.

288. Cheng, T.O. (2004) References to sudden cardiac death by Hippocrates. *Int J Cardiol* **96**, 117.

289. Cheryan, M. (1980) Phytic acid interactions in food systems. *Crit Rev Food Sci Nutr* **13**, 297–335.

290. Cheung, N.W., McElduff, A. & Ross, G.P. (2005) Type 2 diabetes in pregnancy: a wolf in sheep's clothing. *Aust N Z J Obstet Gynaecol* **45**, 479–83.

291. Chevalley, T., Bonjour, J.P., Ferrari, S., Hans, D. & Rizzoli, R. (2005) Skeletal site selectivity in the effects of calcium supplementation on areal bone mineral density gain: a randomized, double-blind, placebo-controlled trial in prepubertal boys. *J Clin Endocrinol Metab* **90**, 3342–9.

292. Chiang, J.Y., Kimmel, R. & Stroup, D. (2001) Regulation of cholesterol 7alpha-hydroxylase gene (CYP7A1) transcription by the liver orphan receptor (LXRalpha). *Gene* **262**, 257–65.

293. Chiba, T., Shinozaki, S., Nakazawa, T., *et al.* (2008) Leptin deficiency suppresses progression of atherosclerosis in apoE-deficient mice. *Atherosclerosis* **196**, 68–75.

294. Chlebowski, R.T., Blackburn, G.L., Thomson, C.A., *et al.* (2006) Dietary fat reduction and breast cancer outcome: interim efficacy results from the Women's Intervention Nutrition Study. *J Natl Cancer Inst* **98**, 1767–76.

295. Chobanian, A.V., Bakris, G.L., Black, H.R., *et al.* (2003) The Seventh Report of the Joint National Committee on Prevention, Detection, Evaluation, and Treatment of High Blood Pressure: the JNC 7 report. *JAMA* **289**, 2560–72.

296. Choi, H.K., Willett, W.C., Stampfer, M.J., Rimm, E. & Hu, F.B. (2005) Dairy consumption and risk of type 2 diabetes mellitus in men: a prospective study. *Arch Intern Med* **165**, 997–1003.

297. Chokkalingam, A.P., Pollak, M., Fillmore, C.M., *et al.* (2001) Insulin-like growth factors and prostate cancer: a population-based case-control study in China. *Cancer Epidemiol Biomarkers Prev* **10**, 421–7.

298. Chou, P., Lin, K.C., Lin, H.Y. & Tsai, S.T. (2001) Gender differences in the relationships of serum uric acid with fasting serum insulin and plasma glucose in patients without diabetes. *J Rheumatol* **28**, 571–6.

299. Chrispeels, M.J. & Raikhel, N.V. (1991) Lectins, lectin genes, and their role in plant defense. *Plant Cell* **3**, 1–9.

300. Cigolini, M., Targher, G., Tonoli, M., *et al.* (1995) Hyperuricaemia: relationships to body fat distribution and other components of the insulin resistance syndrome in 38-year-old healthy men and women. *Int J Obes Relat Metab Disord* **19**, 92–6.

301. Claudel, T., Leibowitz, M.D., Fievet, C., *et al.* (2001) Reduction of atherosclerosis in apolipoprotein E knockout mice by activation of the retinoid X receptor. *Proc Natl Acad Sci USA* **98**, 2610–5.

302. Clements, F.W. (1936) A medical survey in Papua: report of the first expedition by the school of public health and tropical medicine to Papua, 1935. *Med J Aust* **1**, 451–463.

302a. Clevers, H.C., De Bresser, A., Kleinveld, H., Gmelig-Meyling, F.H.J. & Ballieux, R.E. (1986) Wheat germ agglutinin activates human T lymphocytes by stimulation of phosphoinositide hydrolysis. *J Immunol* **136**, 3180–83.

303. Clifton, P.M., Kestin, M., Abbey, M., Drysdale, M. & Nestel, P.J. (1990) Relationship between sensitivity to dietary fat and dietary cholesterol. *Arteriosclerosis* **10**, 394–401.

304. Clifton, P.M., Noakes, M., Keogh, J. & Foster, P. (2003) Effect of an energy reduced high protein red meat diet on weight loss and metabolic parameters in obese women. *Asia Pac J Clin Nutr* **12** (Suppl), S10.

305. Clinical Evidence writers on primary prevention (2002) Primary prevention. *Clinical Evidence* **7**, 91–123.

306. Cobb, M.M., Teitelbaum, H.S. & Breslow, J.L. (1991) Lovastatin efficacy in reducing low-density lipoprotein cholesterol levels on high- vs low-fat diets. *JAMA* **265**, 997–1001.

307. Cockburn, A., Cockburn, E. & Reyman, T.A. (1998) *Mummies, disease & ancient cultures.* Cambridge University Press, Cambridge.

308. Coetzee, M.J., Badenhorst, P.N., de Wet, J.I. & Joubert, G. (1994) Haematological condition of the San (Bushmen) relocated from Namibia to South Africa. *S Afr Med J* **84**, 416–20.

309. Coffey, D.S. (2001) Similarities of prostate and breast cancer: evolution, diet, and estrogens. *Urology* **57**, 31–8.

310. Cohen, A.J. & Roe, F.J. (2000) Review of risk factors for osteoporosis with particular reference to a possible aetiological role of dietary salt. *Food Chem Toxicol* **38**, 237–53.

311. Cohen, H.W., Hailpern, S.M., Fang, J. & Alderman, M.H. (2006) Sodium intake and mortality in the NHANES II follow-up study. *Am J Med* **119**, 275.e7–14.

312. Cohen, M.N. (1989) *Health and the rise of civilization.* Yale University Press, New Haven.

313. Colangelo, L.A., Gapstur, S.M., Gann, P.H., Dyer, A.R. & Liu, K. (2002) Colorectal cancer mortality and factors related to the insulin resistance syndrome. *Cancer Epidemiol Biomarkers Prev* **11**, 385–91.

314. Cole, B.F., Baron, J.A., Sandler, R.S., *et al.* (2007) Folic acid for the prevention of colorectal adenomas: a randomized clinical trial. *JAMA* **297**, 2351–9.

315. Collins, V., Dowse, G. & Zimmet, P. (1990) Prevalence of obesity in Pacific and Indian Ocean populations. *Diabetes Res Clin Pract* **10**, S29–32.

316. Colucci, W.S. & Braunwald, E. (2001) Pathophysiology of Heart Failure. In: *Heart disease. A textbook of cardiovascular medicine* (E. Braunwald, D.P. Zipes & P. Libby eds). Saunders, London, pp. 503–33.

317. Colussi, G., Catena, C., Lapenna, R., *et al.* (2007) Insulin resistance and hyperinsulinemia are related to plasma aldosterone levels in hypertensive patients. *Diabetes Care* **30**, 2349–54.

318. Compston, A. & Coles, A. (2008) Multiple sclerosis. *Lancet* **372**, 1502–17.

319. Conlin, P.R. (2001) Dietary modification and changes in blood pressure. *Curr Opin Nephrol Hypertens* **10**, 359–63.

320. Connor, W.E., Cerqueira, M.T., Connor, R.W., *et al.* (1978) The plasma lipids, lipoproteins, and diet of the Tarahumara Indians of Mexico. *Am J Clin Nutr* **31**, 1131–42.

321. Constantinou, A.I., White, B.E., Tonetti, D., *et al.* (2005) The soy isoflavone daidzein improves the capacity of tamoxifen to prevent mammary tumours. *Eur J Cancer* **41**, 647–54.

322. Contaldo, F., Scalfi, L. & Pasanisi, F. (2004) Ancel Keys centenary and the definition of healthy diet. *Clin Nutr* **23**, 435–6.

323. Convit, A., Wolf, O.T., Tarshish, C. & de Leon, M.J. (2003) Reduced glucose tolerance is associated with poor memory performance and hippocampal atrophy among normal elderly. *Proc Natl Acad Sci USA* **100**, 2019–22.

324. Conyers, R.A. (1971) Myocardial infarction in a New Guinean. *Med J Aust* **2**, 412–7.

325. Cook, N.R., Albert, C.M., Gaziano, J.M., *et al.* (2007) A randomized factorial trial of vitamins C and E and beta carotene in the secondary prevention of cardiovascular events in women: results from the Women's Antioxidant Cardiovascular Study. *Arch Intern Med* **167**, 1610–8.

326. Cooper, C., O'Neill, T. & Silman, A. (1993) The epidemiology of vertebral fractures. European Vertebral Osteoporosis Study Group. *Bone* **14**, S89–97.

327. Cooper, R.S., Rotimi, C.N., Kaufman, J.S., *et al.* (1997) Prevalence of NIDDM among populations of the African diaspora. *Diabetes Care* **20**, 343–8.

328. Corbett, W.T., Kuller, L.H., Blaine, E.H. & Damico, F.J. (1979) Utilization of swine to study the risk factor of an elevated salt diet on blood pressure. *Am J Clin Nutr* **32**, 2068–75.

329. Cordain, L. (1999) Cereal grains: humanity's double-edged sword. *World Rev Nutr Diet* **84**, 19–73.

330. Cordain, L. (2001) Syndrom X – det metabola syndromet. Hyperinsulinemin bakom en mångfald sjukdomar. *Medikament* **6**, 48–51.

331. Cordain, L. (2002) *The Paleo Diet*. Wiley, New York.

332. Cordain, L. (2006) Saturated fat consumption in ancestral human diets: implications for contemporary intakes. In: *Phytochemicals: nutrient-gene interactions* (M.S. Meskin, W.R. Bidlack & R.K. Randolph eds). Taylor & Francis, London, pp. 115–26.

333. Cordain, L., Eades, M.R. & Eades, M.D. (2003) Hyperinsulinemic diseases of civilization: more than just Syndrome X. *Comp Biochem Physiol A Mol Integr Physiol* **136**, 95–112.

334. Cordain, L., Eaton, S.B., Brand Miller, J., Lindeberg, S. & Jensen, C. (2002) An evolutionary analysis of the aetiology and pathogenesis of juvenile-onset myopia. *Acta Ophthalmol Scand* **80**, 125–35.

335. Cordain, L., Eaton, S.B., Sebastian, A., *et al.* (2005) Origins and evolution of the Western diet: health implications for the 21st century. *Am J Clin Nutr* **81**, 341–54.

336. Cordain, L., Gotshall, R.W., Eaton, S.B. & Eaton, S.B., 3rd (1998) Physical activity, energy expenditure and fitness: an evolutionary perspective. *Int J Sports Med* **19**, 328–35.

337. Cordain, L., Lindeberg, S., Hurtado, M., *et al.* (2002) Acne vulgaris: a disease of civilization. *Arch Dermatol* **138**, 1584–90.

338. Cordain, L., Miller, J.B., Eaton, S.B., *et al.* (2000) Plant-animal subsistence ratios and macronutrient energy estimations in worldwide hunter-gatherer diets. *Am J Clin Nutr* **71**, 682–92.

339. Cordain, L., Toohey, L., Smith, M.J. & Hickey, M.S. (2000) Modulation of immune function by dietary lectins in rheumatoid arthritis. *Br J Nutr* **83**, 207–17.

340. Cordain, L., Watkins, B.A., Florant, G.L., *et al.* (2002) Fatty acid analysis of wild ruminant tissues: evolutionary implications for reducing diet-related chronic disease. *Eur J Clin Nutr* **56**, 181–91.

341. Corthesy-Theulaz, I., den Dunnen, J.T., Ferre, P., *et al.* (2005) Nutrigenomics: the impact of biomics technology on nutrition research. *Ann Nutr Metab* **49**, 355–65.

342. Courteix, D., Jaffre, C., Lespessailles, E. & Benhamou, L. (2005) Cumulative effects of calcium supplementation and physical activity on bone accretion in premenarchal children: a double-blind randomised placebo-controlled trial. *Int J Sports Med* **26**, 332–8.

343. Coutinho, M., Gerstein, H.C., Wang, Y. & Yusuf, S. (1999) The relationship between glucose and incident cardiovascular events. A metaregression analysis of published data from 20 studies of 95,783 individuals followed for 12.4 years. *Diabetes Care* **22**, 233–240.

344. Cowley, A.W., Jr. (1997) Genetic and nongenetic determinants of salt sensitivity and blood pressure. *Am J Clin Nutr* **65**, 587S–93S.

345. Cox, B.D. & Whichelow, M. (1996) Ratio of waist circumference to height is better predictor of death than body mass index. *BMJ* **313**, 1487.

346. Craft, S., Asthana, S., Schellenberg, G., *et al.* (2000) Insulin effects on glucose metabolism, memory, and plasma amyloid precursor protein in Alzheimer's disease differ according to apolipoprotein-E genotype. *Ann N Y Acad Sci* **903**, 222–8.

347. Crawford, D.H., Powell, L.W., Leggett, B.A., *et al.* (1995) Evidence that the ancestral haplotype in Australian hemochromatosis patients may be associated with a common mutation in the gene. *Am J Hum Genet* **57**, 362–7.

348. Crews, D.E. & MacKeen, P.C. (1982) Mortality related to cardiovascular disease and diabetes mellitus in a modernizing population. *Soc Sci Med* **16**, 175–81.

349. Crovetti, R., Porrini, M., Santangelo, A. & Testolin, G. (1998) The influence of thermic effect of food on satiety. *Eur J Clin Nutr* **52**, 482–8.

350. Cruickshank, J.K., Mbanya, J.C., Wilks, R., *et al.* (2001) Sick genes, sick individuals or sick populations with chronic disease? The emergence of diabetes and high blood pressure in African-origin populations. *Int J Epidemiol* **30**, 111–7.

351. Cruz, M.L., Evans, K. & Frayn, K.N. (2001) Postprandial lipid metabolism and insulin sensitivity in young Northern Europeans, South Asians and Latin Americans in the UK. *Atherosclerosis* **159**, 441–9.

352. Cruz-Coke, R., Etcheverry, R. & Nagel, R. (1964) Influence of migration on blood pressure of Easter Islanders. *Lancet* **i**, 697–9.

353. Cuatrecasas, P. (1973) Interaction of wheat germ agglutinin and concanavalin A with isolated fat cells. *Biochemistry* **12**, 1312–23.

354. Cuatrecasas, P. & Tell, G.P. (1973) Insulin-like activity of concanavalin A and wheat germ agglutinin – direct interactions with insulin receptors. *Proc Natl Acad Sci USA* **70**, 485–9.

355. Cuchel, M. & Rader, D.J. (2006) Macrophage reverse cholesterol transport: key to the regression of atherosclerosis? *Circulation* **113**, 2548–55.

356. Cummings, S.R. & Melton, L.J. (2002) Epidemiology and outcomes of osteoporotic fractures. *Lancet* **359**, 1761–7.

357. Cunnane, S.C. & Crawford, M.A. (2003) Survival of the fattest: fat babies were the key to evolution of the large human brain. *Comp Biochem Physiol A Mol Integr Physiol* **136**, 17–26.

358. Curioni, C., Andre, C. & Veras, R. (2006) Weight reduction for primary prevention of stroke in adults with overweight or obesity. *Cochrane Database Syst Rev*, CD006062.

359. Cyrus, T., Tang, L.X., Rokach, J., FitzGerald, G.A. & Pratico, D. (2001) Lipid peroxidation and platelet activation in murine atherosclerosis. *Circulation* **104**, 1940–45.

360. D'Agostino, R.B., Jr., Burke, G., O'Leary, D., *et al.* (1996) Ethnic differences in carotid wall thickness. The Insulin Resistance Atherosclerosis Study. *Stroke* **27**, 1744–9.

361. Dahl-Jørgensen, K., Joner, G. & Hanssen, K.F. (1991) Relationship between cows' milk consumption and incidence of IDDM in childhood. *Diabetes Care* **14**, 1081–3.

362. Dai, Z., Xu, Y.C. & Niu, L. (2007) Obesity and colorectal cancer risk: a meta-analysis of cohort studies. *World J Gastroenterol* **13**, 4199–206.

363. Daly, M.E., Paisey, R., Paisey, R., *et al.* (2006) Short-term effects of severe dietary carbohydrate-restriction advice in Type 2 diabetes – a randomized controlled trial. *Diabet Med* **23**, 15–20.

364. Damasceno, N.R., Gidlund, M.A., Goto, H., *et al.* (2001) Casein and soy protein isolate in experimental atherosclerosis: influence on hyperlipidemia and lipoprotein oxidation. *Ann Nutr Metab* **45**, 38–46.

365. Damasceno, N.R., Goto, H., Rodrigues, F.M., *et al.* (2000) Soy protein isolate reduces the oxidizability of LDL and the generation of oxidized LDL autoantibodies in rabbits with diet-induced atherosclerosis. *J Nutr* **130**, 2641–7.

366. Dandona, P., Aljada, A., Chaudhuri, A., Mohanty, P. & Garg, R. (2005) Metabolic syndrome: a comprehensive perspective based on interactions between obesity, diabetes, and inflammation. *Circulation* **111**, 1448–54.

367. Danesh, J. & Appleby, P. (1999) Coronary heart disease and iron status: meta-analyses of prospective studies. *Circulation* **99**, 852–4.

368. Dang, A., Zheng, D., Wang, B., *et al.* (1999) The role of the renin-angiotensin and cardiac sympathetic nervous systems in the development of hypertension and left ventricular hypertrophy in spontaneously hypertensive rats. *Hypertens Res* **22**, 217–21.

369. Daniel, K.T. (2005) *The whole soy story. The dark side of America's favorite health food.* New Trends Publishing, Washington, DC.

370. Dannenberger, D., Nuernberg, G., Scollan, N., *et al.* (2004) Effect of diet on the deposition of n-3 fatty acids, conjugated linoleic and C18:1trans fatty acid isomers in muscle lipids of German Holstein bulls. *J Agric Food Chem* **52**, 6607–15.

371. Dansinger, M.L., Gleason, J.A., Griffith, J.L., Selker, H.P. & Schaefer, E.J. (2005) Comparison of the Atkins, Ornish, Weight Watchers, and Zone diets for weight loss and heart disease risk reduction: a randomized trial. *JAMA* **293**, 43–53.

372. Darwin, C. (1998) *The origin of species.* Wadsworth, London.

373. Davidson, A. & Diamond, B. (2001) Autoimmune diseases. *N Engl J Med* **345**, 340–50.

374. Davidson, M.H., Hunninghake, D., Maki, K.C., Kwiterovich, P.O., Jr. & Kafonek, S. (1999) Comparison of the effects of lean red meat vs lean white meat on serum lipid levels among free-living persons with hypercholesterolemia: a long-term, randomized clinical trial. *Arch Intern Med* **159**, 1331–8.

375. Davies, J. (1948) Pathology of central African natives. IX. Cardiovscular diseases. *East Afr Med J* **25**, 454–67.

376. Davis, H.R. & Glagov, S. (1986) Lectin binding to distinguish cell types in fixed atherosclerotic arteries. *Atherosclerosis* **61**, 193–203.

377. Davis, J., Higginbotham, A., O'Connor, T., *et al.* (2007) Soy protein and isoflavones influence adiposity and development of metabolic syndrome in the obese male ZDF rat. *Ann Nutr Metab* **51**, 42–52.

378. Davis, M.A., Neuhaus, J.M., Ettinger, W.H. & Mueller, W.H. (1990) Body fat distribution and osteoarthritis. *Am J Epidemiol* **132**, 701–7.

379. Dawson-Hughes, B., Heaney, R.P., Holick, M.F., *et al.* (2005) Estimates of optimal vitamin D status. *Osteoporos Int* **16**, 713–6.

380. Day, J., Carruthers, M., Bailey, A. & Robinson, D. (1976) Anthropometric, physiological and biochemical differences between urban and rural Maasai. *Atherosclerosis* **23**, 357–61.

381. Dayi, S.U., Kasikcioglu, H., Uslu, N., *et al.* (2006) Influence of weight loss on myocardial performance index. *Heart Vessels* **21**, 84–8.

382. De Backer, G., Ambrosioni, E., Borch-Johnsen, K., *et al.* (2003) European guidelines on cardiovascular disease prevention in clinical practice. Third Joint Task Force of European and Other Societies on cardiovascular disease prevention in clinical practice. *Eur Heart J* **24**, 1601–10.

383. de Jongh, R.T., Serne, E.H., RG, I.J. & Stehouwer, C.D. (2007) Microvascular function: a potential link between salt sensitivity, insulin resistance and hypertension. *J Hypertens* **25**, 1887–93.

384. de la Torre, J.C. (2004) Is Alzheimer's disease a neurodegenerative or a vascular disorder? Data, dogma, and dialectics. *Lancet Neurol* **3**, 184–90.

385. De Laet, C., Kanis, J.A., Oden, A., *et al.* (2005) Body mass index as a predictor of fracture risk: a meta-analysis. *Osteoporos Int* **16**, 1330–8.

386. de Lorgeril, M., Renaud, S., Mamelle, N., *et al.* (1994) Mediterranean alpha-linolenic acid-rich diet in secondary prevention of coronary heart disease. *Lancet* **ii**, 1454–9.

387. de Lorgeril, M. & Salen, P. (2000) Modified Cretan Mediterranean diet in the prevention of coronary heart disease and cancer. *World Rev Nutr Diet* **87**, 1–23.

388. de Lorgeril, M., Salen, P., Martin, J.L., *et al.* (1999) Mediterranean diet, traditional risk factors, and the rate of cardiovascular complications after myocardial infarction: final report of the Lyon Diet Heart Study [see comments]. *Circulation* **99**, 779–85.

389. De Luca, F., Uyeda, J.A., Mericq, V., *et al.* (2000) Retinoic acid is a potent regulator of growth plate chondrogenesis. *Endocrinology* **141**, 346–53.

390. de Maat, M.P., Pijl, H., Kluft, C. & Princen, H.M. (2000) Consumption of black and green tea had no effect on inflammation, haemostasis and endothelial markers in smoking healthy individuals. *Eur J Clin Nutr* **54**, 757–63.

391. de Rooij, S.R., Painter, R.C., Holleman, F., Bossuyt, P.M. & Roseboom, T.J. (2007) The metabolic syndrome in adults prenatally exposed to the Dutch famine. *Am J Clin Nutr* **86**, 1219–24.

392. de Roos, N.M., Bots, M.L. & Katan, M.B. (2001) Replacement of dietary saturated fatty acids by trans fatty acids lowers serum HDL cholesterol and impairs endothelial function in healthy men and women. *Arterioscler Thromb Vasc Biol* **21**, 1233–7.

393. De Wolfe, M.S. & Whyte, H.M. (1958) Serum cholesterol and lipoproteins in natives of New Guinea and Australians. *Aust Ann Med* **7**, 47–54.

394. DeFoliart, G.R. (1999) Insects as food: why the western attitude is important. *Annu Rev Entomol* **44**, 21–50.

395. DeFronzo, R.A. (2004) Dysfunctional fat cells, lipotoxicity and type 2 diabetes. *Int J Clin Pract Suppl*, 9–21.

396. Del Puente, A., Knowler, W.C., Pettitt, D.J. & Bennett, P.H. (1989) High incidence and prevalence of rheumatoid arthritis in Pima Indians. *Am J Epidemiol* **129**, 1170–8.

397. Delange, F., Van Onderbergen, A., Shabana, W., *et al.* (2000) Silent iodine prophylaxis in Western Europe only partly corrects iodine deficiency; the case of Belgium. *Eur J Endocrinol* **143**, 189–96.

398. DeLucia, M.C. & Carpenter, T.O. (2002) Rickets in the sunshine? *Nutrition* **18**, 97–9.

399. Demaison, L. & Moreau, D. (2002) Dietary n-3 polyunsaturated fatty acids and coronary heart disease- related mortality: a possible mechanism of action. *Cell Mol Life Sci* **59**, 463–77.

400. Denke, M.A. (1993) Dietary determinants of high-density-lipoprotein-cholesterol levels. *Cardiovascular Risk Factors* **3**, 274–8.

401. Department of Health (1991) *Dietary reference values for food, energy and nutrients for the United Kingdom.* HMSO, London.

402. Department of Health Nova Scotia (1989) *A diet manual for Papua New Guinea.* Department of Health, Papua New Guinea, Port Moresby.

403. Dessein, P.H., Shipton, E.A., Stanwix, A.E., Joffe, B.I. & Ramokgadi, J. (2000) Beneficial effects of weight loss associated with moderate calorie/carbohydrate restriction, and increased proportional intake of protein and unsaturated fat on serum urate and lipoprotein levels in gout: a pilot study. *Ann Rheum Dis* **59**, 539–43.

404. Devereux, R.B. (1988) Echocardiography, hypertension, and left ventricular mass. *Health Psychol* **7**, 89–104.

405. Devine, A., Criddle, R.A., Dick, I.M., Kerr, D.A. & Prince, R.L. (1995) A longitudinal study of the effect of sodium and calcium intakes on regional bone density in postmenopausal women. *Am J Clin Nutr* **62**, 740–5.

406. Devine, A., Dick, I.M., Islam, A.F., Dhaliwal, S.S. & Prince, R.L. (2005) Protein consumption is an important predictor of lower limb bone mass in elderly women. *Am J Clin Nutr* **81**, 1423–8.

407. Devine, H.D. (1946) Rheumatic Heart Disease in New Guinea: Including a Cardiovascular Survey of 200 Native Papuans. *Ann Intern Med* **24**, 826–36.

408. Dewdney, J.C.H. (1965) Maprik Hospital – a review of 3888 consecutive admissions, February 1963 to July 1964. *Papua New Guinea Med J* **8**, 89–96.

409. Dewell, A., Hollenbeck, P.L. & Hollenbeck, C.B. (2006) Clinical review: a critical evaluation of the role of soy protein and isoflavone supplementation in the control of plasma cholesterol concentrations. *J Clin Endocrinol Metab* **91**, 772–80.

410. Dewey, C.E. (1999) Diseases of the nervous system and locomotor system. In: *Diseases of swine* (B.E. Straw, S. D'Allaire, W.L. Mengeling & D.J. Taylor eds). Blackwell Science, Oxford, pp. 861–82.

411. Di Buono, M., Hannah, J.S., Katzel, L.I. & Jones, P.J. (1999) Weight loss due to energy restriction suppresses cholesterol biosynthesis in overweight, mildly hypercholesterolemic men. *J Nutr* **129**, 1545–8.

412. Di Castelnuovo, A., Rotondo, S., Iacoviello, L., Donati, M.B. & De Gaetano, G. (2002) Meta-analysis of wine and beer consumption in relation to vascular risk. *Circulation* **105**, 2836–44.

413. Diamanti-Kandarakis, E., Paterakis, T. & Kandarakis, H.A. (2006) Indices of low-grade inflammation in polycystic ovary syndrome. *Ann N Y Acad Sci* **1092**, 175–86.

414. Diamond, J. (2002) Evolution, consequences and future of plant and animal domestication. *Nature* **418**, 700–7.

415. Diamond, J. (2003) The double puzzle of diabetes. *Nature* **423**, 599–602.

416. Diaz-Arjonilla, M., Schwarcz, M., Swerdloff, R.S. & Wang, C. (2009) Obesity, low testosterone levels and erectile dysfunction. *Int J Impot Res* **21**, 89–98.

417. Dichtl, W., Ares, M.P., Jonson, A.N., *et al.* (2002) Linoleic acid-stimulated vascular adhesion molecule-1 expression in endothelial cells depends on nuclear factor-kappaB activation. *Metabolism* **51**, 327–33.

418. Dickinson, H.O., Nicolson, D.J., Campbell, F., Beyer, F.R. & Mason, J. (2006) Potassium supplementation for the management of primary hypertension in adults. *Cochrane Database Syst Rev* **3**, CD004641.

419. Dickinson, H.O., Nicolson, D.J., Campbell, F., *et al.* (2006) Magnesium supplementation for the management of essential hypertension in adults. *Cochrane Database Syst Rev* **3**, CD004640.

420. Dietler, M. (2006) Alcohol: anthropological/archaeological perspectives. *Annu Rev Anthropol* **35**, 229–49.

421. Diez, M., Nguyen, P., Jeusette, I., *et al.* (2002) Weight loss in obese dogs: evaluation of a high-protein, low-carbohydrate diet. *J Nutr* **132**, 1685S–7S.

422. DiFrancesco, L., Allen, O.B. & Mercer, N.H. (1990) Long-term feeding of casein or soy protein with or without cholesterol in Mongolian gerbils. II. Plasma lipid and liver cholesterol responses. *Acta Cardiol* **45**, 273–90.

423. DiFrancesco, L., Percy, D.H. & Mercer, N.H. (1990) Long-term feeding of casein or soy protein with or without cholesterol in Mongolian gerbils. I. Morphologic effects. *Acta Cardiol* **45**, 257–71.

424. Dignam, J.J., Polite, B.N., Yothers, G., *et al.* (2006) Body mass index and outcomes in patients who receive adjuvant chemotherapy for colon cancer. *J Natl Cancer Inst* **98**, 1647–54.

425. Dikow, R., Adamczak, M., Henriquez, D.E. & Ritz, E. (2002) Strategies to decrease cardiovascular mortality in patients with end-stage renal disease. *Kidney Int* **61** (Suppl 80), 5–10.

426. Distante, S., Robson, K.J., Graham-Campbell, J., *et al.* (2004) The origin and spread of the HFE-C282Y haemochromatosis mutation. *Hum Genet* **115**, 269–79.

427. Divi, R.L. & Doerge, D.R. (1996) Inhibition of thyroid peroxidase by dietary flavonoids. *Chem Res Toxicol* **9**, 16–23.

428. Dobson, J.E. (1998) The iodine factor in health and evolution. *Geograph Rev* **88**, 1–28.

429. Dodu, S. (1972) Clinical aspects of ischaemic heart disease (IHD) in Ghana. *Ghana Med J* **11**, 203–214.

430. Doehner, W., Anker, S.D. & Coats, A.J. (2000) Defects in insulin action in chronic heart failure. *Diabetes Obes Metab* **2**, 203–12.

431. Doerge, D.R. & Sheehan, D.M. (2002) Goitrogenic and estrogenic activity of soy isoflavones. *Environ Health Perspect* **110** (Suppl 3), 349–53.

432. Dolfini, E., Elli, L., Ferrero, S., *et al.* (2003) Bread wheat gliadin cytotoxicity: a new three-dimensional cell model. *Scand J Clin Lab Invest* **63**, 135–41.

433. Doll, R., Peto, R., Boreham, J. & Sutherland, I. (2004) Mortality in relation to smoking: 50 years' observations on male British doctors. *BMJ* **328**, 1519.

434. Donnison, C.P. (1929) Blood pressure in the African native. Its bearing upon the ætiology of hyperpiesia and arterio-sclerosis. *Lancet* **i**, 6–7.

435. Donovan, D.S., Solomon, C.G., Seely, E.W., Williams, G.H. & Simonson, D.C. (1993) Effect of sodium intake on insulin sensitivity. *Am J Physiol* **264**, E730–34.

436. Douglas, M.W., Parsons, C.M. & Hymowitz, T. (1999) Nutritional evaluation of lectin-free soybeans for poultry. *Poult Sci* **78**, 91–5.

437. Doyle, C., Kushi, L.H., Byers, T., *et al.* (2006) Nutrition and physical activity during and after cancer treatment: an American Cancer Society guide for informed choices. *CA Cancer J Clin* **56**, 323–53.

438. Drago, S., El Asmar, R., Di Pierro, M., *et al.* (2006) Gliadin, zonulin and gut permeability: effects on celiac and non-celiac intestinal mucosa and intestinal cell lines. *Scand J Gastroenterol* **41**, 408–19.

439. Draper, H.H. (1977) The aboriginal Eskimo diet in modern perspective. *Am Anthropol* **79**, 309–16.

440. Dreux, A.C., Lamb, D.J., Modjtahedi, H. & Ferns, G.A. (2006) The epidermal growth factor receptors and their family of ligands: their putative role in atherogenesis. *Atherosclerosis* **186**, 38–53.

441. Drøyvold, W.B., Nilsen, T.I.L., Lydersen, S., *et al.* (2005) Weight change and mortality – The Nord-Trøndelag Health Study. *J Intern Med* **257**, 338–45.

442. Duckworth, W., Abraira, C., Moritz, T., *et al.* (2008) Glucose control and vascular complications in veterans with type 2 diabetes. *N Engl J Med* **360**, 129–39.

443. Dudeja, V., Misra, A., Pandey, R.M., *et al.* (2001) BMI does not accurately predict overweight in Asian Indians in northern India. *Br J Nutr* **86**, 105–12.

444. Dudley, R. (2002) Fermenting fruit and the historical ecology of ethanol ingestion: is alcoholism in modern humans an evolutionary hangover? *Addiction* **97**, 381–8.

445. Due, A., Larsen, T.M., Hermansen, K., *et al.* (2008) Comparison of the effects on insulin resistance and glucose tolerance of 6-mo high-monounsaturated-fat, low-fat, and control diets. *Am J Clin Nutr* **87**, 855–62.

446. Due, A., Larsen, T.M., Mu, H., *et al.* (2008) Comparison of 3 ad libitum diets for weight-loss maintenance, risk of cardiovascular disease, and diabetes: a 6-mo randomized, controlled trial. *Am J Clin Nutr* **88**, 1232–41.

447. Duffy, C., Perez, K. & Partridge, A. (2007) Implications of phytoestrogen intake for breast cancer. *CA Cancer J Clin* **57**, 260–77.

448. Duffy, S.J., Keaney, J.F., Jr., Holbrook, M., *et al.* (2001) Short- and long-term black tea consumption reverses endothelial dysfunction in patients with coronary artery disease. *Circulation* **104**, 151–6.

449. Dumartheray, E.W., Lanham-New, S.A., Whittamore, D.R., Krieg, M. & Burckhardt, P. (2007) Low estimates of PRAL (nutritional acid load) correlates with bone ultrasound measurements in elderly fractured women. *Calcif Tissue Internat* **80**, S172–3.

450. Dunne, F.P., Brydon, P.A., Proffitt, M., *et al.* (2000) Fetal and maternal outcomes in Indo-Asian compared to Caucasian women with diabetes in pregnancy. *QJM* **93**, 813–8.

451. Durga, J., van Boxtel, M.P., Schouten, E.G., *et al.* (2007) Effect of 3-year folic acid supplementation on cognitive function in older adults in the FACIT trial: a randomised, double blind, controlled trial. *Lancet* **369**, 208–16.

452. Dwyer, J. (1999) Convergence of plant-rich and plant-only diets. *Am J Clin Nutr* **70**, 620S–2S.

453. Dwyer, J.H., Navab, M., Dwyer, K.M., *et al.* (2001) Oxygenated carotenoid lutein and progression of early atherosclerosis: the Los Angeles atherosclerosis study. *Circulation* **103**, 2922–7.

454. Dyerberg, J. (1989) Coronary heart disease in Greenland Inuit: a paradox. Implications for western diet patterns. *Arctic Med Res* **48**, 47–54.

455. Dyson, P.A. (2008) A review of low and reduced carbohydrate diets and weight loss in type 2 diabetes. *J Hum Nutr Diet* **21**, 530–8.

456. Dzhangaliev, A.D., Salova, T.N. & Turekhanova, P.M. (2003) The wild fruit and nut plants of Kazakhstan. *Horticultural Rev* **29**, 305–71.

457. Eason, R.J., Pada, J., Wallace, R., Henry, A. & Thornton, R. (1987) Changing patterns of hypertension, diabetes, obesity and diet among Melanesians and Micronesians in the Solomon Islands. *Med J Aust* **146**, 465–9.

458. Eastwood, M. & Kritchevsky, D. (2005) Dietary fiber: how did we get where we are? *Annu Rev Nutr* **25**, 1–8.

459. Eaton, S. & Konner, M. (1985) Paleolithic nutrition. A consideration of its nature and current implications. *N Engl J Med* **312**, 283–9.

460. Eaton, S.B., Cordain, L. & Lindeberg, S. (2002) Evolutionary health promotion: a consideration of common counterarguments. *Prev Med* **34**, 119–23.

461. Eaton, S.B. & Eaton, S.B., 3rd (2000) Paleolithic vs. modern diets-selected pathophysiological implications. *Eur J Nutr* **39**, 67–70.

462. Eaton, S.B. & Nelson, D.A. (1991) Calcium in evolutionary perspective. *Am J Clin Nutr* **54**, 281S–7S.

463. Eaton, S.B., Strassman, B.I., Nesse, R.M., *et al.* (2002) Evolutionary health promotion. *Prev Med* **34**, 109–18.

464. Ebbeling, C.B., Leidig, M.M., Feldman, H.A., Lovesky, M.M. & Ludwig, D.S. (2007) Effects of a low-glycemic load vs low-fat diet in obese young adults: a randomized trial. *JAMA* **297**, 2092–102.

465. Ebbeling, C.B., Leidig, M.M., Sinclair, K.B., *et al.* (2005) Effects of an ad libitum low-glycemic load diet on cardiovascular disease risk factors in obese young adults. *Am J Clin Nutr* **81**, 976–82.

466. Ebbesson, S.O., Roman, M.J., Devereux, R.B., *et al.* (2008) Consumption of omega-3 fatty acids is not associated with a reduction in carotid atherosclerosis: the Genetics of Coronary Artery Disease in Alaska Natives study. *Atherosclerosis* **199**, 346–53.

467. Ebbing, M., Bleie, O., Ueland, P.M., *et al.* (2008) Mortality and cardiovascular events in patients treated with homocysteine-lowering B vitamins after coronary angiography: a randomized controlled trial. *JAMA* **300**, 795–804.

468. Ebert, D. (1999) The evolution and expression of parasite virulence. In: *Evolution in health and disease* (S.C. Stearns ed). Oxford University Press, Oxford, pp. 161–72.

469. Eckel, R.H. (2004) Diabetes and dietary macronutrients: is carbohydrate all that bad? *Am J Clin Nutr* **80**, 537–8.

470. Edginton, M.E., Hodkinson, J. & Seftel, H.C. (1972) Disease patterns in a South African rural Bantu population, including a commentary on comparisons with the pattern in urbanized Johannesburg Bantu. *S Afr Med J* **46**, 968–76.

471. Edwards, C.A., Tomlin, J. & Read, N.W. (1988) Fibre and constipation. *Br J Clin Pract* **42**, 26–32.

472. Edwards, F.M., Wise, P.H., Thomas, D.W., Murchland, J.B. & Craig, R.J. (1976) Blood pressures and electrocardiographic findings in the South Australian Aborigines. *Aust N Z J Med* **6**, 197–205.

473. Egan, B.M., Greene, E.L. & Goodfriend, T.L. (2001) Insulin resistance and cardiovascular disease. *Am J Hypertens* **14**, 116S–25S.

474. Egan, M.B., Fragodt, A., Raats, M.M., Hodgkins, C. & Lumbers, M. (2007) The importance of harmonizing food composition data across Europe. *Eur J Clin Nutr* **61**, 813–21.

475. Egger, M., Davey Smith, G., Schneider, M. & Minder, C. (1997) Bias in meta-analysis detected by a simple, graphical test. *BMJ* **315**, 629–34.

476. el Hag, A.I. & Karrar, Z.A. (1995) Nutritional vitamin D deficiency rickets in Sudanese children. *Ann Trop Paediatr* **15**, 69–76.

477. el Hassan, A.M. & Wasfi, A. (1972) Cardiovascular disease in Khartoum. Post-mortem and clinical evidence. *Trop Geogr Med* **24**, 118–23.

478. Elford, J., Phillips, A., Thomson, A.G. & Shaper, A.G. (1990) Migration and geographic variations in blood pressure in Britain. *BMJ* **300**, 291–5.

479. Eliassen, A.H., Colditz, G.A., Rosner, B., Willett, W.C. & Hankinson, S.E. (2006) Adult weight change and risk of postmenopausal breast cancer. *JAMA* **296**, 193–201.

480. Eliasson, B., Attvall, S., Taskinen, M.R. & Smith, U. (1997) Smoking cessation improves insulin sensitivity in healthy middle-aged men. *Eur J Clin Invest* **27**, 450–6.

481. Elin, R.J. & Hosseini, J.M. (1993) Is the magnesium content of nuts a factor for coronary heart disease? *Arch Intern Med* **153**, 779–80.

482. Ellervik, C., Tybjaerg-Hansen, A., Appleyard, M., *et al.* (2007) Hereditary hemochromatosis genotypes and risk of ischemic stroke. *Neurology* **68**, 1025–31.

483. Ellervik, C., Tybjaerg-Hansen, A., Grande, P., Appleyard, M. & Nordestgaard, B.G. (2005) Hereditary hemochromatosis and risk of ischemic heart disease: a prospective study and a case-control study. *Circulation* **112**, 185–93.

484. Elliott, P., Stamler, J., Dyer, A.R., *et al.* (2006) Association between protein intake and blood pressure: the INTERMAP Study. *Arch Intern Med* **166**, 79–87.

485. Elliott, P., Walker, L.L., Little, M.P., *et al.* (2007) Change in salt intake affects blood pressure of chimpanzees. Implications for human populations. *Circulation* **116**, 1563–8.

486. Elliott, R.B., Harris, D.P., Hill, J.P., Bibby, N.J. & Wasmuth, H.E. (1999) Type I (insulin-dependent) diabetes mellitus and cow milk: casein variant consumption. *Diabetologia* **42**, 292–6.

487. Elliott, S.S., Keim, N.L., Stern, J.S., Teff, K. & Havel, P.J. (2002) Fructose, weight gain, and the insulin resistance syndrome. *Am J Clin Nutr* **76**, 911–22.

488. Ellis, R., Kelsay, J.L., Reynolds, R.D., *et al.* (1987) Phytate:zinc and phytate X calcium:zinc millimolar ratios in self-selected diets of Americans, Asian Indians, and Nepalese. *J Am Diet Assoc* **87**, 1043–7.

489. Elsayed, E.F., Sarnak, M.J., Tighiouart, H., *et al.* (2008) Waist-to-hip ratio, body mass index, and subsequent kidney disease and death. *Am J Kidney Dis* **52**, 29–38.

490. Elwood, P.C., Pickering, J.E., Hughes, J., Fehily, A.M. & Ness, A.R. (2004) Milk drinking, ischaemic heart disease and ischaemic stroke II. Evidence from cohort studies. *Eur J Clin Nutr* **58**, 718–24.

491. Elwood, P.C., Strain, J.J., Robson, P.J., *et al.* (2005) Milk consumption, stroke, and heart attack risk: evidence from the Caerphilly cohort of older men. *J Epidemiol Community Health* **59**, 502–5.

492. Emanuel, M.B. (1988) Hay fever, a post industrial revolution epidemic: a history of its growth during the 19th century. *Clin Allergy* **18**, 295–304.

493. Emerson, H. & Larimore, L.D. (1924) Diabetes mellitus: a contribution to its epidemiology based chiefly on mortality statistics. *Arch Intern Med* **34**, 585–630.

494. Eneli, I.U., Skybo, T. & Camargo, C.A., Jr. (2008) Weight loss and asthma: a systematic review. *Thorax* **63**, 671–6.

495. Engelmann, M.D., Sandstrom, B. & Michaelsen, K.F. (1998) Meat intake and iron status in late infancy: an intervention study. *J Pediatr Gastroenterol Nutr* **26**, 26–33.

496. Englyst, H.N. & Hudson, G.J. (2000) Carbohydrates. In: *Human Nutrition and Dietetics* (J.S. Garrow & W.P.T. James eds). Churchill Livingstone, Edinburgh, pp. 61–76.

497. Ennezat, P.V., Houel, R., Heloire, F., *et al.* (1998) [Effects of high sodium intake on ventricular remodeling in mice]. *Arch Mal Coeur Vaiss* **91**, 935–9.

498. Ercan, N., Nuttall, F.Q., Gannon, M.C., *et al.* (1993) Plasma glucose and insulin responses to bananas of varying ripeness in persons with noninsulin-dependent diabetes mellitus. *J Am Coll Nutr* **12**, 703–9.

499. Ercan, N., Nuttall, F.Q., Gannon, M.C., Redmon, J.B. & Sheridan, K.J. (1993) Effects of glucose, galactose, and lactose ingestion on the plasma glucose and insulin response in persons with non-insulin-dependent diabetes mellitus. *Metabolism* **42**, 1560–7.

500. Erkkila, A.T. & Lichtenstein, A.H. (2006) Fiber and cardiovascular disease risk: how strong is the evidence? *J Cardiovasc Nurs* **21**, 3–8.

501. Evans, C. & Eastell, R. (1995) Adaptation to high dietary sodium intake. In: Nutritional aspects of osteoporosis '94, Vol. 7 (P. Burckhardt & R.P. Heaney eds). Ares-Serono Symposia, Rome, pp. 413–8.

502. Evans, T.R. & Kaye, S.B. (1999) Retinoids: present role and future potential. *Br J Cancer* **80**, 1–8.

503. Evans, W.J. (1995) What is sarcopenia? *J Gerontol A Biol Sci Med Sci* **50** Spec No, 5–8.

504. Evans, W.J. (1996) Reversing sarcopenia: how weight training can build strength and vitality. *Geriatrics* **51**, 46–7.

505. Fagerberg, B., Berglund, A., Andersson, O.K., Berglund, G. & Wikstrand, J. (1991) Cardiovascular effects of weight reduction versus antihypertensive drug treatment: a comparative, randomized, 1-year study of obese men with mild hypertension. *J Hypertens* **9**, 431–9.

506. Fairweather, T.S. & Wright, A.J. (1990) The effects of sugar-beet fibre and wheat bran on iron and zinc absorption in rats. *Br J Nutr* **64**, 547–52.

507. Falsetti, L. & Eleftheriou, G. (1996) Hyperinsulinemia in the polycystic ovary syndrome: a clinical, endocrine and echographic study in 240 patients. *Gynecol Endocrinol* **10**, 319–26.

508. Fang, J. & Alderman, M.H. (2000) Serum uric acid and cardiovascular mortality the NHANES I epidemiologic follow-up study, 1971–1992. National Health and Nutrition Examination Survey. *JAMA* **283**, 2404–10.

509. Farnworth, E.R. (1975) Areca catechu and Piper betle in Papua New Guinea: an elemental analysis. *Sci N Guinea* **3**, 211–4.

510. Fava, D., Leslie, R.D. & Pozzilli, P. (1994) Relationship between dairy product consumption and incidence of IDDM in childhood in Italy. *Diabetes Care* **17**, 1488–90.

511. Feigin, V.L., Lawes, C.M.M., Bennett, D.A. & Anderson, C.S. (2003) Stroke epidemiology: a review of population-based studies of incidence, prevalence, and case-fatality in the late 20th century. *Lancet Neurol* **2**, 43–53.

512. Feldhahn, J.R., Rand, J.S. & Martin, G. (1999) Insulin sensitivity in normal and diabetic cats. *J Feline Med Surg* **1**, 107–15.

513. Felson, D.T., Zhang, Y., Anthony, J.M., Naimark, A. & Anderson, J.J. (1992) Weight loss reduces the risk for symptomatic knee osteoarthritis in women. The Framingham Study. *Ann Intern Med* **116**, 535–9.

514. Fendri, S., Roussel, B., Lormeau, B., Tribout, B. & Lalau, J.D. (1998) Insulin sensitivity, insulin action, and fibrinolysis activity in nondiabetic and diabetic obese subjects. *Metabolism* **47**, 1372–5.

515. Fenton, T.R., Eliasziw, M., Lyon, A.W., Tough, S.C. & Hanley, D.A. (2008) Meta-analysis of the quantity of calcium excretion associated with the net acid excretion of the modern diet under the acid-ash diet hypothesis. *Am J Clin Nutr* **88**, 1159–66.

516. Fernandez, M.L. (2001) Soluble fiber and nondigestible carbohydrate effects on plasma lipids and cardiovascular risk. *Curr Opin Lipidol* **12**, 35–40.

517. Fernandez, M.L. (2006) Dietary cholesterol provided by eggs and plasma lipoproteins in healthy populations. *Curr Opin Clin Nutr Metab Care* **9**, 8–12.

518. Ferry, R.J., Jr., Cerri, R.W. & Cohen, P. (1999) Insulin-like growth factor binding proteins: new proteins, new functions. *Horm Res* **51**, 53–67.

519. Fiennes, R.N. (1965) Atherosclerosis in wild animals. In: *Comparative atherosclerosis. The morphology of spontaneous and induced atherosclerotic lesions in animals and its relation to human disease* (J. Roberts & R. Straus eds). Harper & Row, New York, pp. 113–26.

520. Finck, B.N., Han, X., Courtois, M., *et al.* (2003) A critical role for PPARalpha-mediated lipotoxicity in the pathogenesis of diabetic cardiomyopathy: modulation by dietary fat content. *Proc Natl Acad Sci USA* **100**, 1226–31.

521. Finlayson, P.J., Caterson, L.D., Rhodes, K.M., *et al.* (1988) Diabetes, obesity and hypertension in Vanuatu. *P N G Med J* **31**, 9–18.

521a. Firestein, G.S., Alvaro-Gracia, J.M. & Maki, R. (1990) Quantitative analysis of cytokine gene expression in rheumatoid arthritis. *J Immunol* **144**, 33347–53.

522. Fisman, E.Z., Motro, M., Tenenbaum, A., *et al.* (2001) Impaired fasting glucose concentrations in nondiabetic patients with ischemic heart disease: a marker for a worse prognosis. *Am Heart J* **141**, 485–90.

523. FitzGerald, R.J., Murray, B.A. & Walsh, D.J. (2004) Hypotensive peptides from milk proteins. *J Nutr* **134**, 980S–8S.

524. Flegal, K.M., Graubard, B.I., Williamson, D.F. & Gail, M.H. (2005) Excess deaths associated with underweight, overweight, and obesity. *JAMA* **293**, 1861–7.

525. Flint, A., Moller, B.K., Raben, A., *et al.* (2006) Glycemic and insulinemic responses as determinants of appetite in humans. *Am J Clin Nutr* **84**, 1365–73.

526. Fogelholm, M. & Kukkonen-Harjula, K. (2000) Does physical activity prevent weight gain – a systematic review. *Obes Rev* **1**, 95–111.

527. Foley, R.N., Parfrey, P.S. & Sarnak, M.J. (1998) Epidemiology of cardiovascular disease in chronic renal disease. *J Am Soc Nephrol* **9**, S16–23.

528. Fontana, L. & Klein, S. (2007) Aging, adiposity, and calorie restriction. *JAMA* **297**, 986–94.

529. Fontana, L., Meyer, T.E., Klein, S. & Holloszy, J.O. (2004) Long-term calorie restriction is highly effective in reducing the risk for atherosclerosis in humans. *Proc Natl Acad Sci USA* **101**, 6659–63.

530. Ford, E.S. & Liu, S. (2001) Glycemic index and serum high-density lipoprotein cholesterol concentration among us adults. *Arch Intern Med* **161**, 572–6.

531. Ford, J.A., Colhoun, E.M., McIntosh, W.B. & Dunnigan, M.G. (1972) Biochemical response of late rickets and osteomalacia to a chupatty-free diet. *Br Med J* **3**, 446–7.

532. Formicola, V. & Giannecchini, M. (1999) Evolutionary trends of stature in upper Paleolithic and Mesolithic Europe. *J Hum Evol* **36**, 319–33.

533. Forsberg, G., Fahlgren, A., Horstedt, P., *et al.* (2004) Presence of bacteria and innate immunity of intestinal epithelium in childhood celiac disease. *Am J Gastroenterol* **99**, 894–904.

534. Fouque, D., Wang, P., Laville, M. & Boissel, J.P. (2000) Low protein diets delay end-stage renal disease in non-diabetic adults with chronic renal failure. *Nephrol Dial Transplant* **15**, 1986–92.

535. Fox, C., Esparza, J., Nicolson, M., *et al.* (1999) Plasma leptin concentrations in Pima Indians living in drastically different environments. *Diabetes Care* **22**, 413–7.

536. Franconi, F., Di Leo, M.A., Bennardini, F. & Ghirlanda, G. (2004) Is taurine beneficial in reducing risk factors for diabetes mellitus? *Neurochem Res* **29**, 143–50.

537. Fransen, H.P., de Jong, N., Wolfs, M., *et al.* (2007) Customary use of plant sterol and plant stanol enriched margarine is associated with changes in serum plant sterol and stanol concentrations in humans. *J Nutr* **137**, 1301–6.

538. Franz, M.J., Bantle, J.P., Beebe, C.A., *et al.* (2002) Evidence-based nutrition principles and recommendations for the treatment and prevention of diabetes and related complications. *Diabetes Care* **25**, 148–98.

539. Fraser, G.E., Sabate, J., Beeson, W.L. & Strahan, T.M. (1992) A possible protective effect of nut consumption on risk of coronary heart disease. The Adventist Health Study [see comments]. *Arch Intern Med* **152**, 1416–24.

540. Frassetto, L., Morris, R.C., Jr. & Sebastian, A. (2005) Long-term persistence of the urine calcium-lowering effect of potassium bicarbonate in postmenopausal women. *J Clin Endocrinol Metab* **90**, 831–4.

541. Frassetto, L., Morris, R.C., Jr., Sellmeyer, D.E., Todd, K. & Sebastian, A. (2001) Diet, evolution and aging – the pathophysiologic effects of the post-agricultural inversion of the potassium-to-sodium and base-to-chloride ratios in the human diet. *Eur J Nutr* **40**, 200–13.

542. Fredlund, K. (2002) *Inhibition of calcium and zinc absorption by phytate in man*, Göteborg, Göteborg.

543. Freed, D.L. (1999) Do dietary lectins cause disease? *BMJ* **318**, 1023–4.

544. Freed, D.L.J. (1991) Lectins in food: their importance in health and disease. *J Nutr Med* **2**, 45–64.

545. Freedland, S.J. & Platz, E.A. (2007) Obesity and prostate cancer: making sense out of apparently conflicting data. *Epidemiol Rev* **29**, 88–97.

546. Freis, E.D. (1992) The role of salt in hypertension. *Blood Press* **1**, 196–200.

547. Freyre, E.A., Rebaza, R.M., Sami, D.A. & Lozada, C.P. (1998) The prevalence of facial acne in Peruvian adolescents and its relation to their ethnicity. *J Adolesc Health* **22**, 480–4.

548. Frid, A.H., Nilsson, M., Holst, J.J. & Bjorck, I.M. (2005) Effect of whey on blood glucose and insulin responses to composite breakfast and lunch meals in type 2 diabetic subjects. *Am J Clin Nutr* **82**, 69–75.

549. Friedenreich, C.M. (2001) Review of anthropometric factors and breast cancer risk. *Eur J Cancer Prev* **10**, 15–32.

550. Frohlich, E.D., Chien, Y., Sesoko, S. & Pegram, B.L. (1993) Relationship between dietary sodium intake, hemodynamics, and cardiac mass in SHR and WKY rats. *Am J Physiol* **264**, R30–4.

551. Frostegard, J. (2005) Atherosclerosis in patients with autoimmune disorders. *Arterioscler Thromb Vasc Biol* **25**, 1776–85.

552. Frystyk, J. (2004) Free insulin-like growth factors – measurements and relationships to growth hormone secretion and glucose homeostasis. *Growth Horm IGF Res* **14**, 337–75.

553. Fukudome, S., Shimatsu, A., Suganuma, H. & Yoshikawa, M. (1995) Effect of gluten exorphins A5 and B5 on the postprandial plasma insulin level in conscious rats. *Life Sci* **57**, 729–34.

554. Fulton, B., Wagstaff, A.J. & Sorkin, E.M. (1995) Doxazosin. An update of its clinical pharmacology and therapeutic applications in hypertension and benign prostatic hyperplasia. *Drugs* **49**, 295–320.

555. Fulzele, K., DiGirolamo, D.J., Liu, Z., *et al.* (2007) Disruption of the insulin-like growth factor type 1 receptor in osteoblasts enhances insulin signaling and action. *J Biol Chem* **282**, 25649–58.

556. Furushima, M., Imaizumi, M. & Nakatsuka, K. (1999) Changes in refraction caused by induction of acute hyperglycemia in healthy volunteers. *Jpn J Ophthalmol* **43**, 398–403.

557. Futuyama, D.J. (1986) *Evolutionary biology*. Sinauer, Sunderland, Mass.

558. Gabor, F., Klausegger, U. & Wirth, M. (2001) The interaction between wheat germ agglutinin and other plant lectins with prostate cancer cells Du-145. *Int J Pharm* **221**, 35–47.

559. Gabor, F., Schwarzbauer, A. & Wirth, M. (2002) Lectin-mediated drug delivery: binding and uptake of BSA-WGA conjugates using the Caco-2 model. *Int J Pharm* **237**, 227–39.

560. Gaitan, E. (1990) Goitrogens in food and water. *Annu Rev Nutr* **10**, 21–39.

561. Gallagher, C.J., Gordon, C.J., Langefeld, C.D., *et al.* (2006) Association of the mu-opioid receptor gene with type 2 diabetes mellitus in an African American population. *Mol Genet Metab* **87**, 54–60.

562. Gallagher, D., Ruts, E., Visser, M., *et al.* (2000) Weight stability masks sarcopenia in elderly men and women. *Am J Physiol Endocrinol Metab* **279**, E366–75.

563. Gamerith, A. (1958) *Ehrfurcht vor Korn und Brot*. Bad Goisern, Austria.

564. Gann, P.H. (2009) Randomized trials of antioxidant supplementation for cancer prevention: first bias, now chance – next, cause. *JAMA* **301**, 102–3.

565. Gannon, M.C. & Nuttall, F.Q. (2006) Control of blood glucose in type 2 diabetes without weight loss by modification of diet composition. *Nutr Metab (Lond)* **3**, 16.

566. Gannon, M.C., Nuttall, F.Q., Krezowski, P.A., Billington, C.J. & Parker, S. (1986) The serum insulin and plasma glucose responses to milk and fruit products in type 2 (non-insulin-dependent) diabetic patients. *Diabetologia* **29**, 784–91.

567. Gardiner, P.A. (1954) The relation of myopia to growth. *Lancet* i, 476–9.

568. Gardiner, P.A. (1956) Observations on the food habits of myopic children. *BMJ* **2**, 699–700.

569. Gardiner, P.A. (1956) The diet of growing myopes. *Trans Ophthalmol Soc* **76**, 171–80.

570. Gardiner, P.A. (1958) Dietary treatment of myopia in children. *Lancet* i, 1152–5.

571. Gardiner, P.A. & MacDonald, I. (1957) Relationship between refraction of the eye and nutrition. *Clin Sci* **16**, 435–42.

572. Gardner, C.D., Kiazand, A., Alhassan, S., *et al.* (2007) Comparison of the Atkins, Zone, Ornish, and LEARN diets for change in weight and related risk factors among overweight premenopausal women: the A TO Z Weight Loss Study: a randomized trial. *JAMA* **297**, 969–77.

573. Garmendia, M.L., Pereira, A., Alvarado, M.E. & Atalah, E. (2007) Relation between insulin resistance and breast cancer among Chilean women. *Ann Epidemiol* **17**, 403–9.

574. Garnsey, P. (1988) *Famine and food supply in the Graeco-Roman world: Responses to risk and crisis.* Cambridge University Press, Cambridge.

575. Gaziano, J.M., Glynn, R.J., Christen, W.G., *et al.* (2009) Vitamins E and C in the prevention of prostate and total cancer in men: the Physicians' Health Study II Randomized Controlled Trial. *JAMA* **301**, 52–62.

576. Gee, R.W. (1983) The epidemiology of hypertension in the South Pacific. *P N G Med J* **26**, 55–8.

577. Gelber, R.P., Kurth, T., Manson, J.E., Buring, J.E. & Gaziano, J.M. (2007) Body mass index and mortality in men: evaluating the shape of the association. *Int J Obes (Lond)* **31**, 1240–47.

578. Gelfand, M. & Kaplan, M. (1958) Bantu coronary insufficiency. Report of a possible case. *Central Afr J Med* **4**, 157–9.

579. Gentner, D. & Holyoak, K.J. (1997) Reasoning and learning by analogy. *Am Psychol* **52**, 32–4.

580. Gerhard, G.T., Ahmann, A., Meeuws, K., *et al.* (2004) Effects of a low-fat diet compared with those of a high-monounsaturated fat diet on body weight, plasma lipids and lipoproteins, and glycemic control in type 2 diabetes. *Am J Clin Nutr* **80**, 668–73.

581. German, J.B. & Dillard, C.J. (2004) Saturated fats: what dietary intake? *Am J Clin Nutr* **80**, 550–9.

582. Gerstein, H.C., Miller, M.E., Byington, R.P., *et al.* (2008) Effects of intensive glucose lowering in type 2 diabetes. *N Engl J Med* **358**, 2545–59.

583. Gerstein, H.C., Pais, P., Pogue, J. & Yusuf, S. (1999) Relationship of glucose and insulin levels to the risk of myocardial infarction: a case-control study. *J Am Coll Cardiol* **33**, 612–9.

584. Gerstenblith, G., Frederiksen, J., Yin, F.C., *et al.* (1977) Echocardiographic assessment of a normal adult aging population. *Circulation* **56**, 273–8.

585. Getahun, D., Ananth, C.V., Peltier, M.R., Salihu, H.M. & Scorza, W.E. (2007) Changes in prepregnancy body mass index between the first and second pregnancies and risk of large-for-gestational-age birth. *Am J Obstet Gynecol* **196**, 530 e1–8.

586. Ghali, J.K., 3rd, Liao, Y. & Cooper, R.S. (1997) Left ventricular hypertrophy in the elderly. *Am J Geriatr Cardiol* **6**, 38–49.

587. Ghali, J.K., Tam, S.W., Ferdinand, K.C., *et al.* (2007) Effects of ACE inhibitors or beta-blockers in patients treated with the fixed-dose combination of isosorbide dinitrate/hydralazine in the African-American Heart Failure Trial. *Am J Cardiovasc Drugs* **7**, 373–80.

588. Ghosh, S. & Rodrigues, B. (2006) Cardiac cell death in early diabetes and its modulation by dietary fatty acids. *Biochim Biophys Acta* **1761**, 1148–62.

589. Gibbs, D. (1994) Rickets and the crippled child: an historical perspective [see comments]. *J R Soc Med* **87**, 729–32.

590. Gibson, R.S. (1994) Content and bioavailability of trace elements in vegetarian diets. *Am J Clin Nutr* **59** (5 Suppl), 1223S–32S.

591. Gillies, C.L., Abrams, K.R., Lambert, P.C., *et al.* (2007) Pharmacological and lifestyle interventions to prevent or delay type 2 diabetes in people with impaired glucose tolerance: systematic review and meta-analysis. *BMJ* **334**, 299.

592. Gillman, M.W., Cupples, L.A., Millen, B.E., Ellison, R.C. & Wolf, P.A. (1997) Inverse association of dietary fat with development of ischemic stroke in men. *JAMA* **278**, 2145–50.

593. Gimble, J.M., Zvonic, S., Floyd, Z.E., Kassem, M. & Nuttall, M.E. (2006) Playing with bone and fat. *J Cell Biochem* **98**, 251–66.

594. Glagov, S., Bassiouny, H.S., Sakaguchi, Y., Goudet, C.A. & Vito, R.P. (1997) Mechanical determinants of plaque modeling, remodeling and disruption. *Atherosclerosis* **131** (Suppl), S13–4.

595. Glass, C.K. & Witztum, J.L. (2001) Atherosclerosis. the road ahead. *Cell* **104**, 503–16.

596. Gleadow, R.M. & Woodrow, I.E. (2002) Constraints on effectiveness of cyanogenic glycosides in herbivore defense. *J Chem Ecol* **28**, 1301–13.

597. Godlee, F. (1999) *Clinical Evidence*, BMJ Publishing Group, ACP/ASIM, London.

598. Godsland, I.F. & Stevenson, J.C. (1995) Insulin resistance: syndrome or tendency? *Lancet* **346**, 100–3.

599. Goldstein, L.B., Adams, R., Alberts, M.J., *et al.* (2006) Primary prevention of ischemic stroke: a guideline from the American Heart Association/American Stroke Association Stroke Council: cosponsored by the Atherosclerotic Peripheral Vascular Disease Interdisciplinary Working Group; Cardiovascular Nursing Council; Clinical Cardiology Council; Nutrition, Physical Activity, and Metabolism Council; and the Quality of Care and Outcomes Research Interdisciplinary Working Group. *Circulation* **113**, e873–923.

600. Goldstein, L.B., Adams, R., Alberts, M.J., *et al.* (2006) Primary prevention of ischemic stroke: a guideline from the American Heart Association/American Stroke Association Stroke Council: cosponsored by the Atherosclerotic Peripheral Vascular Disease Interdisciplinary Working Group; Cardiovascular Nursing Council; Clinical Cardiology Council; Nutrition, Physical Activity, and Metabolism Council; and the Quality of Care and Outcomes Research Interdisciplinary Working Group: the American Academy of Neurology affirms the value of this guideline. *Stroke* **37**, 1583–633.

601. Good, C.K., Holschuh, N., Albertson, A.M. & Eldridge, A.L. (2008) Whole grain consumption and body mass index in adult women: an analysis of NHANES 1999–2000 and the USDA pyramid servings database. *J Am Coll Nutr* **27**, 80–7.

602. Goodman, J.M. (2008) The gregarious lipid droplet. *J Biol Chem* **283**, 28005–9.

603. Goto, Y. & Satoh, J. (1988) Childhood insulin-dependent diabetes. *Adv Exp Med Biol* **246**, 215–9.

604. Gould, E. & Goulding, A. (1995) High dietary salt intakes lower bone mineral density in ovariectomised rats: a dual x-ray absorptiometry study. *Bone* **16**, 115S (abstr).

605. Goulding, A. & Campbell, D.R. (1984) Effects of oral loads of sodium chloride on bone composition in growing rats consuming ample dietary calcium. *Miner Electrolyte Metab* **10**, 58–62.

606. Goulding, A., Rockell, J.E., Black, R.E., *et al.* (2004) Children who avoid drinking cow's milk are at increased risk for prepubertal bone fractures. *J Am Diet Assoc* **104**, 250–3.

607. Gower, B.A. (1999) Syndrome X in children: Influence of ethnicity and visceral fat. *Am J Human Biol* **11**, 249–57.

608. Graham, G.G., MacLean, W.C., Jr., Brown, K.H., *et al.* (1996) Protein requirements of infants and children: growth during recovery from malnutrition. *Pediatrics* **97**, 499–505.

609. Grant, G., More, L.J., McKenzie, N.H. & Pusztai, A. (1982) The effect of heating on the haemagglutinating activity and nutritional properties of bean (Phaseolus vulgaris) seeds. *J Sci Food Agric* **33**, 1324–6.

610. Grant, W.B. (1999) An ecologic study of dietary links to prostate cancer. *Altern Med Rev* **4**, 162–9.

611. Grant, W.B. (2000) The role of meat in the expression of rheumatoid arthritis. *Br J Nutr* **84**, 589–95.

612. Grant, W.D. (1997) Dietary links to Alzheimer's disease. *Alz Dis Rev* **2**, 42–55.

613. Gräslund, B. (2005) *Early humans and their world*. Routledge, London.

614. Green, D.M., Ropper, A.H., Kronmal, R.A., Psaty, B.M. & Burke, G.L. (2002) Serum potassium level and dietary potassium intake as risk factors for stroke. *Neurology* **59**, 314–20.

615. Greene, W.C., Goldman, C.K., Marshall, S.T., Fleisher, T.A. & Waldmann, T.A. (1981) Stimulation of immunoglobulin biosynthesis in human B cells by wheat germ agglutinin. I. Evidence that WGA can produce both a positive and negative signal for activation of human lymphocytes. *J Immunol* **127**, 799–804.

616. Greer, F. & Pusztai, A. (1985) Toxicity of kidney bean (Phaseolus vulgaris) in rats: changes in intestinal permeability. *Digestion* **32**, 42–6.

617. Gregersen, S., Rasmussen, O., Larsen, S. & Hermansen, K. (1992) Glycaemic and insulinaemic responses to orange and apple compared with white bread in non-insulin-dependent diabetic subjects. *Eur J Clin Nutr* **46**, 301–3.

618. Gresl, T.A., Colman, R.J., Havighurst, T.C., *et al.* (2003) Insulin sensitivity and glucose effectiveness from three minimal models: effects of energy restriction and body fat in adult male rhesus monkeys. *Am J Physiol Regul Integr Comp Physiol* **285**, R1340–54.

619. Grodzicki, T., Michalewicz, L. & Messerli, F.H. (1998) Aging and essential hypertension: effect of left ventricular hypertrophy on cardiac function. *Am J Hypertens* **11**, 425–9.

620. Groom, D. (1971) Cardiovascular observations on Tarahumara Indian runners – the modern Spartans. *Am Heart J* **81**, 304–14.

621. Gruber, A., Horwood, F., Sithole, J., Ali, N.J. & Idris, I. (2006) Obstructive sleep apnoea is independently associated with the metabolic syndrome but not insulin resistance state. *Cardiovasc Diabetol* **5**, 22.

622. Grundy, S.M., Barrett-Connor, E., Rudel, L.L., Miettinen, T. & Spector, A.A. (1988) Workshop on the impact of dietary cholesterol on plasma lipoproteins and atherogenesis. *Arteriosclerosis* **8**, 95–101.

623. Grundy, S.M. & Denke, M.A. (1990) Dietary influences on serum lipids and lipoproteins. *J Lipid Res* **31**, 1149–72.

624. Gubitz, G. & Sandercock, P. (2000) Prevention of ischaemic stroke. *BMJ* **321**, 1455–9.

625. Guggenmos, J., Schubart, A.S., Ogg, S., *et al.* (2004) Antibody cross-reactivity between myelin oligodendrocyte glycoprotein and the milk protein butyrophilin in multiple sclerosis. *J Immunol* **172**, 661–8.

626. Gunter, M.J. & Leitzmann, M.F. (2006) Obesity and colorectal cancer: epidemiology, mechanisms and candidate genes. *J Nutr Biochem* **17**, 145–56.

627. Gunther, T. & Schule, R. (2007) Fat or bone? A non-canonical decision. *Nat Cell Biol* **9**, 1229–31.

628. Gunton, J.E., Hitchman, R. & McElduff, A. (2001) Effects of ethnicity on glucose tolerance, insulin resistance and beta cell function in 223 women with an abnormal glucose challenge test during pregnancy. *Aust N Z J Obstet Gynaecol* **41**, 182–6.

629. Guo, T.L., White, K.L., Jr., Brown, R.D., *et al.* (2002) Genistein modulates splenic natural killer cell activity, antibody-forming cell response, and phenotypic marker expression in F(0) and F(1) generations of Sprague-Dawley rats. *Toxicol Appl Pharmacol* **181**, 219–27.

630. Gupta, R.A. & Dubois, R.N. (2002) Controversy: PPARgamma as a target for treatment of colorectal cancer. *Am J Physiol Gastrointest Liver Physiol* **283**, G266–9.

631. Gustafson, D., Rothenberg, E., Blennow, K., Steen, B. & Skoog, I. (2003) An 18-year follow-up of overweight and risk of Alzheimer disease. *Arch Intern Med* **163**, 1524–8.

632. Gustafsson, M. & Boren, J. (2004) Mechanism of lipoprotein retention by the extracellular matrix. *Curr Opin Lipidol* **15**, 505–14.

633. Guyard-Dangremont, V., Desrumaux, C., Gambert, P., Lallemant, C. & Lagrost, L. (1998) Phospholipid and cholesteryl ester transfer activities in plasma from 14 vertebrate species. Relation to atherogenesis susceptibility. *Comp Biochem Physiol B Biochem Mol Biol* **120**, 517–25.

634. Gyftopoulos, K., Sotiropoulou, G., Varakis, I. & Barbalias, G.A. (2000) Cellular distribution of retinoic acid receptor-alpha in benign hyperplastic and malignant human prostates: comparison with androgen, estrogen and progesterone receptor status. *Eur Urol* **38**, 323–30.

635. Hadjivassiliou, M., Grunewald, R.A., Chattopadhyay, A.K., *et al.* (1998) Clinical, radiological, neurophysiological, and neuropathological characteristics of gluten ataxia. *Lancet* **352**, 1582–5.

636. Hadjivassiliou, M., Grunewald, R.A. & Davies-Jones, G.A. (2002) Gluten sensitivity as a neurological illness. *J Neurol Neurosurg Psychiatry* **72**, 560–3.

637. Hadjivassiliou, M., Grunewald, R.A., Lawden, M., *et al.* (2001) Headache and CNS white matter abnormalities associated with gluten sensitivity. *Neurology* **56**, 385–8.

638. Hadjivassiliou, M., Kandler, R.H., Chattopadhyay, A.K., *et al.* (2006) Dietary treatment of gluten neuropathy. *Muscle Nerve* **34**, 762–6.

639. Haffner, S.M. (1998) The importance of hyperglycemia in the nonfasting state to the development of cardiovascular disease. *Endocr Rev* **19**, 583–92.

640. Hafstrom, I., Ringertz, B., Spangberg, A., *et al.* (2001) A vegan diet free of gluten improves the signs and symptoms of rheumatoid arthritis: the effects on arthritis correlate with a reduction in antibodies to food antigens. *Rheumatology (Oxford)* **40**, 1175–9.

641. Hagen, A. (1992) *A handbook of Anglo-Saxon food: Processing and consumption*. Anglo-Saxon Books, Middlesex.

642. Hagen, K.B., Byfuglien, M.G., Falzon, L., Olsen, S.U. & Smedslund, G. (2009) Dietary interventions for rheumatoid arthritis. *Cochrane Database Syst Rev*, CD006400.

643. Hajjar, I., Kotchen, J.M. & Kotchen, T.A. (2006) Hypertension: trends in prevalence, incidence, and control. *Annu Rev Public Health* **27**, 465–90.

644. Hakkak, R., Korourian, S., Ronis, M.J., Johnston, J.M. & Badger, T.M. (2001) Dietary whey protein protects against azoxymethane-induced colon tumors in male rats. *Cancer Epidemiol Biomarkers Prev* **10**, 555–8.

645. Hales, C.N. & Barker, D.J.P. (1992) Type 2 (non-insulin-dependent) diabetes mellitus: the thrifty phenotype hypothesis. *Diabetologia* **35**, 595–601.

646. Hallberg, L. & Hulthen, L. (2002) Perspectives on iron absorption. *Blood Cells Mol Dis* **29**, 562–73.

647. Hallberg, L., Sandström, B., Ralph, A. & Arthur, J. (2000) Iron, zinc and other trace elements. In: *Human Nutrition and Dietetics* (J.S. Garrow & W.P.T. James eds). Churchill Livingstone, Edinburgh, pp. 177–209.

648. Halperin, E.C. (2004) Paleo-oncology: the role of ancient remains in the study of cancer. *Perspect Biol Med* **47**, 1–14.

649. Hamann, I., Seidlova-Wuttke, D., Wuttke, W. & Köhrle, J. (2006) Effects of isoflavonoids and other plant-derived compounds on the hypothalamus–pituitary–thyroid hormone axis. *Maturitas* **55S**, S14–25.

650. Hamberg, O., Nielsen, K. & Vilstrup, H. (1992) Effects of an increase in protein intake on hepatic efficacy for urea synthesis in healthy subjects and in patients with cirrhosis. *J Hepatol* **14**, 237–43.

651. Hamer, M. (2006) Coffee and health: explaining conflicting results in hypertension. *J Hum Hypertens* **20**, 909–12.

652. Hamman, R.F., Wing, R.R., Edelstein, S.L., *et al.* (2006) Effect of weight loss with lifestyle intervention on risk of diabetes. *Diabetes Care* **29**, 2102–7.

653. Hammarsten, J. (2002) Klinisk prostatacancer bör ses som en livsstilssjukdom. *Medikament* **6**, 23–4.

654. Hammarsten, J. & Hogstedt, B. (1999) Clinical, anthropometric, metabolic and insulin profile of men with fast annual growth rates of benign prostatic hyperplasia. *Blood Press* **8**, 29–36.

655. Hammarsten, J. & Hogstedt, B. (2001) Hyperinsulinaemia as a risk factor for developing benign prostatic hyperplasia. *Eur Urol* **39**, 151–8.

656. Hammarsten, J. & Hogstedt, B. (2005) Hyperinsulinaemia: a prospective risk factor for lethal clinical prostate cancer. *Eur J Cancer* **41**, 2887–95.

657. Hammarsten, J., Hogstedt, B., Holthuis, N. & Mellstrom, D. (1998) Components of the metabolic syndrome-risk factors for the development of benign prostatic hyperplasia. *Prostate Cancer Prostatic Dis* **1**, 157–62.

658. Han, D., Nie, J., Bonner, M.R., *et al.* (2006) Lifetime adult weight gain, central adiposity, and the risk of pre- and postmenopausal breast cancer in the Western New York exposures and breast cancer study. *Int J Cancer* **119**, 2931–7.

659. Hanglow, A.C., Welsh, C.J., Conn, P. & Coombs, R.R. (1985) Early rheumatoid-like synovial lesions in rabbits drinking cow's milk. II. Antibody responses to bovine serum proteins. *Int Arch Allergy Appl Immunol* **78**, 152–60.

660. Haniu, M., Arakawa, T., Bures, E.J., *et al.* (1998) Human leptin receptor. Determination of disulfide structure and N-glycosylation sites of the extracellular domain. *J Biol Chem* **273**, 28691–9.

661. Hannan, M.T., Tucker, K.L., Dawson-Hughes, B., *et al.* (2000) Effect of dietary protein on bone loss in elderly men and women: the Framingham Osteoporosis Study. *J Bone Miner Res* **15**, 2504–12.

662. Hansen, H.P., Tauber-Lassen, E., Jensen, B.R. & Parving, H.H. (2002) Effect of dietary protein restriction on prognosis in patients with diabetic nephropathy. *Kidney Int* **62**, 220–8.

663. Hansson, G.K. (2005) Inflammation, atherosclerosis, and coronary artery disease. *N Engl J Med* **352**, 1685–95.

664. Hansson, G.K., Libby, P., Schonbeck, U. & Yan, Z.Q. (2002) Innate and adaptive immunity in the pathogenesis of atherosclerosis. *Circ Res* **91**, 281–91.

665. Hansson, L., Zanchetti, A., Carruthers, S.G., *et al.* (1998) Effects of intensive blood-pressure lowering and low-dose aspirin in patients with hypertension: principal results of the Hypertension Optimal Treatment (HOT) randomised trial. *Lancet* **351**, 1755–62.

666. Harding, S.A., Anscombe, R., Weatherall, M., *et al.* (2006) Abnormal glucose metabolism and features of the metabolic syndrome are common in patients presenting for elective cardiac catheterization. *Intern Med J* **36**, 759–64.

667. Hardy, J. & Selkoe, D.J. (2002) The amyloid hypothesis of Alzheimer's disease: progress and problems on the road to therapeutics. *Science* **297**, 353–6.

668. Harland, B.F. (1989) Dietary fibre and mineral bioavailability. *Nutr Res Rev* **2**, 133–47.

669. Harland, B.F., Smith, S.A., Howard, M.P., Ellis, R. & Smith, J.J. (1988) Nutritional status and phytate:zinc and phytate × calcium:zinc dietary molar ratios of lacto-ovo vegetarian Trappist monks: 10 years later. *J Am Diet Assoc* **88**, 1562–6.

670. Harland, J.I. & Haffner, T.A. (2008) Systematic review, meta-analysis and regression of randomised controlled trials reporting an association between an intake of circa 25g soya protein per day and blood cholesterol. *Atherosclerosis* **200**, 13–27.

671. Harper, A.B., Laughlin, W.S. & Mazess, R.B. (1984) Bone mineral content in St. Lawrence Island Eskimos. *Hum Biol* **56**, 63–78.

672. Harris, S.S. & Dawson-Hughes, B. (2007) Reduced sun exposure does not explain the inverse association of 25-hydroxyvitamin D with percent body fat in older adults. *J Clin Endocrinol Metab* **92**, 3155–7.

673. Harrison, D. & Mellanby, E. (1934) Phytic acid and the rickets-producing action of cereals. *Biochem J* **28**, 517–28.

674. Harrison, E., Adjei, A., Ameho, C., Yamamoto, S. & Kono, S. (1998) The effect of soybean protein on bone loss in a rat model of postmenopausal osteoporosis. *J Nutr Sci Vitaminol (Tokyo)* **44**, 257–68.

675. Harrison, G.J. & Harrison, L.R. (1986) Nutritional diseases. In: *Clinical Avian Medicine and Surgery* (G.J. Harrison & L.R. Harrison eds). Saunders, Philadelphia, pp. 397–407.

676. Harrison, L.C. & Honeyman, M.C. (1999) Cow's milk and type 1 diabetes: the real debate is about mucosal immune function. *Diabetes* **48**, 1501–7.

677. Harvie, M., Howell, A., Vierkant, R.A., *et al.* (2005) Association of gain and loss of weight before and after menopause with risk of postmenopausal breast cancer in the Iowa women's health study. *Cancer Epidemiol Biomarkers Prev* **14**, 656–61.

678. Hashimoto, K., Ikewaki, K., Yagi, H., *et al.* (2005) Glucose intolerance is common in Japanese patients with acute coronary syndrome who were not previously diagnosed with diabetes. *Diabetes Care* **28**, 1182–6.

679. Haslam, D. (2007) Obesity: a medical history. *Obes Rev* **8** (Suppl 1), 31–6.

680. Hasserius, R., Redlund-Johnell, I., Mellstrom, D., *et al.* (2001) Vertebral deformation in urban Swedish men and women: prevalence based on 797 subjects. *Acta Orthop Scand* **72**, 273–8.

681. Haugen, M.A., Kjeldsen-Kragh, J. & Forre, O. (1994) A pilot study of the effect of an elemental diet in the management of rheumatoid arthritis. *Clin Exp Rheumatol* **12**, 275–9.

682. Hauser, S.L. & Goodkin, D.E. (2001) Multiple sclerosis and other demyelinating diseases. In: Harrison's principles of internal medicine (E. Braunwald, A.S. Fauci, D.L. Kasper, S.L. Hauser, D.L. Longo & J.L. Jameson eds). McGraw-Hill, New York, pp. 2452–61.

683. Hawrylewicz, E.J., Huang, H.H. & Blair, W.H. (1991) Dietary soybean isolate and methionine supplementation affect mammary tumor progression in rats. *J Nutr* **121**, 1693–8.

684. Hayashi, T., Boyko, E.J., McNeely, M.J., *et al.* (2007) Minimum waist and visceral fat values for identifying Japanese Americans at risk for the metabolic syndrome. *Diabetes Care* **30**, 120–7.

685. Hayden, B. (1981) Subsistence and ecological adaptations of modern hunter-gatherers. In: *Omnivorous primates: gathering and hunting in human evolution* (R.D.S. Harding & G. Teleki eds). Columbia University Press, New York, pp. 344–421.

686. Hays, J.H., Gorman, R.T. & Shakir, K.M. (2002) Results of use of metformin and replacement of starch with saturated fat in diets of patients with type 2 diabetes. *Endocr Pract* **8**, 177–83.

687. He, F.J. & MacGregor, G.A. (2001) Fortnightly review: Beneficial effects of potassium. *BMJ* **323**, 497–501.

688. He, F.J. & MacGregor, G.A. (2004) Effect of longer-term modest salt reduction on blood pressure. *Cochrane Database Syst Rev*, CD004937.

689. He, F.J., Nowson, C.A. & MacGregor, G.A. (2006) Fruit and vegetable consumption and stroke: meta-analysis of cohort studies. *Lancet* **367**, 320–6.

690. He, J., Klag, M.J., Whelton, P.K., *et al.* (1991) Migration, blood pressure pattern, and hypertension: the Yi Migrant Study. *Am J Epidemiol* **134**, 1085–101.

691. He, J., Ogden, L.G., Bazzano, L.A., *et al.* (2001) Risk factors for congestive heart failure in US men and women: NHANES I epidemiologic follow-up study. *Arch Intern Med* **161**, 996–1002.

692. He, J., Ogden, L.G., Bazzano, L.A., *et al.* (2002) Dietary sodium intake and incidence of congestive heart failure in overweight US men and women: first National Health and Nutrition Examination Survey Epidemiologic Follow-up Study. *Arch Intern Med* **162**, 1619–24.

693. He, J., Ogden, L.G., Vupputuri, S., *et al.* (1999) Dietary sodium intake and subsequent risk of cardiovascular disease in overweight adults. *JAMA* **282**, 2027–34.

694. He, J., Streiffer, R.H., Muntner, P., Krousel-Wood, M.A. & Whelton, P.K. (2004) Effect of dietary fiber intake on blood pressure: a randomized, double-blind, placebo-controlled trial. *J Hypertens* **22**, 73–80.

695. He, J., Tell, G.S., Tang, Y.C., Mo, P.S. & He, G.Q. (1991) Effect of migration on blood pressure: the Yi People Study. *Epidemiology* **2**, 88–97.

696. He, J. & Whelton, P.K. (1997) Role of sodium reduction in the treatment and prevention of hypertension. *Curr Opin Cardiol* **12**, 202–7.

697. He, J. & Whelton, P.K. (1999) Effect of dietary fiber and protein intake on blood pressure: a review of epidemiologic evidence. *Clin Exp Hypertens* **21**, 785–96.

698. He, K., Merchant, A., Rimm, E.B., *et al.* (2003) Dietary fat intake and risk of stroke in male US healthcare professionals: 14 year prospective cohort study. *BMJ* **327**, 777–82.

699. Heaney, R.P. (2001) Protein intake and bone health: the influence of belief systems on the conduct of nutritional science. *Am J Clin Nutr* **73**, 5–6.

700. Heaney, R.P. (2006) Role of dietary sodium in osteoporosis. *J Am Coll Nutr* **25**, 271S–6S.

701. Heaney, R.P. & Layman, D.K. (2008) Amount and type of protein influences bone health. *Am J Clin Nutr* **87**, 1567S–70S.

702. Heart Protection Study Collaborative Group. (2002) MRC/BHF Heart Protection Study of cholesterol lowering with simvastatin in 20,536 high-risk individuals: a randomised placebo-controlled trial. *Lancet* **360**, 7–22.

703. Heaton, K.W. (1981) Gallstones. In: *Western Diseases: their Emergence and Prevention* (H.C. Trowell & D.P. Burkitt eds). Edward Arnold, London, pp. 47–59.

704. Heaton, K.W. (2000) Review article: epidemiology of gall-bladder disease–role of intestinal transit. *Aliment Pharmacol Ther* **14** (Suppl 2), 9–13.

705. Hedo, J.A., Harrison, L.C. & Roth, J. (1981) Binding of insulin receptors to lectins: evidence for common carbohydrate determinants on several membrane receptors. *Biochemistry* **20**, 3385–93.

706. Heidler, S., Temml, C., Broessner, C., *et al.* (2007) Is the metabolic syndrome an independent risk factor for erectile dysfunction? *J Urol* **177**, 651–4.

707. Heilbronn, L.K. & Ravussin, E. (2003) Calorie restriction and aging: review of the literature and implications for studies in humans. *Am J Clin Nutr* **78**, 361–9.

708. Hein, G.E. (2006) Glycation endproducts in osteoporosis – is there a pathophysiologic importance? *Clin Chim Acta* **371**, 32–6.

709. Heintz, A.P., Hacker, N.F. & Lagasse, L.D. (1985) Epidemiology and etiology of ovarian cancer: a review. *Obstet Gynecol* **66**, 127–35.

710. Held, C., Gerstein, H.C., Yusuf, S., *et al.* (2007) Glucose levels predict hospitalization for congestive heart failure in patients at high cardiovascular risk. *Circulation* **115**, 1371–5.

711. Hemberg, P. (1987) *Ett läkardistrikt berättar. Om gångna tiders sjukvård i Bo och Svennevads socknar*. Country Life AB, Södertälje.

712. Henderson, B.E. & Aiken, G.H. (1979) Cancer in Papua New Guinea. *Natl Cancer Inst Monogr* **53**, 67–72.

713. Hennig, B., Meerarani, P., Ramadass, P., *et al.* (1999) Zinc nutrition and apoptosis of vascular endothelial cells: implications in atherosclerosis. *Nutrition* **15**, 744–8.

714. Henschen, F. (1962) *Sjukdomarnas historia och geografi*. Bonniers, Stockholm.

715. Henschen, F. (1966) *The history and geography of diseases*. Delacorte Press, New York.

716. Herbert, V. (1988) Vitamin B-12: plant sources, requirements, and assay. *Am J Clin Nutr* **48**, 852–8.

717. Hermansen, K., Rasmussen, O., Gregersen, S. & Larsen, S. (1992) Influence of ripeness of banana on the blood glucose and insulin response in type 2 diabetic subjects. *Diabet Med* **9**, 739–43.

718. Hermansen, K., Sondergaard, M., Hoie, L., Carstensen, M. & Brock, B. (2001) Beneficial effects of a soy-based dietary supplement on lipid levels and cardiovascular risk markers in type 2 diabetic subjects. *Diabetes Care* **24**, 228–33.

719. Hernandez, C.J. & Keaveny, T.M. (2006) A biomechanical perspective on bone quality. *Bone* **39**, 1173–81.

720. Hernigou, P. (1995) Historical overview of rickets, osteomalacia, and vitamin D. *Rev Rhum Engl Ed* **62**, 261–70.

721. Herrera, C.M. & Pellmyr, O. (2002) *Plant-animal interactions. An evolutionary approach.* Blackwell, Oxford.

722. Hertog, M.G., Sweetnam, P.M., Fehily, A.M., Elwood, P.C. & Kromhout, D. (1997) Antioxidant flavonols and ischemic heart disease in a Welsh population of men: the Caerphilly Study. *Am J Clin Nutr* **65**, 1489–94.

723. Hertog, M.G.L., Feskens, E.J.M., Hollman, P.C.H., Katan, M.B. & Kromhout, D. (1993) Dietary antioxidant flavonoids and risk of coronary heart disease: the Zutphen Study. *Lancet* **ii**, 1007–11.

724. Hession, M., Rolland, C., Kulkarni, U., Wise, A. & Broom, J. (2009) Systematic review of randomized controlled trials of low-carbohydrate vs. low-fat/low-calorie diets in the management of obesity and its comorbidities. *Obes Rev* **10**, 36–50.

725. Hetzel, B.S. (1994) Iodine deficiency and fetal brain damage. *N Engl J Med* **331**, 1770–1.

726. Heymsfield, S.B., Harp, J.B., Reitman, M.L., *et al.* (2007) Why do obese patients not lose more weight when treated with low-calorie diets? A mechanistic perspective. *Am J Clin Nutr* **85**, 346–54.

727. Higginson, J. (1979) Cancer and environment: Higginson speaks out. *Science* **205**, 1363–4, 1366.

728. Higginson, J. & Pepler, W.J. (1954) Fat intake, serum cholesterol, and atherosclerosis in the South African Bantu. Part II. Atherosclerosis and coronary artery disease. *J Clin Invest* **33**, 1366–71.

729. Hill, M. (2002) Meat, cancer and dietary advice to the public. *Eur J Clin Nutr* **56** (Suppl 1), S36–41.

730. Hirose, K., Takezaki, T., Hamajima, N., Miura, S. & Tajima, K. (2003) Dietary factors protective against breast cancer in Japanese premenopausal and postmenopausal women. *Int J Cancer* **107**, 276–82.

731. Ho, K.J., Biss, K., Mikkelson, B., Lewis, L.A. & Taylor, C.B. (1971) The Masai of East Africa: some unique biological characteristics. *Arch Pathol* **91**, 387–410.

732. Ho, S.C., Chen, Y.M., Woo, J.L., *et al.* (2001) Sodium is the leading dietary factor associated with urinary calcium excretion in Hong Kong Chinese adults. *Osteoporos Int* **12**, 723–31.

733. Ho, S.F., O'Mahony, M.S., Steward, J.A., *et al.* (2001) Dyspnoea and quality of life in older people at home. *Age Ageing* **30**, 155–9.

734. Hobbs, C.J., Plymate, S.R., Rosen, C.J. & Adler, R.A. (1993) Testosterone administration increases insulin-like growth factor-I levels in normal men. *J Clin Endocrinol Metab* **77**, 776–9.

735. Hodgson, J.M., Burke, V., Beilin, L.J. & Puddey, I.B. (2006) Partial substitution of carbohydrate intake with protein intake from lean red meat lowers blood pressure in hypertensive persons. *Am J Clin Nutr* **83**, 780–7.

736. Hodgson, J.M., Wahlqvist, M.L., Boxall, J.A. & Balazs, D. (1993) Can linoleic acid contribute to coronary artery disease? *Am J Clin Nutr* **58**, 228–34.

737. Hodgson, J.M., Ward, N.C., Burke, V., Beilin, L.J. & Puddey, I.B. (2007) Increased lean red meat intake does not elevate markers of oxidative stress and inflammation in humans. *J Nutr* **137**, 363–7.

738. Hoefle, G., Saely, C.H., Risch, L., *et al.* (2007) Leptin, leptin soluble receptor and coronary atherosclerosis. *Eur J Clin Invest* **37**, 629–36.

739. Hofbauer, L.C., Brueck, C.C., Shanahan, C.M., Schoppet, M. & Dobnig, H. (2007) Vascular calcification and osteoporosis – from clinical observation towards molecular understanding. *Osteoporos Int* **18**, 251–9.

740. Hofbauer, L.C., Brueck, C.C., Singh, S.K. & Dobnig, H. (2007) Osteoporosis in patients with diabetes mellitus. *J Bone Miner Res* **22**, 1317–28.

741. Hoidrup, S., Gronbaek, M., Gottschau, A., Lauritzen, J.B. & Schroll, M. (1999) Alcohol intake, beverage preference, and risk of hip fracture in men and women. Copenhagen Centre for Prospective Population Studies. *Am J Epidemiol* **149**, 993–1001.

742. Hokin, B.D. & Butler, T. (1999) Cyanocobalamin (vitamin B-12) status in Seventh-day Adventist ministers in Australia. *Am J Clin Nutr* **70**, 576S–8S.

743. Holick, M.F. (1999) Vitamin D. In: *Modern nutrition in health and disease* (M.E. Shils, J.A. Olson, M. Shike & A.C. Ross eds). Lippincott Williams & Wilkins, Philadelphia, PA, pp. 329–45.

744. Holland, T.D. & O'Brien, M.J. (1997) Parasites, porotic hyperostosis, and the implications of changing perspectives. *American Antiquity* **62**, 183–93.

745. Hollander, M., Bots, M.L., Del Sol, A.I., *et al.* (2002) Carotid plaques increase the risk of stroke and subtypes of cerebral infarction in asymptomatic elderly: the Rotterdam study. *Circulation* **105**, 2872–7.

746. Hollenberg, N.K. (2006) The influence of dietary sodium on blood pressure. *J Am Coll Nutr* **25**, 240S–6S.

747. Hollingsworth, K.G., Abubacker, M.Z., Joubert, I., Allison, M.E. & Lomas, D.J. (2006) Low-carbohydrate diet induced reduction of hepatic lipid content observed with a rapid non-invasive MRI technique. *Br J Radiol* **79**, 712–5.

748. Holm, S. (1937) The ocular refractive state of the Palae-Negroids in Gabon, French Equatorial Africa. *Acta Ophtalmol* (Suppl 13), 1–299.

749. Holman, R.R., Paul, S.K., Bethel, M.A., Matthews, D.R. & Neil, H.A. (2008) 10-year follow-up of intensive glucose control in type 2 diabetes. *N Engl J Med* **359**, 1577–89.

750. Holst-Jensen, S.E., Pfeiffer-Jensen, M., Monsrud, M., *et al.* (1998) Treatment of rheumatoid arthritis with a peptide diet: a randomized, controlled trial. *Scand J Rheumatol* **27**, 329–36.

751. Homma, S., Hirose, N., Ishida, H., Ishii, T. & Araki, G. (2001) Carotid plaque and intima-media thickness assessed by b-mode ultrasonography in subjects ranging from young adults to centenarians. *Stroke* **32**, 830–5.

752. Homma, S., Ishii, T., Tsugane, S. & Hirose, N. (1997) Different effects of hypertension and hypercholesterolemia on the natural history of aortic atherosclerosis by the stage of intimal lesions. *Atherosclerosis* **128**, 85–95.

753. Hooper, L., Bartlett, C., Davey, S.G. & Ebrahim, S. (2004) Advice to reduce dietary salt for prevention of cardiovascular disease. *Cochrane Database Syst Rev*, CD003656.

754. Hooper, L., Kroon, P.A., Rimm, E.B., *et al.* (2008) Flavonoids, flavonoid-rich foods, and cardiovascular risk: a meta-analysis of randomized controlled trials. *Am J Clin Nutr* **88**, 38–50.

755. Hooper, L., Summerbell, C.D., Higgins, J.P., *et al.* (2000) Reduced or modified dietary fat for prevention of cardiovascular disease. *Cochrane Database Syst Rev*, CD002137.

756. Hooper, L., Thompson, R.L., Harrison, R.A., *et al.* (2004) Omega 3 fatty acids for prevention and treatment of cardiovascular disease. *Cochrane Database Syst Rev*, CD003177.

757. Hooper, L., Thompson, R.L., Harrison, R.A., *et al.* (2006) Risks and benefits of omega 3 fats for mortality, cardiovascular disease, and cancer: systematic review. *BMJ* **332**, 752–60.

758. Hopkins, P.N. (1992) Effects of dietary cholesterol on serum cholesterol: a meta-analysis and review. *Am J Clin Nutr* **55**, 1060–70.

759. Hoppe, C., Molgaard, C., Juul, A. & Michaelsen, K.F. (2004) High intakes of skimmed milk, but not meat, increase serum IGF-I and IGFBP-3 in eight-year-old boys. *Eur J Clin Nutr* **58**, 1211–16.

760. Hoppe, C., Molgaard, C. & Michaelsen, K.F. (2006) Cow's milk and linear growth in industrialized and developing countries. *Annu Rev Nutr* **26**, 131–73.

761. Hoppe, C., Molgaard, C., Vaag, A., Barkholt, V. & Michaelsen, K.F. (2005) High intakes of milk, but not meat, increase s-insulin and insulin resistance in 8-year-old boys. *Eur J Clin Nutr* **59**, 393–8.

762. Hoppe, C., Udam, T.R., Lauritzen, L., *et al.* (2004) Animal protein intake, serum insulin-like growth factor I, and growth in healthy 2.5-y-old Danish children. *Am J Clin Nutr* **80**, 447–52.

763. Hornabrook, R.W. (1975) Editorial: neurology in Papua New Guinea. *P N G Med J* **18**, 193–6.

764. Hornabrook, R.W., Crane, G.G. & Stanhope, J.M. (1974) Karkar and Lufa: an epidemiological and health background to the human adaptability studies of the International Biological Programme. *Philos Trans R Soc Lond Biol* **268**, 293–308.

765. Horton, J.D., Shimomura, I., Ikemoto, S., Bashmakov, Y. & Hammer, R.E. (2003) Overexpression of sterol regulatory element-binding protein-1a in mouse adipose tissue produces adipocyte hypertrophy, increased fatty acid secretion, and fatty liver. *J Biol Chem* **278**, 36652–60.

766. Horton, R. (2005) Expression of concern: Indo-Mediterranean Diet Heart Study. *Lancet* **366**, 354–6.

767. Hou, Y.L., Wu, X.P., Luo, X.H., *et al.* (2007) Differences in age-related bone mass of proximal femur between Chinese women and different ethnic women in the United States. *J Bone Miner Metab* **25**, 243–52.

768. Howard, B.V., Van Horn, L., Hsia, J., *et al.* (2006) Low-fat dietary pattern and risk of cardiovascular disease: the Women's Health Initiative Randomized Controlled Dietary Modification Trial. *JAMA* **295**, 655–66.

769. Howarth, N.C., Saltzman, E. & Roberts, S.B. (2001) Dietary fiber and weight regulation. *Nutr Rev* **59**, 129–39.

770. Hsueh, W.A. & Law, R.E. (2001) PPARgamma and atherosclerosis: effects on cell growth and movement. *Arterioscler Thromb Vasc Biol* **21**, 1891–5.

771. Hu, D.Y., Pan, C.Y. & Yu, J.M. (2006) The relationship between coronary artery disease and abnormal glucose regulation in China: the China Heart Survey. *Eur Heart J* **27**, 2573–9.

772. Hu, F.B., Manson, J.E. & Willett, W.C. (2001) Types of dietary fat and risk of coronary heart disease: a critical review. *J Am Coll Nutr* **20**, 5–19.

773. Hu, F.B., Rimm, E.B., Stampfer, M.J., *et al.* (2000) Prospective study of major dietary patterns and risk of coronary heart disease in men. *Am J Clin Nutr* **72**, 912–21.

774. Hu, F.B., Stampfer, M.J., Haffner, S.M., *et al.* (2002) Elevated Risk of Cardiovascular Disease Prior to Clinical Diagnosis of Type 2 Diabetes. *Diabetes Care* **25**, 1129–34.

775. Hu, F.B., Stampfer, M.J., Manson, J.E., *et al.* (1998) Frequent nut consumption and risk of coronary heart disease in women: prospective cohort study. *BMJ* **317**, 1341–5.

776. Huff, M.W., Roberts, D.C. & Carroll, K.K. (1982) Long-term effects of semipurified diets containing casein or soy protein isolate on atherosclerosis and plasma lipoproteins in rabbits. *Atherosclerosis* **41**, 327–36.

777. Hugi, D., Gut, S.H. & Blum, J.W. (1997) Blood metabolites and hormones – especially glucose and insulin – in veal calves: effects of age and nutrition. *Zentralbl Veterinarmed A* **44**, 407–16.

778. Hugi, D., Tappy, L., Sauerwein, R.M., Bruckmaier, R.M. & Blum, J.W. (1998) Insulin-dependent glucose utilization in intensively milk-fed veal calves is modulated by supplementing lactose in an age-dependent manner. *J Nutr* **128**, 1023–30.

779. Hulshof, K.F., van Erp-Baart, M.A., Anttolainen, M., *et al.* (1999) Intake of fatty acids in western Europe with emphasis on trans fatty acids: the TRANSFAIR Study. *Eur J Clin Nutr* **53**, 143–57.

780. Hulthe, J., Bokemark, L., Wikstrand, J. & Fagerberg, B. (2000) The metabolic syndrome, LDL particle size, and atherosclerosis: the Atherosclerosis and Insulin Resistance (AIR) study. *Arterioscler Thromb Vasc Biol* **20**, 2140–7.

781. Hulthe, J. & Fagerberg, B. (2002) Circulating oxidized LDL is associated with subclinical atherosclerosis development and inflammatory cytokines (AIR Study). *Arterioscler Thromb Vasc Biol* **22**, 1162–7.

782. Hunninghake, D.B., Maki, K.C., Kwiterovich, P.O., Jr., *et al.* (2000) Incorporation of lean red meat into a National Cholesterol Education Program Step I diet: a long-term, randomized clinical trial in free-living persons with hypercholesterolemia. *J Am Coll Nutr* **19**, 351–60.

783. Hunt, C.D. & Johnson, L.K. (2007) Calcium requirements: new estimations for men and women by cross-sectional statistical analyses of calcium balance data from metabolic studies. *Am J Clin Nutr* **86**, 1054–63.

784. Hunt, S.A., Abraham, W.T., Chin, M.H., *et al.* (2005) ACC/AHA 2005 Guideline Update for the Diagnosis and Management of Chronic Heart Failure in the Adult: a report of the American College of Cardiology/American Heart Association Task Force on Practice Guidelines (Writing Committee to Update the 2001 Guidelines for the Evaluation and Management of Heart Failure): developed in collaboration with the American College of Chest Physicians and the International Society for Heart and Lung Transplantation: endorsed by the Heart Rhythm Society. *Circulation* **112**, e154–235.

785. Hunter, J.D. (1962) Diet, body build, blood pressure, and serum cholesterol levels in coconut-eating Polynesians. *Fed Proc* **21**, 36–43.

786. Hutton, P.W. (1956) Neurological disease in Uganda. *East Afr Med J* **33**, 209–223.

787. Hyder, J.A., Allison, M.A., Criqui, M.H. & Wright, C.M. (2007) Association between systemic calcified atherosclerosis and bone density. *Calcif Tissue Int* **80**, 301–6.

788. Ibanez, L., Dimartino-Nardi, J., Potau, N. & Saenger, P. (2000) Premature adrenarche – normal variant or forerunner of adult disease? *Endocr Rev* **21**, 671–96.

789. Ibanez, L., Potau, N., Chacon, P., Pascual, C. & Carrascosa, A. (1998) Hyperinsulinaemia, dyslipaemia and cardiovascular risk in girls with a history of premature pubarche. *Diabetologia* **41**, 1057–63.

790. Ilich, J.Z. & Kerstetter, J.E. (2000) Nutrition in bone health revisited: a story beyond calcium. *J Am Coll Nutr* **19**, 715–37.

791. Ingelsson, E., Arnlov, J., Sundstrom, J., *et al.* (2005) Novel metabolic risk factors for heart failure. *J Am Coll Cardiol* **46**, 2054–60.

792. Ingelsson, E., Schaefer, E.J., Contois, J.H., *et al.* (2007) Clinical utility of different lipid measures for prediction of coronary heart disease in men and women. *JAMA* **298**, 776–85.

793. Ingram, C.J., Mulcare, C.A., Itan, Y., Thomas, M.G. & Swallow, D.M. (2009) Lactose digestion and the evolutionary genetics of lactase persistence. *Hum Genet* **124**, 579–91.

794. INTERHEALTH Steering Committee. (1991) Demonstration projects for the integrated prevention and control of noncommunicable diseases (INTERHEALTH programme): epidemiological background and rationale. *World Health Stat Q* **44**, 48–54.

795. INTERSALT (1988) Intersalt: an international study of electrolyte excretion and blood pressure. Results for 24 hour urinary sodium and potassium excretion. Intersalt Cooperative Research Group. *BMJ* **297**, 319–28.

796. Ip, M.S., Lam, B., Ng, M.M., *et al.* (2002) Obstructive sleep apnea is independently associated with insulin resistance. *Am J Respir Crit Care Med* **165**, 670–6.

797. Iqbal, T.H., Lewis, K.O. & Cooper, B.T. (1994) Phytase activity in the human and rat small intestine. *Gut* **35**, 1233–6.

798. Isaacson, C. (1977) The changing pattern of heart disease in South African Blacks. *S Afr Med J* **52**, 793–8.

799. Isaksson, H., Danielsson, M., Rosenhamer, G., Konarski-Svensson, J.C. & Ostergren, J. (1991) Characteristics of patients resistant to antihypertensive drug therapy. *J Intern Med* **229**, 421–6.

800. Iscan, M.Y. & Kennedy, K.A.R. (1989) *Reconstruction of life from the human skeleton.* Wiley-Liss, New York.

801. Ishihara, M., Inoue, I., Kawagoe, T., *et al.* (2006) Is admission hyperglycaemia in non-diabetic patients with acute myocardial infarction a surrogate for previously undiagnosed abnormal glucose tolerance? *Eur Heart J* **27**, 2413–9.

802. Ishikawa, H., Akedo, I., Otani, T., *et al.* (2005) Randomized trial of dietary fiber and *Lactobacillus casei* administration for prevention of colorectal tumors. *Int J Cancer* **116**, 762–7.

803. ISIS-4 Collaborative Group (1995) ISIS-4: A randomized factorial trial assessing early oral captopril, oral mononitrate, and intravenous magnesium sulphate in 58,050 patients with suspected acute myocardial infarction. *Lancet* **345**, 669–85.

804. Iso, H., Kobayashi, M., Ishihara, J., *et al.* (2006) Intake of fish and n3 fatty acids and risk of coronary heart disease among Japanese: the Japan Public Health Center-Based (JPHC) Study Cohort I. *Circulation* **113**, 195–202.

805. Iso, H., Stampfer, M.J., Manson, J.E., *et al.* (2001) Prospective study of fat and protein intake and risk of intraparenchymal hemorrhage in women. *Circulation* **103**, 856–63.

806. Itami, S., Kurata, S. & Takayasu, S. (1995) Androgen induction of follicular epithelial cell growth is mediated via insulin-like growth factor-I from dermal papilla cells. *Biochem Biophys Res Commun* **212**, 988–94.

807. Ito, M., Lang, T.F., Jergas, M., *et al.* (1997) Spinal trabecular bone loss and fracture in American and Japanese women. *Calcif Tissue Int* **61**, 123–8.

808. Ito, M., Toda, T., Kummerow, F.A. & Nishimori, I. (1986) Effect of magnesium deficiency on ultrastructural changes in coronary arteries of swine. *Acta Pathol Jpn* **36**, 225–34.

809. Itoh, R., Suyama, Y., Oguma, Y. & Yokota, F. (1999) Dietary sodium, an independent determinant for urinary deoxypyridinoline in elderly women. A cross-sectional study on the effect of dietary factors on deoxypyridinoline excretion in 24-h urine specimens from 763 free-living healthy Japanese. *Eur J Clin Nutr* **53**, 886–90.

810. Iuliano-Burns, S., Saxon, L., Naughton, G., Gibbons, K. & Bass, S.L. (2003) Regional specificity of exercise and calcium during skeletal growth in girls: a randomized controlled trial. *J Bone Miner Res* **18**, 156–62.

811. Jackes, M. (1992) Paleodemography: problems and techniques. In: *Skeletal biology of past peoples: research methods* (S.R. Saunders & A. Katzenberg eds). Wiley-Liss, New York, pp. 189–224.

812. Jackson, L.F.C. (1991) Secondary compounds in plants (allelochemicals) as promoters of human biological variability. *Annu Rev Anthropol* **20**, 505–46.

813. Jackson, R., Broad, J., Connor, J. & Wells, S. (2005) Alcohol and ischaemic heart disease: probably no free lunch. *Lancet* **366**, 1911–2.

814. Jacobs, E.T., Alberts, D.S., Foote, J.A., *et al.* (2008) Vitamin D insufficiency in southern Arizona. *Am J Clin Nutr* **87**, 608–13.

815. Jacobsen, N., Jensen, H. & Goldschmidt, E. (2007) Prevalence of myopia in Danish conscripts. *Acta Ophthalmol Scand* **85**, 165–70.

816. James, G.D. & Baker, P.T. (1990) Human Population Biology and Hypertension: Evolutionary and Ecological Aspects of Blood Pressure. In: *Hypertension: Pathophysiology, Diagnosis, and Management* (J.H. Laragh & B.M. Brenner eds). Raven Press, Ltd, New York, pp. 137–45.

817. Järvi, A.E., Karlstrom, B.E., Granfeldt, Y.E., *et al.* (1999) Improved glycemic control and lipid profile and normalized fibrinolytic activity on a low-glycemic index diet in type 2 diabetic patients. *Diabetes Care* **22**, 10–18.

818. Jebb, S.A. (2007) Dietary determinants of obesity. *Obes Rev* **8**, 93–7.

819. Jehle, S., Zanetti, A., Muser, J., Hulter, H.N. & Krapf, R. (2006) Partial neutralization of the acidogenic Western diet with potassium citrate increases bone mass in postmenopausal women with osteopenia. *J Am Soc Nephrol* **17**, 3213–22.

820. Jenab, M., Riboli, E., Cleveland, R.J., *et al.* (2007) Serum C-peptide, IGFBP-1 and IGFBP-2 and risk of colon and rectal cancers in the European Prospective Investigation into Cancer and Nutrition. *Int J Cancer* **121**, 368–76.

821. Jenkins, C. (1987) Medical anthropology in the Western Scrader range, Papua New Guinea. *Nat Geogr Res* 3, 412–30.
822. Jenkins, D.J. & Kendall, C.W. (2006) The garden of Eden: plant-based diets, the genetic drive to store fat and conserve cholesterol, and implications for epidemiology in the 21st century. *Epidemiology* 17, 128–30.
823. Jenkins, D.J., Kendall, C.W., Faulkner, D.A., *et al.* (2006) Assessment of the longer-term effects of a dietary portfolio of cholesterol-lowering foods in hypercholesterolemia. *Am J Clin Nutr* 83, 582–91.
824. Jenkins, D.J., Kendall, C.W., Marchie, A., *et al.* (2005) Direct comparison of dietary portfolio vs statin on C-reactive protein. *Eur J Clin Nutr* 59, 851–60.
825. Jenkins, D.J., Kendall, C.W., Marchie, A., *et al.* (2003) Effects of a dietary portfolio of cholesterol-lowering foods vs lovastatin on serum lipids and C-reactive protein. *JAMA* 290, 502–10.
826. Jenkins, D.J., Kendall, C.W., McKeown-Eyssen, G., *et al.* (2008) Effect of a low-glycemic index or a high-cereal fiber diet on type 2 diabetes: a randomized trial. *JAMA* 300, 2742–53.
827. Jenkins, D.J., Kendall, C.W., Popovich, D.G., *et al.* (2001) Effect of a very-high-fiber vegetable, fruit, and nut diet on serum lipids and colonic function. *Metabolism* 50, 494–503.
828. Jenkins, D.J., Popovich, D.G., Kendall, C.W., *et al.* (1997) Effect of a diet high in vegetables, fruit, and nuts on serum lipids. *Metabolism* 46, 530–37.
829. Jeppesen, J., Hansen, T.W., Rasmussen, S., *et al.* (2007) Insulin resistance, the metabolic syndrome, and risk of incident cardiovascular disease: a population-based study. *J Am Coll Cardiol* 49, 2112–19.
830. Jialal, I., Naiker, P., Reddi, K., Moodley, J. & Joubert, S.M. (1987) Evidence for insulin resistance in nonobese patients with polycystic ovarian disease. *J Clin Endocrinol Metab* 64, 1066–9.
831. Jobling, M.A., Hurles, M. & Tyler-Smith, C. (2004) *Human evolutionary genetics: origins, peoples & disease.* Garland Science, New York.
832. Joffe, B.I., Jackson, W.P., Thomas, M.E., *et al.* (1971) Metabolic responses to oral glucose in the Kalahari Bushmen. *BMJ* 4, 206–8.
833. Johansen, O.E., Birkeland, K.I., Brustad, E., *et al.* (2006) Undiagnosed dysglycaemia and inflammation in cardiovascular disease. *Eur J Clin Invest* 36, 544–51.
834. John, J.H., Ziebland, S., Yudkin, P., Roe, L.S. & Neil, H.A. (2002) Effects of fruit and vegetable consumption on plasma antioxidant concentrations and blood pressure: a randomised controlled trial. *Lancet* 359, 1969–74.
835. Johnell, O., Borgstrom, F., Jonsson, B. & Kanis, J. (2007) Latitude, socioeconomic prosperity, mobile phones and hip fracture risk. *Osteoporos Int* 18, 333–7.
836. Johnell, O. & Kanis, J.A. (2006) An estimate of the worldwide prevalence and disability associated with osteoporotic fractures. *Osteoporos Int* 17, 1726–33.
837. Johnson, A. & Behrens, C.A. (1982) Nutritional criteria in Machiguenga food production decisions: a linear-programming analysis. *Human Ecology* 10, 167–89.
838. Johnson, D.W. (2006) Dietary protein restriction as a treatment for slowing chronic kidney disease progression: the case against. *Nephrology (Carlton)* 11, 58–62.
839. Johnson, G.L. & Smith, E. (1901) Contributions to the comparative anatomy of the mammalian eye, based chiefly on ophthalmoscopic examination. *Phil Trans Royal Soc* B194, 1–82.
840. Johnson, I.T. & Lund, E.K. (2007) Review article: nutrition, obesity and colorectal cancer. *Aliment Pharmacol Ther* 26, 161–81.
841. Johnson, R.J., Perez-Pozo, S.E., Sautin, Y.Y., *et al.* (2009) Hypothesis: could excessive fructose intake and uric acid cause type 2 diabetes? *Endocr Rev* 30, 96–116.
842. Johnston, C.S., Day, C.S. & Swan, P.D. (2002) Postprandial thermogenesis is increased 100% on a high-protein, low-fat diet versus a high-carbohydrate, low-fat diet in healthy, young women. *J Am Coll Nutr* 21, 55–61.

843. Johnston, S.C., Mendis, S. & Mathers, C.D. (2009) Global variation in stroke burden and mortality: estimates from monitoring, surveillance, and modelling. *Lancet Neurol* 8, 345–54.

844. Jokinen, M.P., Clarkson, T.B. & Prichard, R.W. (1985) Animal models in atherosclerosis research. *Exp Mol Pathol* 42, 1–28.

845. Jones, G., Riley, M.D. & Whiting, S. (2001) Association between urinary potassium, urinary sodium, current diet, and bone density in prepubertal children. *Am J Clin Nutr* 73, 839–44.

846. Jones, J.L., Daley, B.J., Enderson, B.L., Zhou, J.R. & Karlstad, M.D. (2002) Genistein inhibits tamoxifen effects on cell proliferation and cell cycle arrest in T47D breast cancer cells. *Am Surg* 68, 575–7; discussion 577–8.

847. Jönsson, L. (1972) Coronary arterial lesions and myocardial infarcts in the dog. A pathologic and microangiographic study. *Acta Vet Scand Suppl* 38, 1–80.

848. Jönsson, T., Ahren, B., Pacini, G., *et al.* (2006) A Paleolithic diet confers higher insulin sensitivity, lower C-reactive protein and lower blood pressure than a cereal-based diet in domestic pigs. *Nutr Metab (Lond)* 3, 39.

848a. Jönsson, T., Granfeldt, Y., Ahren, B., *et al.* (2009). Beneficial effects of a Paleolithic diet on cardiovascular risk factors in type 2 diabetes: a randomized cross-over pilot study. *Cardiovasc Diabetol* 8, 35.

849. Jönsson, T., Olsson, S., Ahrén, B., *et al.* (2005) Agrarian diet and diseases of affluence – do evolutionary novel dietary lectins cause leptin resistance? *BMC Endocr Discord* 5, 10.

850. Joosten, M.M., Beulens, J.W., Kersten, S. & Hendriks, H.F. (2008) Moderate alcohol consumption increases insulin sensitivity and ADIPOQ expression in postmenopausal women: a randomised, crossover trial. *Diabetologia* 51, 1375–81.

851. Joshipura, K.J., Hu, F.B., Manson, J.E., *et al.* (2001) The effect of fruit and vegetable intake on risk for coronary heart disease. *Ann Intern Med* 134, 1106–14.

852. Ju, Y.H., Doerge, D.R., Allred, K.F., Allred, C.D. & Helferich, W.G. (2002) Dietary genistein negates the inhibitory effect of tamoxifen on growth of estrogen-dependent human breast cancer (MCF-7) cells implanted in athymic mice. *Cancer Res* 62, 2474–7.

853. Jula, A.M. & Karanko, H.M. (1994) Effects on left ventricular hypertrophy of long-term nonpharmacological treatment with sodium restriction in mild-to-moderate essential hypertension. *Circulation* 89, 1023–31.

854. Junqueira, L.C., Carneiro, J. & Kelley, R.O. (1995) *Basic Histology*. Lange.

855. Jüptner, H. & Quinell, C. (1965) Epidemiological observations during a measles epidemic in the Trobriand Islands (Papua). *Med J Aust* 1, 538–40.

856. Jurmain, R.D. & Kilgore, L. (1995) Skeletal evidence of osteoarthritis: a palaeopathological perspective. *Ann Rheum Dis* 54, 443–50.

857. Juul, A., Scheike, T., Nielsen, C.T., *et al.* (1995) Serum insulin-like growth factor I (IGF-I) and IGF-binding protein 3 levels are increased in central precocious puberty: effects of two different treatment regimens with gonadotropin-releasing hormone agonists, without or in combination with an antiandrogen (cyproterone acetate). *J Clin Endocrinol Metab* 80, 3059–67.

858. Kaaks, R. & Lukanova, A. (2001) Energy balance and cancer: the role of insulin and insulin-like growth factor-I. *Proc Nutr Soc* 60, 91–106.

859. Kafatos, A., Verhagen, H., Moschandreas, J., Apostolaki, I. & Van Westerop, J.J. (2000) Mediterranean diet of Crete: foods and nutrient content. *J Am Diet Assoc* 100, 1487–93.

860. Kagami, H., Uryu, K., Okamoto, K., *et al.* (1991) Differential lectin binding on walls of thoraco-cervical blood vessels and lymphatics in rats. *Okajimas Folia Anat Jpn* 68, 161–70.

861. Kahn, H.S. & Williamson, D.F. (1994) Abdominal obesity and mortality risk among men in nineteenth-century North America. *Int J Obes Relat Metab Disord* 18, 686–91.

862. Kahn, S.E., Hull, R.L. & Utzschneider, K.M. (2006) Mechanisms linking obesity to insulin resistance and type 2 diabetes. *Nature* 444, 840–6.

863. Kaiyala, K.J., Prigeon, R.L., Kahn, S.E., *et al.* (1999) Reduced beta-cell function contributes to impaired glucose tolerance in dogs made obese by high-fat feeding. *Am J Physiol* **277**, E659–67.

864. Kalhan, R., Puthawala, K., Agarwal, S., Amini, S.B. & Kalhan, S.C. (2001) Altered lipid profile, leptin, insulin, and anthropometry in offspring of South Asian immigrants in the United States. *Metabolism* **50**, 1197–202.

865. Kalkwarf, H.J., Khoury, J.C. & Lanphear, B.P. (2003) Milk intake during childhood and adolescence, adult bone density, and osteoporotic fractures in US women. *Am J Clin Nutr* **77**, 257–65.

866. Kalmijn, S., Launer, L.J., Ott, A., *et al.* (1997) Dietary fat intake and the risk of incident dementia in the Rotterdam Study. *Ann Neurol* **42**, 776–82.

867. Kamikubo, Y., Dellas, C., Loskutoff, D.J., Quigley, J.P. & Ruggeri, Z.M. (2008) Contribution of leptin receptor N-linked glycans to leptin binding. *Biochem J* **410**, 595–604.

868. Kaminer, B. & Lutz, W.P.W. (1960) Blood pressure in Bushmen of the Kalahari desert. *Circulation* **22**, 289–95.

869. Kang, J.H., Yu, B.Y. & Youn, D.S. (2007) Relationship of serum adiponectin and resistin levels with breast cancer risk. *J Korean Med Sci* **22**, 117–21.

870. Kanis, J.A., Johnell, O., De Laet, C., *et al.* (2002) International variations in hip fracture probabilities: implications for risk assessment. *J Bone Miner Res* **17**, 1237–44.

871. Kanis, J.A., Johnell, O., Oden, A., *et al.* (2000) Long-term risk of osteoporotic fracture in Malmo. *Osteoporos Int* **11**, 669–74.

872. Kant, A.K., Graubard, B.I. & Kumanyika, S.K. (2007) Trends in black-white differentials in dietary intakes of U.S. adults, 1971–2002. *Am J Prev Med* **32**, 264–72.

873. Kantanen, J., Olsaker, I., Holm, L.E., *et al.* (2000) Genetic diversity and population structure of 20 North European cattle breeds. *J Hered* **91**, 446–57.

874. Kaplan, J.R., Manuck, S.B., Adams, M.R., *et al.* (1993) Plaque changes and arterial enlargement in atherosclerotic monkeys after manipulation of diet and social environment. *Arterioscler Thromb* **13**, 254–63.

875. Kariks, J. & McGovern, V.J. (1967) Heart disease in the territory of Papua-New Guinea: a preliminary report based on a necropsy study. *Med J Aust* **1**, 176–7.

876. Karppanen, H. & Mervaala, E. (2006) Sodium intake and hypertension. *Prog Cardiovasc Dis* **49**, 59–75.

877. Karsenty, G. (2006) Convergence between bone and energy homeostases: leptin regulation of bone mass. *Cell Metab* **4**, 341–8.

878. Katan, M.B. (2000) Trans fatty acids and plasma lipoproteins. *Nutr Rev* **58**, 188–91.

879. Katan, M.B. (2009) Weight-loss diets for the prevention and treatment of obesity. *N Engl J Med* **360**, 923–5.

880. Katzmarzyk, P.T. & Craig, C.L. (2006) Independent effects of waist circumference and physical activity on all-cause mortality in Canadian women. *Appl Physiol Nutr Metab* **31**, 271–6.

881. Katzmarzyk, P.T., Janssen, I., Ross, R., Church, T.S. & Blair, S.N. (2006) The importance of waist circumference in the definition of metabolic syndrome: prospective analyses of mortality in men. *Diabetes Care* **29**, 404–9.

882. Kavanaghi, R., Workman, E., Nash, P., *et al.* (1995) The effects of elemental diet and subsequent food reintroduction on rheumatoid arthritis. *Br J Rheumatol* **34**, 270–73.

883. Kavantzas, N., Chatziioannou, A., Yanni, A.E., *et al.* (2006) Effect of green tea on angiogenesis and severity of atherosclerosis in cholesterol-fed rabbit. *Vascul Pharmacol* **44**, 461–3.

884. Kazerouni, N., Sinha, R., Hsu, C.H., Greenberg, A. & Rothman, N. (2001) Analysis of 200 food items for benzo[a]pyrene and estimation of its intake in an epidemiologic study. *Food Chem Toxicol* **39**, 423–36.

885. Kean, B.H. & Hamill, J.F. (1949) Anthropology of arterial tension. *Arch Intern Med* **83**, 355–62.

886. Kearney, J., Thomas, J. & Haddad, L. (2005) Food and nutritents. In: *Human Nutrition* (C.A. Geissler & H.J. Powers eds). Elsevier Churchill Livingstone, London, pp. 1–23.

887. Keenan, J.M. & Morris, D.H. (1995) Hypercholesterolemia. Dietary advice for patients regarding meat [see comments]. *Postgrad Med* **98**, 113–14, 117–18, 120–21 passim.

888. Kelley, G.A. & Kelley, K.S. (2006) Exercise and bone mineral density at the femoral neck in postmenopausal women: a meta-analysis of controlled clinical trials with individual patient data. *Am J Obstet Gynecol* **194**, 760–67.

889. Kelly, S., Frost, G., Whittaker, V. & Summerbell, C. (2004) Low glycaemic index diets for coronary heart disease. *Cochrane Database Syst Rev*, CD004467.

890. Kemkes-Grottenthaler, A. (2005) The short die young: the interrelationship between stature and longevity-evidence from skeletal remains. *Am J Phys Anthropol* **128**, 340–47.

891. Kenchaiah, S., Evans, J.C., Levy, D., *et al.* (2002) Obesity and the risk of heart failure. *N Engl J Med* **347**, 305–13.

892. Kennedy, R.L., Chokkalingam, K. & Farshchi, H.R. (2005) Nutrition in patients with Type 2 diabetes: are low-carbohydrate diets effective, safe or desirable? *Diabet Med* **22**, 821–32.

893. Kernan, W.N., Inzucchi, S.E., Viscoli, C.M., *et al.* (2002) Insulin resistance and risk for stroke. *Neurology* **59**, 809–15.

894. Kerstetter, J.E., O'Brien, K.O. & Insogna, K.L. (2003) Dietary protein, calcium metabolism, and skeletal homeostasis revisited. *Am J Clin Nutr* **78**, 584S–92S.

895. Kerstetter, J.E., Svastisalee, C.M., Caseria, D.M., Mitnick, M.E. & Insogna, K.L. (2000) A threshold for low-protein-diet-induced elevations in parathyroid hormone. *Am J Clin Nutr* **72**, 168–73.

896. Kestin, M., Rouse, I.L., Correll, R.A. & Nestel, P.J. (1989) Cardiovascular disease risk factors in free-living men: comparison of two prudent diets, one based on lactoovovegetarianism and the other allowing lean meat. *Am J Clin Nutr* **50**, 280–87.

897. Kevau, I.H. (1990) Cardiology in Papua New Guinea in the twenty-first century [editorial]. *P N G Med J* **33**, 271–4.

898. Kevau, I.H. (1990) Clinical documentation of twenty cases of acute myocardial infarction in Papua New Guineans. *P N G Med J* **33**, 275–80.

899. Key, T.J. (2005) Cancers. In: *Human nutrition* (C.A. Geissler & H.J. Powers eds). Elsevier Churchill Livingstone, London, pp. 415–28.

900. Key, T.J., Fraser, G.E., Thorogood, M., *et al.* (1999) Mortality in vegetarians and nonvegetarians: detailed findings from a collaborative analysis of 5 prospective studies. *Am J Clin Nutr* **70**, 516S–24S.

901. Keys, A. (1953) Prediction and possible prevention of coronary disease. *Am J Public Health Nations Health* **43**, 1399–407.

902. Keys, A. (1980) *Seven countries. A multivariate analysis of death and coronary heart disease*. Harvard University Press, Cambridge, Mass.

903. Khandekar, R., Al Harby, S. & Mohammed, A.J. (2005) Determinants of myopia among Omani school children: a case-control study. *Ophthalmic Epidemiol* **12**, 207–13.

904. Khaw, K.T. & Barrett, C.E. (1987) Dietary potassium and stroke-associated mortality. A 12-year prospective population study. *N Engl J Med* **316**, 235–40.

905. Kiens, B. & Richter, E.A. (1996) Types of carbohydrate in an ordinary diet affect insulin action and muscle substrates in humans. *Am J Clin Nutr* **63**, 47–53.

906. Kilander, L., Nyman, H., Boberg, M., Hansson, L. & Lithell, H. (1998) Hypertension is related to cognitive impairment: a 20-year follow-up of 999 men. *Hypertension* **31**, 780–86.

907. Kim, S.P., Ellmerer, M., Van Citters, G.W. & Bergman, R.N. (2003) Primacy of hepatic insulin resistance in the development of the metabolic syndrome induced by an isocaloric moderate-fat diet in the dog. *Diabetes* **52**, 2453–60.

908. Kim, Y.I. (2007) Folate and colorectal cancer: an evidence-based critical review. *Mol Nutr Food Res* **51**, 267–92.

909. King, H., Finch, C., Koki, G., *et al.* (1991) Glucose tolerance in Papua New Guinea: comparison of Austronesian and non-Austronesian communities of Karkar Island. *Diabet Med* **8**, 481–8.

910. King, H. & Rewers, M. (1993) Global estimates for prevalence of diabetes mellitus and impaired glucose tolerance in adults. WHO Ad Hoc Diabetes Reporting Group. *Diabetes Care* **16**, 157–77.

911. Kinjo, M., Setoguchi, S. & Solomon, D.H. (2007) Bone mineral density in adults with the metabolic syndrome: analysis in a population-based U.S. Sample. *J Clin Endocrinol Metab* **92**, 4161–4.

912. Kirby, C.R. & Convertino, V.A. (1986) Plasma aldosterone and sweat sodium concentrations after exercise and heat acclimation. *J Appl Physiol* **61**, 967–70.

913. Kirk, J.K., Graves, D.E., Craven, T.E., *et al.* (2008) Restricted-carbohydrate diets in patients with type 2 diabetes: a meta-analysis. *J Am Diet Assoc* **108**, 91–100.

914. Kitabchi, A.E. & Shea, J.J. (1975) Diabetes mellitus in fluctuant hearing loss. *Otolaryngol Clin North Am* **8**, 357–68.

915. Kitabchi, A.E., Shea, J.J., Duckworth, W.C. & Adams, F. (1971) High incidence of diabetes and glucose intolerance in fluctuant hearing loss. *J Lab Clin Med* **78**, 995–6.

916. Kitamura, A., Iso, H., Iida, M., *et al.* (2002) Trends in the incidence of coronary heart disease and stroke and the prevalence of cardiovascular risk factors among Japanese men from 1963 to 1994. *Am J Med* **112**, 104–9.

917. Kitamura, A., Iso, H., Nai to, Y., *et al.* (1994) High-density lipoprotein cholesterol and premature coronary heart disease in urban Japanese men. *Circulation* **89**, 2533–9.

918. Kivipelto, M., Ngandu, T., Fratiglioni, L., *et al.* (2005) Obesity and vascular risk factors at midlife and the risk of dementia and Alzheimer disease. *Arch Neurol* **62**, 1556–60.

919. Kjaergard, L.L. & Als-Nielsen, B. (2002) Association between competing interests and authors' conclusions: epidemiological study of randomised clinical trials published in the BMJ. *BMJ* **325**, 249.

920. Kjeldsen-Kragh, J., Haugen, M., Borchgrevink, C.F., *et al.* (1991) Controlled trial of fasting and one-year vegetarian diet in rheumatoid arthritis. *Lancet* **338**, 899–902.

921. Klein, G.L. & Simmons, D.J. (1993) Nutritional rickets: thoughts about pathogenesis. *Ann Med* **25**, 379–84.

922. Klinger, B., Anin, S., Silbergeld, A., Eshet, R. & Laron, Z. (1998) Development of hyperandrogenism during treatment with insulin-like growth factor-I (IGF-I) in female patients with Laron syndrome. *Clin Endocrinol (Oxf)* **48**, 81–7.

923. Klompmaker, T.R. (2005) Lifetime high calcium intake increases osteoporotic fracture risk in old age. *Med Hypotheses* **65**, 552–8.

924. Kloner, R.A. & Rezkalla, S.H. (2007) To drink or not to drink? That is the question. *Circulation* **116**, 1306–17.

925. Kluger, M.J., Kozak, W., Conn, C.A., Leon, L.R. & Soszynski, D. (1996) The adaptive value of fever. *Infect Dis Clin North Am* **10**, 1–20.

926. Knoke, J.D. & Barrett-Connor, E. (2003) Weight loss: a determinant of hip bone loss in older men and women. The Rancho Bernardo Study. *Am J Epidemiol* **158**, 1132–8.

927. Knopp, R.H., Retzlaff, B., Walden, C., *et al.* (2000) One-year effects of increasingly fat-restricted, carbohydrate-enriched diets on lipoprotein levels in free-living subjects. *Proc Soc Exp Biol Med* **225**, 191–9.

928. Knowler, W.C., Barrett-Connor, E., Fowler, S.E., *et al.* (2002) Reduction in the incidence of type 2 diabetes with lifestyle intervention or metformin. *N Engl J Med* **346**, 393–403.

929. Knudson, J.D., Dincer, U.D., Dick, G.M., *et al.* (2005) Leptin resistance extends to the coronary vasculature in prediabetic dogs and provides a protective adaptation against endothelial dysfunction. *Am J Physiol Heart Circ Physiol* **289**, H1038–46.

930. Knudtson, M.D., Klein, B.E., Klein, R. & Shankar, A. (2005) Associations with weight loss and subsequent mortality risk. *Ann Epidemiol* **15**, 483–91.

931. Knuiman, J.T., West, C.E., Katan, M.B. & Hautvast, J.G. (1987) Total cholesterol and high density lipoprotein cholesterol levels in populations differing in fat and carbohydrate intake. *Arteriosclerosis* **7**, 612–19.

932. Ko, I.W.P., Corlett, R.T. & Xu, R.-J. (1998) Sugar composition of wild fruits in Hong Kong, China. *J Tropical Ecol* **14**, 381–7.

933. Kobayashi, S. & Venkatachalam, M.A. (1992) Differential effects of calorie restriction on glomeruli and tubules of the remnant kidney. *Kidney Int* **42**, 710–7.

933a. Koch, A.E., Shah, M.R., Harlow, L.A., Lovis, R.M. & Pope, R.M. (1994) Soluble inter-cellular adhesion molecule-1 in arthritis. *Clin Immunol Immunopathol* **71**, 208–15.

934. Koebnick, C., Hoffmann, I., Dagnelie, P.C., *et al.* (2004) Long-term ovo-lacto vegetarian diet impairs vitamin B-12 status in pregnant women. *J Nutr* **134**, 3319–26.

935. Koepke, N. & Baten, J. (2005) The biological standard of living in Europe during the last two millennia. *Europ Rev Econ History* **9**, 61–95.

936. Koklu, E., Ozturk, M.A., Kurtoglu, S., *et al.* (2007) Aortic Intima-Media Thickness, Serum IGF-I, IGFBP-3, and Leptin Levels in Intrauterine Growth-Restricted Newborns of Healthy Mothers. *Pediatr Res* **62**, 704–9.

937. Konradsen, S., Ag, H., Lindberg, F., Hexeberg, S. & Jorde, R. (2008) Serum 1,25-dihydroxy vitamin D is inversely associated with body mass index. *Eur J Nutr* **47**, 87–91.

938. Kontogianni, M.D., Panagiotakos, D.B., Pitsavos, C., Chrysohoou, C. & Stefanadis, C. (2008) Relationship between meat intake and the development of acute coronary syn-dromes: the CARDIO2000 case–control study. *Eur J Clin Nutr* **62**, 171–7.

939. Kopp, W. (2004) Nutrition, evolution and thyroid hormone levels – a link to iodine deficiency disorders? *Med Hypotheses* **62**, 871–5.

940. Korner, N. (1980) Cardiovascular disease in Papua New Guinea. *Med J Aust* **1**, 1–7.

941. Kotronen, A., Westerbacka, J., Bergholm, R., Pietilainen, K.H. & Yki-Jarvinen, H. (2007) Liver fat in the metabolic syndrome. *J Clin Endocrinol Metab* **92**, 3490–7.

942. Kousta, E., Cela, E., Lawrence, N., *et al.* (2000) The prevalence of polycystic ovaries in women with a history of gestational diabetes. *Clin Endocrinol (Oxf)* **53**, 501–7.

943. Koutis, A.D., Isacsson, A., Lionis, C.D., *et al.* (1993) Differences in the diagnose panorama in primary health care in Dalby, Sweden and Spili, Crete. *Scand J Soc Med* **21**, 51–8.

944. Krauss, R.M., Deckelbaum, R.J., Ernst, N., *et al.* (1996) Dietary guidelines for healthy American adults. A statement for health professionals from the Nutrition Committee, American Heart Association. *Circulation* **94**, 1795–800.

945. Krauss, R.M., Eckel, R.H., Howard, B., *et al.* (2000) AHA Dietary Guidelines: revision 2000: A statement for healthcare professionals from the Nutrition Committee of the Amer-ican Heart Association. *Circulation* **102**, 2284–99.

946. Kris-Etherton, P.M. (1999) AHA Science Advisory. Monounsaturated fatty acids and risk of cardiovascular disease. American Heart Association. Nutrition Committee. *Circulation* **100**, 1253–8.

947. Kris-Etherton, P.M., Zhao, G., Binkoski, A.E., Coval, S.M. & Etherton, T.D. (2001) The effects of nuts on coronary heart disease risk. *Nutr Rev* **59**, 103–11.

948. Kritchevsky, D. (1977) Diet and cholesteremia. *Lipids* **12**, 49–52.

949. Kritchevsky, D. (1990) Protein and atherosclerosis. *J Nutr Sci Vitaminol (Tokyo)* **36** (Suppl 2), S81–6.

950. Kritchevsky, D. (1995) Dietary protein, cholesterol and atherosclerosis: a review of the early history. *J Nutr* **125**, 589S–93S.

951. Kritchevsky, D. (1998) History of recommendations to the public about dietary fat. *J Nutr* **128**, 449S–52S.

952. Kritchevsky, D. (2001) Diet and atherosclerosis. *J Nutr Health Aging* **5**, 155–9.

953. Kritchevsky, D. (2002) Dietary fat and atherosclerosis. *J Nutr Biochem* **13**, 391.

954. Kritchevsky, D., Davidson, L.M., Kim, H.K., *et al.* (1980) Influence of type of carbohydrate on atherosclerosis in baboons fed semipurified diets plus 0.1% cholesterol. *Am J Clin Nutr* **33**, 1869–87.

955. Kritchevsky, D., Tepper, S.A., Czarnecki, S.K., Klurfeld, D.M. & Story, J.A. (1981) Experimental atherosclerosis in rabbits fed cholesterol-free diets. Part 9. Beef protein and textured vegetable protein. *Atherosclerosis* **39**, 169–75.

956. Kritchevsky, D., Tepper, S.A., Davidson, L.M., Fisher, E.A. & Klurfeld, D.M. (1989) Experimental atherosclerosis in rabbits fed cholesterol-free diets. 13. Interaction of proteins and fat. *Atherosclerosis* **75**, 123–7.

957. Kritchevsky, D., Tepper, S.A. & Klurfeld, D.M. (1998) Lectin may contribute to the atherogenicity of peanut oil. *Lipids* **33**, 821–3.

958. Kritchevsky, D., Tepper, S.A., Weber, M.M. & Klurfeld, D.M. (1988) Influence of soy protein or casein on pre-established atherosclerosis in rabbits. *Artery* **15**, 163–9.

959. Kritchevsky, D., Tepper, S.A., Williams, D.E. & Story, J.A. (1977) Experimental atherosclerosis in rabbits fed cholesterol-free diets. Part 7. Interaction of animal or vegetable protein with fiber. *Atherosclerosis* **26**, 397–403.

960. Kritchevsky, D., Tepper, S.A., Wright, S., *et al.* (2003) Cholesterol vehicle in experimental atherosclerosis 24: avocado oil. *J Am Coll Nutr* **22**, 52–5.

961. Kromann, N. & Green, A. (1980) Epidemiological studies in the Upernavik district, Greenland. Incidence of some chronic diseases 1950–1974. *Acta Med Scand* **208**, 401–6.

962. Kromhout, D. (2001) Epidemiology of cardiovascular diseases in Europe. *Public Health Nutr* **4**, 441–57.

963. Kuek, A., Hazleman, B.L. & Ostor, A.J. (2007) Immune-mediated inflammatory diseases (IMIDs) and biologic therapy: a medical revolution. *Postgrad Med J* **83**, 251–60.

964. Kuller, L.H. (2004) Ethnic differences in atherosclerosis, cardiovascular disease and lipid metabolism. *Curr Opin Lipidol* **15**, 109–13.

965. Kupari, M., Koskinen, P. & Virolainen, J. (1994) Correlates of left ventricular mass in a population sample aged 36 to 37 years. Focus on lifestyle and salt intake. *Circulation* **89**, 1041–50.

966. Kushi, L.H., Folsom, A.R., Prineas, R.J., *et al.* (1996) Dietary antioxidant vitamins and death from coronary heart disease in postmenopausal women. *N Engl J Med* **334**, 1156–62.

967. Kylin, E. (1923) Studien über das Hypertonie-Hyperglykemie-Hyperurikemie-Syndrom. *Zentralblatt für Innere Medizin* **7**, 105.

968. Laaksonen, D.E., Lindstrom, J., Lakka, T.A., *et al.* (2005) Physical activity in the prevention of type 2 diabetes: the Finnish diabetes prevention study. *Diabetes* **54**, 158–65.

969. Lacroix, M., Gaudichon, C., Martin, A., *et al.* (2004) A long-term high-protein diet markedly reduces adipose tissue without major side effects in Wistar male rats. *Am J Physiol Regul Integr Comp Physiol* **287**, R934–42.

970. Laden, G. & Wrangham, R. (2005) The rise of the hominids as an adaptive shift in fallback foods: plant underground storage organs (USOs) and australopith origins. *J Hum Evol* **49**, 482–98.

971. Laffitte, B.A., Joseph, S.B., Walczak, R., *et al.* (2001) Autoregulation of the human liver X receptor alpha promoter. *Mol Cell Biol* **21**, 7558–68.

972. Laitinen, M.H., Ngandu, T., Rovio, S., *et al.* (2006) Fat intake at midlife and risk of dementia and Alzheimer's disease: a population-based study. *Dement Geriatr Cogn Disord* **22**, 99–107.

973. Lakatta, E.G. (2003) Arterial and cardiac aging: major shareholders in cardiovascular disease enterprises: Part III: cellular and molecular clues to heart and arterial aging. *Circulation* **107**, 490–97.

974. Lakatta, E.G. & Levy, D. (2003) Arterial and cardiac aging: major shareholders in cardiovascular disease enterprises: Part II: the aging heart in health: links to heart disease. *Circulation* **107**, 346–54.

975. Lakka, H.M., Lakka, T.A., Tuomilehto, J. & Salonen, J.T. (2002) Abdominal obesity is associated with increased risk of acute coronary events in men. *Eur Heart J* **23**, 706–13.

976. Lalande, A., Roux, C., Graulet, A.M., Schiavi, P. & De Vernejoul, M.C. (1998) The diuretic indapamide increases bone mass and decreases bone resorption in spontaneously hypertensive rats supplemented with sodium. *J Bone Miner Res* **13**, 1444–50.

977. Lambert, H.L., Eastell, R., Karnik, K., Russell, J.M. & Barker, M.E. (2008) Calcium supplementation and bone mineral accretion in adolescent girls: an 18-mo randomized controlled trial with 2-y follow-up. *Am J Clin Nutr* **87**, 455–62.

978. Lammers, K.M., Lu, R., Brownley, J., *et al.* (2008) Gliadin induces an increase in intestinal permeability and zonulin release by binding to the chemokine receptor CXCR3. *Gastroenterology* **135**, 194–204 e3.

979. Lamounier-Zepter, V., Ehrhart-Bornstein, M. & Bornstein, S.R. (2006) Insulin resistance in hypertension and cardiovascular disease. *Best Pract Res Clin Endocrinol Metab* **20**, 355–67.

980. Lane, M.A., Baer, D.J., Rumpler, W.V., *et al.* (1996) Calorie restriction lowers body temperature in rhesus monkeys, consistent with a postulated anti-aging mechanism in rodents. *Proc Natl Acad Sci USA* **93**, 4159–64.

981. Lanou, A.J., Berkow, S.E. & Barnard, N.D. (2005) Calcium, dairy products, and bone health in children and young adults: a reevaluation of the evidence. *Pediatrics* **115**, 736–43.

982. Lappalainen, R., Mennen, L., van Weert, L. & Mykkanen, H. (1993) Drinking water with a meal: a simple method of coping with feelings of hunger, satiety and desire to eat. *Eur J Clin Nutr* **47**, 815–19.

983. Larsen, C.S. (1995) Biological changes in human populations with agriculture. *Annu Rev Anthropol* **95**, 185–213.

984. Larsson, C.L. & Johansson, G.K. (2002) Dietary intake and nutritional status of young vegans and omnivores in Sweden. *Am J Clin Nutr* **76**, 100–106.

985. Larsson, M. & Sandberg, A.-S. (1991) Phytate reduction in bread containing oat flour, oat bran or rye bran. *J Cereal Sci* **14**, 141–9.

986. Larter, C.Z., Yeh, M.M., Williams, J., Bell-Anderson, K.S. & Farrell, G.C. (2008) MCD-induced steatohepatitis is associated with hepatic adiponectin resistance and adipogenic transformation of hepatocytes. *J Hepatol* **49**, 407–16.

987. Laudet, V. & Gronemeyer, H. (2002) *The nuclear receptor facts book*. Academic Press, San Diego.

988. Lauer, K. (1997) Diet and multiple sclerosis. *Neurology* **49**, S55–61.

989. Laugesen, M. & Elliott, R. (2003) Ischaemic heart disease, Type 1 diabetes, and cow milk A1 beta-casein. *N Z Med J* **116**, U295.

990. Laughlin, R.S., Musch, M.W., Hollbrook, C.J., *et al.* (2000) The key role of Pseudomonas aeruginosa PA-I lectin on experimental gut-derived sepsis. *Ann Surg* **232**, 133–42.

991. Laughlin, W.S., Harper, A.B. & Thompson, D.D. (1979) New approaches to the pre- and post-contact history of Arctic peoples. *Am J Phys Anthropol* **51**, 579–87.

992. Laustiola, K.E. (1991) Atherothrombotic mechanisms in smoking [editorial]. *J Intern Med* **230**, 469–70.

993. Lavigne, C., Tremblay, F., Asselin, G., Jacques, H. & Marette, A. (2001) Prevention of skeletal muscle insulin resistance by dietary cod protein in high fat-fed rats. *Am J Physiol Endocrinol Metab* **281**, E62–71.

994. Law, M. (1998) Lipids and cardiovascular disease. In: *Evidence based cardiology* (S. Yusuf, J.A. Cairns, A.J. Camm, E.L. Fallen & B.J. Gersh eds). BMJ Books, London, pp. 191–205.

995. Law, M.R. (2000) Plant sterol and stanol margarines and health. *West J Med* **173**, 43–7.

996. Law, M.R., Frost, C.D. & Wald, N.J. (1991) By how much does dietary salt reduction lower blood pressure? I–Analysis of observational data among populations. *BMJ* **302**, 811–15.

997. Law, M.R., Frost, C.D. & Wald, N.J. (1991) By how much does dietary salt reduction lower blood pressure? III–Analysis of data from trials of salt reduction [published erratum appears in BMJ 1991 Apr 20;302 (6782):939]. *BMJ* **302**, 819–24.

998. Law, M.R. & Morris, J.K. (1999) By how much does fruit and vegetable consumption reduce the risk of ischaemic heart disease: response to commentary. *Eur J Clin Nutr* **53**, 903–4.

999. Law, M.R. & Wald, N.J. (1994) An ecological study of serum cholesterol and ischaemic heart disease between 1950 and 1990. *Eur J Clin Nutr* **48**, 305–25.

1000. Lawlor, D.A., Davey Smith, G., Kundu, D., Bruckdorfer, K.R. & Ebrahim, S. (2004) Those confounded vitamins: what can we learn from the differences between observational versus randomised trial evidence? *Lancet* **363**, 1724–7.

1001. Lawlor, D.A., Ebrahim, S., Timpson, N. & Davey Smith, G. (2005) Avoiding milk is associated with a reduced risk of insulin resistance and the metabolic syndrome: findings from the British Women's Heart and Health Study. *Diabet Med* **22**, 808–11.

1002. Lea, E. & Worsley, A. (2002) The cognitive contexts of beliefs about the healthiness of meat. *Public Health Nutr* **5**, 37–45.

1003. Leden, I. & Arcini, C. (1994) Doubts about rheumatoid arthritis as a New World disease. *Semin Arthritis Rheum* **23**, 354–6.

1004. Lee, D.H., Lee, I.K., Song, K., *et al.* (2006) A strong dose-response relation between serum concentrations of persistent organic pollutants and diabetes: results from the National Health and Examination Survey 1999–2002. *Diabetes Care* **29**, 1638–44.

1005. Lee, R.B. (1968) What hunters do for a living, or, how to make out on scarce resources. In: *Man the hunter* (R.B. Lee & I. DeVore eds). Aldine, Chicago, pp. 30–48.

1006. Lee, S.H., Park, J.S., Kim, W., *et al.* (2008) Impact of body mass index and waist-to-hip ratio on clinical outcomes in patients with ST-segment elevation acute myocardial infarction (from the Korean Acute Myocardial Infarction Registry). *Am J Cardiol* **102**, 957–65.

1007. Leeds, A.R. (2002) Glycemic index and heart disease. *Am J Clin Nutr* **76**, 286S–9S.

1008. Leenen, F.H. & Yuan, B. (1998) Dietary-sodium-induced cardiac remodeling in spontaneously hypertensive rat versus Wistar-Kyoto rat. *J Hypertens* **16**, 885–92.

1009. Legro, R.S. (2002) Polycystic ovary syndrome: the new millennium. *Mol Cell Endocrinol* **186**, 219–25.

1010. Leighton, G. & Clark, M.L. (1929) Milk consumption and the growth of school-children; second preliminary report on tests to Scottish Board of Health. *Lancet* **1**, 40–3.

1011. Lemaitre, R.N., King, I.B., Raghunathan, T.E., *et al.* (2002) Cell membrane trans-fatty acids and the risk of primary cardiac arrest. *Circulation* **105**, 697–701.

1012. Lemann, J., Jr. (1999) Relationship between urinary calcium and net acid excretion as determined by dietary protein and potassium: a review. *Nephron* **81**, 18–25.

1013. Lemann, J., Jr., Gray, R.W. & Pleuss, J.A. (1989) Potassium bicarbonate, but not sodium bicarbonate, reduces urinary calcium excretion and improves calcium balance in healthy men. *Kidney Int* **35**, 688–95.

1014. Lemann, J., Jr., Pleuss, J.A., Gray, R.W. & Hoffmann, R.G. (1991) Potassium administration reduces and potassium deprivation increases urinary calcium excretion in healthy adults [corrected]. *Kidney Int* **39**, 973–83.

1015. Leosdottir, M., Nilsson, P., Nilsson, J.A., Mansson, H. & Berglund, G. (2004) The association between total energy intake and early mortality: data from the Malmo Diet and Cancer Study. *J Intern Med* **256**, 499–509.

1016. Lerch, C. & Meissner, T. (2007) Interventions for the prevention of nutritional rickets in term born children. *Cochrane Database Syst Rev*, CD006164.

1017. Lesauskaite, V., Tanganelli, P., Bianciardi, G., *et al.* (1999) World Health Organization (WHO) and the World Heart Federation (WHF) Pathobiological Determinants of Atherosclerosis in Youth (PBDAY) Study. Histomorphometric investigation of the aorta and coronary arteries in young people from different geographical locations. *Nutr Metab Cardiovasc Dis* **9**, 266–76.

1018. Leslie, W.D., Lix, L.M., Prior, H.J., *et al.* (2007) Biphasic fracture risk in diabetes: a population-based study. *Bone* **40**, 1595–601.

1019. Lesser, L.I., Ebbeling, C.B., Goozner, M., Wypij, D. & Ludwig, D.S. (2007) Relationship between funding source and conclusion among nutrition-related scientific articles. *PLoS Med* **4**, e5.

1020. Levey, A.S., Andreoli, S.P., DuBose, T., Provenzano, R. & Collins, A.J. (2007) Chronic kidney disease: common, harmful and treatable – World Kidney Day 2007. *Am J Nephrol* **27**, 108–12.

1021. Levin, A. (2001) Prevalence of cardiovascular damage in early renal disease. *Nephrol Dial Transplant* **16**, 7–11.

1022. Levine, H.D. (1946) Rheumatic heart disease in New Guinea: including a Cardiovascular Survey of 200 Native Papuans. *Ann Intern Med* **24**, 826–36.

1023. Lewington, S., Clarke, R., Qizilbash, N., Peto, R. & Collins, R. (2002) Age-specific relevance of usual blood pressure to vascular mortality: a meta-analysis of individual data for one million adults in 61 prospective studies. *Lancet* **360**, 1903–13.

1024. Li, C., Ford, E.S., McGuire, L.C. & Mokdad, A.H. (2007) Association of metabolic syndrome and insulin resistance with congestive heart failure: findings from the Third National Health and Nutrition Examination Survey. *J Epidemiol Community Health* **61**, 67–73.

1025. Li, C.I., Littman, A.J. & White, E. (2007) Relationship between age maximum height is attained, age at menarche, and age at first full-term birth and breast cancer risk. *Cancer Epidemiol Biomarkers Prev* **16**, 2144–9.

1026. Li, D., Siriamornpun, S., Wahlqvist, M.L., Mann, N.J. & Sinclair, A.J. (2005) Lean meat and heart health. *Asia Pac J Clin Nutr* **14**, 113–19.

1027. Li, Y., Eitan, S., Wu, J., *et al.* (2003) Morphine induces desensitization of insulin receptor signaling. *Mol Cell Biol* **23**, 6255–66.

1028. Libby, P. (2005) The pathogenesis of atherosclerosis. In: *Harrison's Principles of Internal Medicine* (D.L. Kasper, E. Braunwald, A.S. Fauci, S.L. Hauser, D.L. Longo & J.L. Jameson eds). McGraw-Hill Co, New York, pp. 1425–30.

1029. Libuda, L., Alexy, U., Remer, T., *et al.* (2008) Association between long-term consumption of soft drinks and variables of bone modeling and remodeling in a sample of healthy German children and adolescents. *Am J Clin Nutr* **88**, 1670–77.

1030. Lichtenstein, A.H., Appel, L.J., Brands, M., *et al.* (2006) Summary of American Heart Association Diet and Lifestyle Recommendations revision 2006. *Arterioscler Thromb Vasc Biol* **26**, 2186–91.

1031. Liebson, P.R., Grandits, G., Prineas, R., *et al.* (1993) Echocardiographic correlates of left ventricular structure among 844 mildly hypertensive men and women in the Treatment of Mild Hypertension Study (TOMHS). *Circulation* **87**, 476–86.

1032. Lien, S., Kantanen, J., Olsaker, I., *et al.* (1999) Comparison of milk protein allele frequencies in Nordic cattle breeds. *Anim Genet* **30**, 85–91.

1033. Liener, I.E. (1986) Nutritional significance of lectins in the diet. In: *The lectins: properties, functions and applications in biology and medicine* (I.E. Liener, N. Sharon & I.J. Goldstein eds). Academic Press, Chichester, pp. 527–52.

1034. Liener, I.E., Donatucci, D.A. & Tarcza, J.C. (1984) Starch blockers: a potential source of trypsin inhibitors and lectins. *Am J Clin Nutr* **39**, 196–200.

1035. Liese, A.D., Schulz, M., Fang, F., *et al.* (2005) Dietary glycemic index and glycemic load, carbohydrate and fiber intake, and measures of insulin sensitivity, secretion, and adiposity in the Insulin Resistance Atherosclerosis Study. *Diabetes Care* **28**, 2832–8.

1036. Liesegang, A., Bürgi, E., Sassi, M.L., Risteli, J. & Wanner, M. (2002) Influence of a vegetarian diet versus a diet with fishmeal on bone in growing pigs. *J Vet Med A* **49**, 230–38.

1037. Lightowler, H.J. & Davies, G.J. (1998) Iodine intake and iodine deficiency in vegans as assessed by the duplicate-portion technique and urinary iodine excretion. *Br J Nutr* **80**, 529–35.

1038. Liljeberg, H. & Bjorck, I. (1998) Delayed gastric emptying rate may explain improved glycaemia in healthy subjects to a starchy meal with added vinegar. *Eur J Clin Nutr* **52**, 368–71.

1039. Lillioja, S. (1996) Impaired glucose tolerance in Pima Indians. *Diabet Med* **13**, S127–32.

1040. Lin, L., Umahara, M., York, D.A. & Bray, G.A. (1998) Beta-casomorphins stimulate and enterostatin inhibits the intake of dietary fat in rats. *Peptides* **19**, 325–31.

1041. Lindeberg, S. (1994) *Apparent absence of cerebrocardiovascular disease in Melanesians. Risk factors and nutritional considerations – the Kitava Study.* M.D., Ph.D., University of Lund.

1042. Lindeberg, S. (2003) Stroke in Papua New Guinea. *Lancet Neurol* **2**, 273.

1043. Lindeberg, S. (2005) Who wants to be normal? *Eur Heart J* **26**, 2605–6.

1044. Lindeberg, S. (2009) Modern human physiology with respect to evolutionary adaptations that relate to diet in the past. In: *The evolution of hominin diets: integrating approaches to the study of Palaeolithic subsistence* (M.P. Richards & J.J. Hublin eds), Springer, Berlin, pp. 43–57.

1045. Lindeberg, S., Berntorp, E., Carlsson, R., Eliasson, M. & Marckmann, P. (1997) Haemostatic variables in Pacific Islanders apparently free from stroke and ischaemic heart disease. *Thromb Haemost* **77**, 94–8.

1046. Lindeberg, S., Berntorp, E., Nilsson-Ehle, P., Terent, A. & Vessby, B. (1997) Age relations of cardiovascular risk factors in a traditional Melanesian society: the Kitava Study. *Am J Clin Nutr* **66**, 845–52.

1047. Lindeberg, S., Cordain, L., Rastam, L. & Ahren, B. (2004) Serum uric acid in traditional Pacific Islanders and in Swedes. *J Intern Med* **255**, 373–8.

1048. Lindeberg, S., Eliasson, M., Lindahl, B. & Ahrén, B. (1999) Low serum insulin in traditional Pacific Islanders – the Kitava Study. *Metabolism* **48**, 1216–19.

1049. Lindeberg, S., Jonsson, T., Granfeldt, Y., *et al.* (2007) A Palaeolithic diet improves glucose tolerance more than a Mediterranean-like diet in individuals with ischaemic heart disease. *Diabetologia* **50**, 1795–807.

1050. Lindeberg, S. & Lundh, B. (1993) Apparent absence of stroke and ischaemic heart disease in a traditional Melanesian island: a clinical study in Kitava. *J Intern Med* **233**, 269–75.

1051. Lindeberg, S., Nilsson-Ehle, P., Terént, A., Vessby, B. & Scherstén, B. (1994) Cardiovascular risk factors in a Melanesian population apparently free from stroke and ischaemic heart disease – the Kitava study. *J Intern Med* **236**, 331–40.

1052. Lindeberg, S., Nilsson-Ehle, P. & Vessby, B. (1996) Lipoprotein composition and serum cholesterol ester fatty acids in nonwesternized Melanesians. *Lipids* **31**, 153–8.

1053. Lindeberg, S., Soderberg, S., Ahren, B. & Olsson, T. (2001) Large differences in serum leptin levels between nonwesternized and westernized populations: the Kitava study. *J Intern Med* **249**, 553–8.

1054. Lindeberg, S. & Terent, A. (2001) [Insufficient standardization of blood pressure measurements is a serious source of error]. *Läkartidningen* **98**, 1429–31.

1055. Lindeberg, S. & Vessby, B. (1995) Fatty acid composition of cholesterol esters and serum tocopherols in Melanesians apparently free from cardiovascular disease – the Kitava study. *Nutr Metab Cardiovasc Dis* **5**, 45–53.

1056. Lindholm, L.H., Koutis, A.D., Lionis, C.D., *et al.* (1992) Risk factors for ischaemic heart disease in a Greek population. A cross-sectional study of men and women living in the village of Spili in Crete. *Eur Heart J* **13**, 291–8.

1057. Lindqvist, P., Andersson, K., Sundh, V., *et al.* (2006) Concurrent and separate effects of body mass index and waist-to-hip ratio on 24-year mortality in the Population Study of Women in Gothenburg: evidence of age-dependency. *Eur J Epidemiol* **21**, 789–94.

1058. Lionis, C., Bathianaki, M., Antonakis, N., Papavasiliou, S. & Philalithis, A. (2001) A high prevalence of diabetes mellitus in a municipality of rural Crete, Greece. *Diabet Med* **18**, 768–9.

1059. Lippe-Stokes, S. (1976) Eskimo story-knife tales: reflections of change in food habits. In: *Food, ecology and culture. Readings in the anthropology of dietary practices* (J.R.K. Robson ed). Gordon and Breach, New York, pp. 75–82.

1060. Lippman, S.M., Klein, E.A., Goodman, P.J., *et al.* (2009) Effect of selenium and vitamin E on risk of prostate cancer and other cancers: the Selenium and Vitamin E Cancer Prevention Trial (SELECT). *JAMA* **301**, 39–51.

1061. Lips, P. (2004) Which circulating level of 25-hydroxyvitamin D is appropriate? *J Steroid Biochem Mol Biol* **89–90**, 611–14.

1062. Lipscombe, L.L. & Hux, J.E. (2007) Trends in diabetes prevalence, incidence, and mortality in Ontario, Canada 1995–2005: a population-based study. *Lancet* **369**, 750–56.

1063. Lipsky, B.A., Pecoraro, R.E., Chen, M.S. & Koepsell, T.D. (1987) Factors affecting staphylococcal colonization among NIDDM outpatients. *Diabetes Care* **10**, 483–6.

1064. Little, D.L. (1996) Reducing the effects of clover disease by strategic grazing of pastures. *Aust Vet J* **73**, 192–3.

1065. Little, M.A., Galvin, K. & Mugambi, M. (1983) Cross-sectional growth of nomadic Turkana pastoralists. *Hum Biol* **55**, 811–30.

1066. Liu, B., Lee, H.Y., Weinzimer, S.A., *et al.* (2000) Direct functional interactions between insulin-like growth factor-binding protein-3 and retinoid X receptor-alpha regulate transcriptional signaling and apoptosis. *J Biol Chem* **275**, 33607–13.

1067. Liu, L., Ikeda, K. & Yamori, Y. (2002) Inverse relationship between urinary markers of animal protein intake and blood pressure in Chinese: results from the WHO Cardiovascular Diseases and Alimentary Comparison (CARDIAC) Study. *Int J Epidemiol* **31**, 227–33.

1068. Liu, S., Buring, J.E., Sesso, H.D., *et al.* (2002) A prospective study of dietary fiber intake and risk of cardiovascular disease among women. *J Am Coll Cardiol* **39**, 49–56.

1069. Liu, S., Choi, H.K., Ford, E., *et al.* (2006) A prospective study of dairy intake and the risk of type 2 diabetes in women. *Diabetes Care* **29**, 1579–84.

1070. Liu, S., Willett, W.C., Manson, J.E., *et al.* (2003) Relation between changes in intakes of dietary fiber and grain products and changes in weight and development of obesity among middle-aged women. *Am J Clin Nutr* **78**, 920–27.

1071. Liu, S., Willett, W.C., Stampfer, M.J., *et al.* (2000) A prospective study of dietary glycemic load, carbohydrate intake, and risk of coronary heart disease in US women. *Am J Clin Nutr* **71**, 1455–61.

1072. Liu, S.K., Tilley, L.P., Tappe, J.P. & Fox, P.R. (1986) Clinical and pathologic findings in dogs with atherosclerosis: 21 cases (1970–1983). *J Am Vet Med Assoc* **189**, 227–32.

1073. Livingston, J.N. & Purvis, B.J. (1981) The effects of wheat germ agglutinin on the adipocyte insulin receptor. *Biochim Biophys Acta* **678**, 194–201.

1074. Liyanage, R., Han, K.H., Watanabe, S., *et al.* (2008) Potato and soy peptide diets modulate lipid metabolism in rats. *Biosci Biotechnol Biochem* **72**, 943–50.

1075. Lizard, G. (2008) Phytosterols: to be or not to be toxic; that is the question. *Br J Nutr* **100**, 1150–51.

1076. Lo, G.S., Evans, R.H., Phillips, K.S., Dahlgren, R.R. & Steinke, F.H. (1987) Effect of soy fiber and soy protein on cholesterol metabolism and atherosclerosis in rabbits. *Atherosclerosis* **64**, 47–54.

1077. Lock, C.A., Lecouturier, J., Mason, J.M. & Dickinson, H.O. (2006) Lifestyle interventions to prevent osteoporotic fractures: a systematic review. *Osteoporos Int* **17**, 20–28.

1078. Loke, Y.K., Singh, S. & Furberg, C.D. (2009) Long-term use of thiazolidinediones and fractures in type 2 diabetes: systematic review and meta-analysis. *CMAJ* **180**, 32–9.

1079. Lonn, E., Yusuf, S., Arnold, M.J., *et al.* (2006) Homocysteine lowering with folic acid and B vitamins in vascular disease. *N Engl J Med* **354**, 1567–77.

1080. Looker, A.C., Pfeiffer, C.M., Lacher, D.A., *et al.* (2008) Serum 25-hydroxyvitamin D status of the US population: 1988–1994 compared with 2000–2004. *Am J Clin Nutr* **88**, 1519–27.

1081. Lopaschuk, G.D., Folmes, C.D. & Stanley, W.C. (2007) Cardiac energy metabolism in obesity. *Circ Res* **101**, 335–47.

1082. Lopez, A.D. (2005) The evolution of the Global Burden of Disease framework for disease, injury and risk factor quantification: developing the evidence base for national, regional and global public health action. *Global Health* **1**, 5.

1083. Lopez, A.D., Mathers, C.D., Ezzati, M., Jamison, D.T. & Murray, C.J. (2006) Global and regional burden of disease and risk factors, 2001: systematic analysis of population health data. *Lancet* **367**, 1747–57.

1084. Lopez-Otin, C. & Diamandis, E.P. (1998) Breast and prostate cancer: an analysis of common epidemiological, genetic, and biochemical features. *Endocr Rev* **19**, 365–96.

1085. Lothrop, C., Harrison, G.J., Schultz, D. & Utteridge, T. (1986) Miscellaneous diseases. In: *Clinical Avian Medicine and Surgery* (G.J. Harrison & L.R. Harrison eds). Saunders, Philadelphia, pp. 525–36.

1086. Lowenstein, F.H. (1961) Blood-pressure in relation to age and sex in the tropics and subtropics. A review of the literature and an investigation in two tribes of Brazil Indians. *Lancet* i, 389–92.

1086a. Lowes, J.R., Radwan, P., Priddle, J.D. & Jewell, D.P. (1992) Characterisation and quantification of mucosal cytokine that induces epithelial histocompatibility locus antigen-DR expression in inflammatory bowel disease. *Gut* **33**, 315–19.

1087. Lucas, P.W., Ang, K.Y., Sui, Z., *et al.* (2006) A brief review of the recent evolution of the human mouth in physiological and nutritional contexts. *Physiol Behav* **89**, 36–8.

1088. Lucca, P., Hurrell, R. & Potrykus, I. (2002) Fighting iron deficiency anemia with iron-rich rice. *J Am Coll Nutr* **21**, 184S–90S.

1089. Luchsinger, J.A., Tang, M.X., Shea, S. & Mayeux, R. (2002) Caloric intake and the risk of Alzheimer disease. *Arch Neurol* **59**, 1258–63.

1090. Luchtenborg, M., Weijenberg, M.P., de Goeij, A.F., *et al.* (2005) Meat and fish consumption, APC gene mutations and hMLH1 expression in colon and rectal cancer: a prospective cohort study (The Netherlands). *Cancer Causes Control* **16**, 1041–54.

1091. Ludwig, D.S., Majzoub, J.A., Al-Zahrani, A., *et al.* (1999) High glycemic index foods, overeating, and obesity. *Pediatrics* **103**, E26.

1092. Luft, F.C. & Weinberger, M.H. (1997) Heterogeneous responses to changes in dietary salt intake: the salt-sensitivity paradigm. *Am J Clin Nutr* **65**, 612S–17S.

1093. Lulseged, S. & Fitwi, G. (1999) Vitamin D deficiency rickets: socio-demographic and clinical risk factors in children seen at a referral hospital in Addis Ababa. *East Afr Med J* **76**, 457–61.

1094. Lundquist, C.W. & Björnwall, J. (1936) Observations of arteriosclerosis in Northern Sweden. *Läkartidningen* **33**, 1209–15.

1095. Lupi, O., Madkan, V. & Tyring, S.K. (2006) Tropical dermatology: bacterial tropical diseases. *J Am Acad Dermatol* **54**, 559–78; quiz 578–80.

1096. Lusis, A.J. (2000) Atherosclerosis. *Nature* **407**, 233–41.

1097. Lusis, A.J., Attie, A.D. & Reue, K. (2008) Metabolic syndrome: from epidemiology to systems biology. *Nat Rev Genet* **9**, 819–30.

1098. Luyken, R. & Jansen, A.A.J. (1960) The cholesterol level in the blood serum of some population groups in New-Guinea. *Trop Geogr Med* **2**, 145–8.

1099. Lynch, S.R., Dassenko, S.A., Cook, J.D., Juillerat, M.A. & Hurrell, R.F. (1994) Inhibitory effect of a soybean-protein-related moiety on iron absorption in humans. *Am J Clin Nutr* **60**, 567–72.

1100. Ma, G., Young, D.B. & Clower, B.R. (1999) Inverse relationship between potassium intake and coronary artery disease in the cholesterol-fed rabbit. *Am J Hypertens* **12**, 821–5.

1101. Ma, J. & Stampfer, M.J. (2002) Body iron stores and coronary heart disease. *Clin Chem* **48**, 601–3.

1102. Macdonald, D. (1984) *The Encyclopedia of Mammals*. Facts on File Publishing, New York.

1103. Macdonald, H.M., New, S.A., Fraser, W.D., Campbell, M.K. & Reid, D.M. (2005) Low dietary potassium intakes and high dietary estimates of net endogenous acid production are associated with low bone mineral density in premenopausal women and increased markers of bone resorption in postmenopausal women. *Am J Clin Nutr* **81**, 923–33.

1104. MacFarlane, A.J., Burghardt, K.M., Kelly, J., *et al.* (2003) A type 1 diabetes-related protein from wheat (triticum aestivum): cDNA clone of a wheat storage globulin, Glb1, linked to islet damage. *J Biol Chem* **278**, 54–63.

1105. Macfarlane, B. & White, D.O. (1972) *Natural history of infectious disease*. Cambridge University Press, Cambridge.

1106. MacLennan, R., Macrae, F., Bain, C., *et al.* (1995) Randomized trial of intake of fat, fiber, and beta carotene to prevent colorectal adenomas. The Australian Polyp Prevention Project. *J Natl Cancer Inst* **87**, 1760–66.

1107. MacLennan, R., Paissat, D., Ring, A. & Thomas, S. (1985) Possible aetiology of oral cancer in Papua New Guinea. *P N G Med J* **28**, 3–8.

1108. Maddocks, I. (1964) Dietary factors in the genesis of hypertension. In: *Proceedings of the Sixth International Congress of Nutrition* (C.F. Mills & R. Passmore eds). Livingstone, Edinburgh, pp. 137–47.

1109. Maddocks, I. (1967) Blood pressures in Melanesians. *Med J Aust* **1**, 1123–6.

1110. Maddox, D.A., Alavi, F.K., Silbernick, E.M. & Zawada, E.T. (2002) Protective effects of a soy diet in preventing obesity-linked renal disease. *Kidney Int* **61**, 96–104.

1111. Maingrette, F. & Renier, G. (2005) Linoleic acid increases lectin-like oxidized LDL receptor-1 (LOX-1) expression in human aortic endothelial cells. *Diabetes* **54**, 1506–13.

1112. Mair, W., Piper, M.D. & Partridge, L. (2005) Calories do not explain extension of life span by dietary restriction in Drosophila. *PLoS Biol* **3**, e223.

1113. Majchrzak, D., Singer, I., Manner, M., *et al.* (2006) B-Vitamin status and concentrations of homocysteine in Austrian omnivores, vegetarians and vegans. *Ann Nutr Metab* **50**, 485–91.

1114. Majed, B., Moreau, T., Senouci, K., *et al.* (2008) Is obesity an independent prognosis factor in woman breast cancer? *Breast Cancer Res Treat* **111**, 329–42.

1115. Maldonado, E.N., Casanave, E.B. & Aveldano, M.I. (2002) Major plasma lipids and fatty acids in four HDL mammals. *Comp Biochem Physiol A Mol Integr Physiol* **132**, 297–303.

1116. Maldonado, E.N., Romero, J.R., Ochoa, B. & Aveldano, M.I. (2001) Lipid and fatty acid composition of canine lipoproteins. *Comp Biochem Physiol B Biochem Mol Biol* **128**, 719–29.

1117. Malhotra, A. & White, D.P. (2002) Obstructive sleep apnoea. *Lancet* **360**, 237–45.

1118. Malinow, M.R. (1983) Experimental models of atherosclerosis regression. *Atherosclerosis* **48**, 105–18.

1119. Malinowski, B. (1916) Baloma: The Spirits of the Dead in the Trobriand Islands. *J Royal Anthropol Inst* **46**, 353–430.

1120. Malinowski, B. (1919) Kula: The Circulating Exchange of Valuables in the Archipelagoes of Eastern New Guinea. *Man* **20**, 97–105.

1121. Malinowski, B. (1922) *Argonauts of the Western Pacific*. Routledge & Kegan Paul Ltd, London.

1122. Malinowski, B. (1925) Magic, science and religion. In: *Science, religion and reality* (J. Needham ed). Routledge & Kegan Paul Ltd, London, pp. 20–84.

1123. Malinowski, B. (1926) *Myth in primitive psychology*. Routledge & Kegan Paul Ltd, London.

1124. Malinowski, B. (1927) *Sex and repression in savage society*. Routledge & Kegan Paul Ltd, London.

1125. Malinowski, B. (1929) *The sexual life of savages in northwestern Melanesia*. Routledge & Kegan Paul Ltd, London.

1126. Malinowski, B. (1935) *Coral gardens and their magic*. George Allen & Unwin Ltd, London.
1127. Maloney, B.K. (1993) Palaeoecology and the origin of the coconut. *GeoJournal* **31**, 355–62.
1128. Malosse, D. & Perron, H. (1993) Correlation analysis between bovine populations, other farm animals, house pets, and multiple sclerosis prevalence. *Neuroepidemiology* **12**, 15–27.
1129. Malosse, D., Perron, H., Sasco, A. & Seigneurin, J.M. (1992) Correlation between milk and dairy product consumption and multiple sclerosis prevalence: a worldwide study. *Neuroepidemiology* **11**, 304–12.
1130. Mancia, G., De Backer, G., Dominiczak, A., *et al.* (2007) 2007 Guidelines for the management of arterial hypertension: The Task Force for the Management of Arterial Hypertension of the European Society of Hypertension (ESH) and of the European Society of Cardiology (ESC). *Eur Heart J* **28**, 1462–536.
1131. Mancilha-Carvalho, J.J. & Crews, D.E. (1990) Lipid profiles of Yanomamo Indians of Brazil. *Prev Med* **19**, 66–75.
1132. Mancilha-Carvalho, J.J., de Oliveira, R. & Esposito, R.J. (1989) Blood pressure and electrolyte excretion in the Yanomamo Indians, an isolated population. *J Hum Hypertens* **3**, 309–14.
1133. Mandayam, S. & Mitch, W.E. (2006) Dietary protein restriction benefits patients with chronic kidney disease. *Nephrology (Carlton)* **11**, 53–7.
1134. Mangels, A.R. & Messina, V. (2001) Considerations in planning vegan diets: infants. *J Am Diet Assoc* **101**, 670–77.
1135. Mann, D.L. (2008) Heart failure and cor pulmonale. In: *Harrison's principles of internal medicine* (A.S. Fauci, E. Braunwald, D.L. Kasper, S.L. Hauser, D.L. Longo, J.L. Jameson & J. Loscalzo eds). McGraw-Hill Co, New York, pp. 1443–55.
1136. Mann, G. (1975) Letter: bone mineral content of North Alaskan Eskimos. *Am J Clin Nutr* **28**, 566–7.
1137. Mann, G.V. (1955) The serum lipoprotein and cholesterol concentrations of Central and North Americans with different dietary habits. *Am J Med* **19**, 25.
1138. Mann, G.V. (1962) The health and nutritional status of Alaskan Eskimos. *Am J Clin Nutr* **11**, 31–40.
1139. Mann, G.V., Roels, O.A., Price, D.L. & Merrill, J.M. (1961) Cardiovascular disease in African Pygmies. A survey of the health status, serum lipids and diet of pygmies in Congo. *J Chron Dis* **15**, 341–71.
1140. Mann, G.V., Spoerry, A., Gray, M. & Jarashow, D. (1972) Atherosclerosis in the Masai. *Am J Epidemiol* **95**, 26–37.
1141. Mann, J. (2000) Diseases of the heart and circulation: the role of dietary factors in aetiology and management. In: *Human nutrition and dietetics* (J.S. Garrow & W.P.T. James eds). Churchill Livingstone, Edinburgh, pp. 689–714.
1142. Mann, J.I., De Leeuw, I., Hermansen, K., *et al.* (2004) Evidence-based nutritional approaches to the treatment and prevention of diabetes mellitus. *Nutr Metab Cardiovasc Dis* **14**, 373–94.
1143. Mann, N. (2000) Dietary lean red meat and human evolution. *Eur J Nutr* **39**, 71–9.
1144. Mann, N.J., Li, D., Sinclair, A.J., *et al.* (1999) The effect of diet on plasma homocysteine concentrations in healthy male subjects. *Eur J Clin Nutr* **53**, 895–9.
1145. Mantzoros, C.S., Tzonou, A., Signorello, L.B., *et al.* (1997) Insulin-like growth factor 1 in relation to prostate cancer and benign prostatic hyperplasia. *Br J Cancer* **76**, 1115–8.
1146. Maor, G., Rochwerger, M., Segev, Y. & Phillip, M. (2002) Leptin acts as a growth factor on the chondrocytes of skeletal growth centers. *J Bone Miner Res* **17**, 1034–43.
1147. Marckmann, P. & Gronbaek, M. (1999) Fish consumption and coronary heart disease mortality. A systematic review of prospective cohort studies. *Eur J Clin Nutr* **53**, 585–90.
1148. Mares, V., Borges, L.F. & Sidman, R.L. (1984) Uptake and transport of lectins from the cerebrospinal fluid by cells of the immature mouse brain. *Acta Histochem* **74**, 11–19.

1149. Marfella, R., Esposito, K., Siniscalchi, M., *et al.* (2004) Effect of weight loss on cardiac synchronization and proinflammatory cytokines in premenopausal obese women. *Diabetes Care* **27**, 47–52.

1150. Marshall, D., Johnell, O. & Wedel, H. (1996) Meta-analysis of how well measures of bone mineral density predict occurrence of osteoporotic fractures [see comments]. *BMJ* **312**, 1254–9.

1151. Martell, N., Rodriguez-Cerrillo, M., Grobbee, D.E., *et al.* (2003) High prevalence of secondary hypertension and insulin resistance in patients with refractory hypertension. *Blood Press* **12**, 149–54.

1152. Martin, S. & Parton, R.G. (2006) Lipid droplets: a unified view of a dynamic organelle. *Nat Rev Mol Cell Biol* **7**, 373–8.

1153. Martin, W.F., Armstrong, L.E. & Rodriguez, N.R. (2005) Dietary protein intake and renal function. *Nutr Metab (Lond)* **2**, 25.

1154. Massey, L.K. (2003) Dietary animal and plant protein and human bone health: a whole foods approach. *J Nutr* **133**, 862S–5S.

1155. Massey, L.K. (2005) Effect of dietary salt intake on circadian calcium metabolism, bone turnover, and calcium oxalate kidney stone risk in postmenopausal women. *Nutr Res* **25**, 891–903.

1156. Massey, L.K. & Kynast-Gales, S.A. (2001) Diets with either beef or plant proteins reduce risk of calcium oxalate precipitation in patients with a history of calcium kidney stones. *J Am Diet Assoc* **101**, 326–31.

1157. Mathews, C.L. (1974) Cardiovascular disease in Lae – a five year review. *P N G Med J* **17**, 251–62.

1158. Matkovic, V., Fontana, D., Tominac, C., Goel, P. & Chesnut, C.H., 3rd (1990) Factors that influence peak bone mass formation: a study of calcium balance and the inheritance of bone mass in adolescent females. *Am J Clin Nutr* **52**, 878–88.

1159. Matkovic, V., Ilich, J.Z., Andon, M.B., *et al.* (1995) Urinary calcium, sodium, and bone mass of young females. *Am J Clin Nutr* **62**, 417–25.

1160. Matlik, L., Savaiano, D., McCabe, G., *et al.* (2007) Perceived milk intolerance is related to bone mineral content in 10- to 13-year-old female adolescents. *Pediatrics* **120**, e669–77.

1161. Matthews, F.E. & Dening, T. (2002) Prevalence of dementia in institutional care. *Lancet* **360**, 225–6.

1162. Matz, K., Keresztes, K., Tatschl, C., *et al.* (2006) Disorders of glucose metabolism in acute stroke patients: an underrecognized problem. *Diabetes Care* **29**, 792–7.

1163. Maurer, M., Riesen, W., Muser, J., Hulter, H.N. & Krapf, R. (2003) Neutralization of Western diet inhibits bone resorption independently of K intake and reduces cortisol secretion in humans. *Am J Physiol Renal Physiol* **284**, F32–40.

1164. Maxwell, A.J. & Bruinsma, K.A. (2001) Uric acid is closely linked to vascular nitric oxide activity. Evidence for mechanism of association with cardiovascular disease. *J Am Coll Cardiol* **38**, 1850–58.

1165. Mayr, E. (2001) *What evolution is*. Weidenfeld & Nicolson, London.

1166. Mazess, R.B. (1966) Bone density in Sadlermiut Eskimo. *Hum Biol* **38**, 42–9.

1167. Mazess, R.B. & Mather, W. (1974) Bone mineral content of North Alaskan Eskimos. *Am J Clin Nutr* **27**, 916–25.

1168. Mazess, R.B. & Mather, W.E. (1975) Bone mineral content in Canadian Eskimos. *Hum Biol* **47**, 44–63.

1169. Maziak, W. (2009) Point-counterpoint. The triumph of the null hypothesis: epidemiology in an age of change. *Int J Epidemiol* **38**, 393–402.

1170. McCance, R., Edgecombe, C. & Widdowson, E. (1942) Mineral metabolism of dephytinized bread. *J Physiol* **101**.

1171. McCance, R. & Widdowsos, E. (1942) Mineral metabolism of healthy adults on white and brown bread dietaries. *J Physiol* **101**, 44–85.

1172. McCarty, C.A., Livingston, P.M. & Taylor, H.R. (1997) Prevalence of myopia in adults: implications for refractive surgeons. *J Refract Surg* **13**, 229–34.

1173. McClenaghan, N.H. (2005) Determining the relationship between dietary carbohydrate intake and insulin resistance. *Nutr Res Rev* **18**, 222–40.

1174. McCormack, J. & Greenhalgh, T. (2000) Seeing what you want to see in randomised controlled trials: versions and perversions of UKPDS data. United Kingdom prospective diabetes study. *BMJ* **320**, 1720–23.

1175. McCormick, D.B. (2006) The dubious use of vitamin-mineral supplements in relation to cardiovascular disease. *Am J Clin Nutr* **84**, 680–81.

1176. McCullagh, K.G. (1972) Arteriosclerosis in the African elephant. *Atherosclerosis* **16**, 307–35.

1177. McCullagh, K.G. (1972) Arteriosclerosis in the African elephant. I. Intimal atherosclerosis and its possible causes. *Atherosclerosis* **16**, 307–35.

1178. McCullough, M.L., Chevaux, K., Jackson, L., *et al.* (2006) Hypertension, the Kuna, and the epidemiology of flavanols. *J Cardiovasc Pharmacol* **47** (Suppl 2), S103–9; discussion 119–21.

1179. McDonald, P., Edwards, R.A., Greenhalgh, J.F.D. & Morgan, C.A. (1995) *Animal Nutrition*. Longman, Harlow.

1180. McGavock, J.M., Victor, R.G., Unger, R.H. & Szczepaniak, L.S. (2006) Adiposity of the heart, revisited. *Ann Intern Med* **144**, 517–24.

1181. McGill, H.C., Jr., McMahan, C.A., Herderick, E.E., *et al.* (2000) Effects of coronary heart disease risk factors on atherosclerosis of selected regions of the aorta and right coronary artery. PDAY Research Group. Pathobiological determinants of atherosclerosis in youth. *Arterioscler Thromb Vasc Biol* **20**, 836–45.

1182. McGill, H.C., Jr., McMahan, C.A., Herderick, E.E., *et al.* (2002) Obesity accelerates the progression of coronary atherosclerosis in young men. *Circulation* **105**, 2712–18.

1183. McGill, H.C., Jr., McMahan, C.A., Kruski, A.W. & Mott, G.E. (1981) Relationship of lipoprotein cholesterol concentrations to experimental atherosclerosis in baboons. *Arteriosclerosis* **1**, 3–12.

1184. McGill, H.C.J., Strong, J.P., Holman, R.L. & Werthessen, N.T. (1960) Arterial lesions in the Kenya baboon. *Circulation Res* **8**, 670–79.

1185. McGill, H.J. (1988) The cardiovascular pathology of smoking. *Am Heart J* **115**, 250–57.

1186. McKeigue, P.M., Pierpoint, T., Ferrie, J.E. & Marmot, M.G. (1992) Relationship of glucose intolerance and hyperinsulinaemia to body fat pattern in south Asians and Europeans. *Diabetologia* **35**, 785–91.

1187. McKelvie, R.S., Benedict, C.R. & Yusuf, S. (1999) Evidence based cardiology: prevention of congestive heart failure and management of asymptomatic left ventricular dysfunction. *BMJ* **318**, 1400–402.

1188. McKeown-Eyssen, G.E., Bright-See, E., Bruce, W.R., *et al.* (1994) A randomized trial of a low fat high fibre diet in the recurrence of colorectal polyps. Toronto Polyp Prevention Group. *J Clin Epidemiol* **47**, 525–36.

1189. McKinnell, R.G., Parchment, R.E., Perantoni, A.O. & Pierce, G.B. (1998) *The biological basis of cancer*. Cambridge University Press, Cambridge.

1190. McLachlan, C.N. (2001) Beta-casein A1, ischaemic heart disease mortality, and other illnesses. *Med Hypotheses* **56**, 262–72.

1191. McLean, R.M. (1994) Magnesium and its therapeutic uses: a review. *Am J Med* **96**, 63–76.

1192. McMillan-Price, J., Petocz, P., Atkinson, F., *et al.* (2006) Comparison of 4 diets of varying glycemic load on weight loss and cardiovascular risk reduction in overweight and obese young adults: a randomized controlled trial. *Arch Intern Med* **166**, 1466–75.

1193. McMurray, J.J. & Pfeffer, M.A. (2005) Heart failure. *Lancet* **365**, 1877–89.

1194. McNamara, D.J. (2000) Dietary cholesterol and atherosclerosis. *Biochim Biophys Acta* **1529**, 310–20.

1195. Mead, M. (1935) *Sex and temperament in three primitive societies*. William Morrow and Company, Inc, New York.

1196. Meisinger, C., Koenig, W., Baumert, J. & Doring, A. (2008) Uric acid levels are associated with all-cause and cardiovascular disease mortality independent of systemic inflammation in men from the general population: the MONICA/KORA cohort study. *Arterioscler Thromb Vasc Biol* **28**, 1186–92.

1197. Melamed, M.L., Michos, E.D., Post, W. & Astor, B. (2008) 25-hydroxyvitamin D levels and the risk of mortality in the general population. *Arch Intern Med* **168**, 1629–37.

1198. Melander, O., Groop, L. & Hulthen, U.L. (2000) Effect of salt on insulin sensitivity differs according to gender and degree of salt sensitivity. *Hypertension* **35**, 827–31.

1199. Melin, A.L., Wilske, J., Ringertz, H. & Saaf, M. (1999) Vitamin D status, parathyroid function and femoral bone density in an elderly Swedish population living at home. *Aging (Milano)* **11**, 200–207.

1200. Mellanby, E. (1950) *A story of nutrition research*. Williams & Wilkins Co, Baltimore.

1201. Mellen, P.B., Walsh, T.F. & Herrington, D.M. (2008) Whole grain intake and cardiovascular disease: a meta-analysis. *Nutr Metab Cardiovasc Dis* **18**, 283–90.

1202. Meloni, C., Morosetti, M., Suraci, C., *et al.* (2002) Severe dietary protein restriction in overt diabetic nephropathy: benefits or risks? *J Ren Nutr* **12**, 96–101.

1203. Meneely, G.R. & Dahl, L.K. (1961) Electrolytes in hypertension: the effects of sodium chloride. The evidence from animal and human studies. *Med Clin North Am* **45**, 271–83.

1204. Menotti, A., Blackburn, H., Kromhout, D., *et al.* (2001) Cardiovascular risk factors as determinants of 25-year all-cause mortality in the seven countries study. *Eur J Epidemiol* **17**, 337–46.

1205. Menotti, A., Blackburn, H., Kromhout, D., *et al.* (1997) The inverse relation of average population blood pressure and stroke mortality rates in the seven countries study: a paradox. *Eur J Epidemiol* **13**, 379–86.

1206. Menotti, A., Keys, A., Blackburn, H., *et al.* (1990) Twenty-year stroke mortality and prediction in twelve cohorts of the Seven Countries Study. *Int J Epidemiol* **19**, 309–15.

1207. Menotti, A., Kromhout, D., Blackburn, H., *et al.* (1999) Food intake patterns and 25-year mortality from coronary heart disease: cross-cultural correlations in the Seven Countries Study. The Seven Countries Study Research Group. *Eur J Epidemiol* **15**, 507–15.

1208. Mensink, R.P. (2006) Dairy products and the risk to develop type 2 diabetes or cardiovascular disease. *Internat Dairy J* **16**, 1001–4.

1209. Mensink, R.P. & Katan, M.B. (1992) Effect of dietary fatty acids on serum lipids and lipoproteins. A meta-analysis of 27 trials. *Arterioscler Thromb* **12**, 911–19.

1210. Mensink, R.P., Zock, P.L., Kester, A.D. & Katan, M.B. (2003) Effects of dietary fatty acids and carbohydrates on the ratio of serum total to HDL cholesterol and on serum lipids and apolipoproteins: a meta-analysis of 60 controlled trials. *Am J Clin Nutr* **77**, 1146–55.

1211. Mente, A., de Koning, L., Shannon, H.S. & Anand, S.S. (2009) A systematic review of the evidence supporting a causal link between dietary factors and coronary heart disease. *Arch Intern Med* **169**, 659–69.

1212. Merbs, C. (1989) Trauma. In: *Reconstruction of life from the skeleton* (M.H. Işcan & K.A.R. Kennedy eds). Wiley-Liss, New York, pp. 161–89.

1213. Merimee, T.J., Rimoin, D.L. & Cavalli, S.L. (1972) Metabolic studies in the African pygmy. *J Clin Invest* **51**, 395–401.

1214. Mertz, J.R. & Wallman, J. (2000) Choroidal retinoic acid synthesis: a possible mediator between refractive error and compensatory eye growth. *Exp Eye Res* **70**, 519–27.

1215. Messina, V. & Mangels, A.R. (2001) Considerations in planning vegan diets: children. *J Am Diet Assoc* **101**, 661–9.

1216. Metz, J.A., Karanja, N., Young, E.W., Morris, C.D. & McCarron, D.A. (1990) Bone mineral density in spontaneous hypertension: differential effects of dietary calcium and sodium. *Am J Med Sci* **300**, 225–30.

1217. Meyer, C., Mueller, M.F., Duncker, G.I. & Meyer, H.J. (1999) Experimental animal myopia models are applicable to human juvenile-onset myopia. *Surv Ophthalmol* **44** (Suppl 1), S93–102.

1218. Meyerhardt, J.A., Niedzwiecki, D., Hollis, D., *et al.* (2007) Association of dietary patterns with cancer recurrence and survival in patients with stage III colon cancer. *JAMA* **298**, 754–64.

1219. Meyers, W.M. & Neafie, R.C. (1991) Tropical phagedenic ulcer. In: *Tropical medicine* (G.T. Strickland ed). W. B. Saunders, Philadelphia, pp. 310–11.

1220. Miall, W.E., Del, C.E., Fodor, J., *et al.* (1972) Longitudinal study of heart disease in a Jamaican rural population. I. Prevalence, with special reference to ECG findings. *Bull World Health Organ* **46**, 429–41.

1221. Michell, A.R. (1989) Physiological aspects of the requirement for sodium in mammals. *Nutr Res Rev* 2, 149–60.

1222. Michels, K.B., Fuchs, C.S., Giovannucci, E., *et al.* (2005) Fiber intake and incidence of colorectal cancer among 76,947 women and 47,279 men. *Cancer Epidemiol Biomarkers Prev* **14**, 842–9.

1223. Miida, T., Takahashi, A. & Ikeuchi, T. (2007) Prevention of stroke and dementia by statin therapy: experimental and clinical evidence of their pleiotropic effects. *Pharmacol Ther* **113**, 378–93.

1224. Mikkelsen, K.L., Heitmann, B.L., Keiding, N. & Sorensen, T.I. (1999) Independent effects of stable and changing body weight on total mortality. *Epidemiology* **10**, 671–8.

1225. Milan, A., Mulatero, P., Rabbia, F. & Veglio, F. (2002) Salt intake and hypertension therapy. *J Nephrol* **15**, 1–6.

1226. Milton, K. (1999) Nutritional characteristics of wild primate foods: do the diets of our closest living relatives have lessons for us? *Nutrition* **15**, 488–98.

1227. Milton, K. (2000) Hunter-gatherer diets-a different perspective. *Am J Clin Nutr* **71**, 665–7.

1228. Minnis, P.E. (1985) *Social adaptations to food stress.* University of Chicago Press, Chicago.

1229. Mittra, S., Bansal, V.S. & Bhatnagar, P.K. (2008) From a glucocentric to a lipocentric approach towards metabolic syndrome. *Drug Discov Today* **13**, 211–18.

1230. Mizushima, S. & Yamori, Y. (1992) Nutritional improvement, cardiovascular diseases and longevity in Japan. *Nutr Health* **8**, 97–105.

1231. Mola, G. & McGoldrick, I. (1982) Epidemiology of gynaecological and female breast neoplasms in Papua New Guinea. *P N G Med J* **25**, 143–50.

1232. Moncada, S., Martin, J.F. & Higgs, A. (1993) Symposium on regression of atherosclerosis. *Eur J Clin Invest* **23**, 385–98.

1233. Monetini, L., Cavallo, M.G., Manfrini, S., *et al.* (2002) Antibodies to bovine beta-casein in diabetes and other autoimmune diseases. *Horm Metab Res* **34**, 455–9.

1234. Montague, S. (1974) *The Trobriand society.* Ph.D., University of Chicago.

1235. Monteiro, I. & Vaz Almeid, M.D. (2007) [Dietary fat and ischemic stroke risk in Northern Portugal]. *Acta Med Port* **20**, 307–18.

1236. Moore, H., Summerbell, C., Hooper, L., *et al.* (2004) Dietary advice for treatment of type 2 diabetes mellitus in adults. *Cochrane Database Syst Rev*, CD004097.

1237. Moorman, P.G. & Terry, P.D. (2004) Consumption of dairy products and the risk of breast cancer: a review of the literature. *Am J Clin Nutr* **80**, 5–14.

1238. Mordes, J.P. & Rossini, A.A. (1981) Animal models of diabetes. *Am J Med* **70**, 353–60.

1239. Morell, M. (1989) *Studier i den svenska livsmedelskonsumtionens historia. Hospitalhjonens livsmedelskonsumtion 1621–1872.* Almqvist & Wiksell, Uppsala.

1240. Morgan, E. (1997) The aquatic ape hypothesis *(Independent Voices Series).* Souvenir Press, London.

1241. Morgan, T., Aubert, J.F. & Brunner, H. (2001) Interaction between sodium intake, angiotensin II, and blood pressure as a cause of cardiac hypertrophy. *Am J Hypertens* **14**, 914–20.

1242. Morimoto, A., Uzu, T., Fujii, T., *et al.* (1997) Sodium sensitivity and cardiovascular events in patients with essential hypertension. *Lancet* **350**, 1734–7.

1243. Morris, E.R. (1986) Phytate and dietary mineral bioavailability. In: *Phytic acid: Chemistry and applications*, Vol. **4** (E. Graf ed). Pilatus Press, Minneapolis, pp. 57–76.

1244. Morris, M.C., Evans, D.A., Bienias, J.L., *et al.* (2003) Dietary fats and the risk of incident Alzheimer disease. *Arch Neurol* **60**, 194–200.

1245. Morris, M.C., Evans, D.A., Tangney, C.C., Bienias, J.L. & Wilson, R.S. (2005) Fish consumption and cognitive decline with age in a large community study. *Arch Neurol* **62**, 1849–53.

1246. Morris, R.C., Jr., Sebastian, A., Forman, A., Tanaka, M. & Schmidlin, O. (1999) Normotensive salt sensitivity: effects of race and dietary potassium. *Hypertension* **33**, 18–23.

1247. Moseson, M., Koenig, K.L., Shore, R.E. & Pasternack, B.S. (1993) The influence of medical conditions associated with hormones on the risk of breast cancer. *Int J Epidemiol* **22**, 1000–1009.

1248. Moss, M. & Freed, D. (2003) The cow and the coronary: epidemiology, biochemistry and immunology. *Int J Cardiol* **87**, 203–16.

1249. Moss, M. & Freed, D.L.J. (1999) Survival trends, coronary event rates, and the MONICA project. *Lancet* **354**, 862.

1250. Motard-Belanger, A., Charest, A., Grenier, G., *et al.* (2008) Study of the effect of trans fatty acids from ruminants on blood lipids and other risk factors for cardiovascular disease. *Am J Clin Nutr* **87**, 593–9.

1251. Mozaffarian, D., Katan, M.B., Ascherio, A., Stampfer, M.J. & Willett, W.C. (2006) Trans fatty acids and cardiovascular disease. *N Engl J Med* **354**, 1601–13.

1252. Mozaffarian, D. & Rimm, E.B. (2006) Fish intake, contaminants, and human health: evaluating the risks and the benefits. *JAMA* **296**, 1885–99.

1253. Mozaffarian, D., Rimm, E.B. & Herrington, D.M. (2004) Dietary fats, carbohydrate, and progression of coronary atherosclerosis in postmenopausal women. *Am J Clin Nutr* **80**, 1175–84.

1254. Mukamal, K.J., Maclure, M., Muller, J.E., Sherwood, J.B. & Mittleman, M.A. (2002) Tea consumption and mortality after acute myocardial infarction. *Circulation* **105**, 2476–81.

1255. Mukamal, K.J., Robbins, J.A., Cauley, J.A., Kern, L.M. & Siscovick, D.S. (2007) Alcohol consumption, bone density, and hip fracture among older adults: the cardiovascular health study. *Osteoporos Int* **18**, 593–602.

1256. Muna, W.F. (1993) Cardiovascular disorders in Africa. *World Health Stat Q* **46**, 125–33.

1257. Munger, R.G., Cerhan, J.R. & Chiu, B.C. (1999) Prospective study of dietary protein intake and risk of hip fracture in postmenopausal women [see comments]. *Am J Clin Nutr* **69**, 147–52.

1258. Muntoni, S., Cocco, P., Aru, G. & Cucca, F. (2000) Nutritional factors and worldwide incidence of childhood type 1 diabetes. *Am J Clin Nutr* **71**, 1525–9.

1259. Murakami, S., Kondo, Y., Sakurai, T., Kitajima, H. & Nagate, T. (2002) Taurine suppresses development of atherosclerosis in Watanabe heritable hyperlipidemic (WHHL) rabbits. *Atherosclerosis* **163**, 79–87.

1260. Muscari, A., Volta, U., Bonazzi, C., *et al.* (1989) Association of serum IgA antibodies to milk antigens with severe atherosclerosis. *Atherosclerosis* **77**, 251–6.

1261. Mutti, D.O., Zadnik, K. & Adams, A.J. (1996) Myopia. The nature versus nurture debate goes on. *Invest Ophthalmol Vis Sci* **37**, 952–7.

1262. Mutti, D.O., Zadnik, K. & Murphy, C.J. (1999) Naturally occurring vitreous chamber-based myopia in the Labrador retriever. *Invest Ophthalmol Vis Sci* **40**, 1577–84.

1263. Muwazi, E. (1944) Neurological disease among African natives of Uganda: a review of 269 cases. *East Afr Med J* **21**, 2–19.

1264. Nachbar, M.S. & Oppenheim, J.D. (1980) Lectins in the United States diet: a survey of lectins in commonly consumed foods and a review of the literature. *Am J Clin Nutr* **33**, 2338–45.

1265. Nadim, A., Amini, H. & Malek-Afzali, H. (1978) Blood pressure and rural–urban migration in Iran. *Int J Epidemiol* 7, 131–8.

1266. Nagaev, I. & Smith, U. (2001) Insulin resistance and type 2 diabetes are not related to resistin expression in human fat cells or skeletal muscle. *Biochem Biophys Res Commun* 285, 561–4.

1267. Nagar, Y. & Hershkovitz, I. (2004) Interrelationship between various aging methods, and their relevance to palaeodemography. *Human Evol* 19, 145–56.

1268. Nagurney, J.T. (1975) Neurological admissions to Goroka Base Hospital – an eight month survey. *P N G Med J* 18, 220–26.

1269. Nair, U.J., Friesen, M., Richard, I., *et al.* (1990) Effect of lime composition on the formation of reactive oxygen species from areca nut extract in vitro. *Carcinogenesis* 11, 2145–8.

1270. Nam, S.Y., Lee, E.J., Kim, K.R., *et al.* (1997) Effect of obesity on total and free insulin-like growth factor (IGF)-1, and their relationship to IGF-binding protein (BP)-1, IGFBP-2, IGFBP-3, insulin, and growth hormone. *Int J Obes Relat Metab Disord* 21, 355–9.

1271. Nan, L., Tuomilehto, J., Dowse, G., Virtala, E. & Zimmet, P. (1994) Prevalence of coronary heart disease indicated by electrocardiogram abnormalities and risk factors in developing countries. *J Clin Epidemiol* 47, 599–611.

1272. Nandhini, A.T., Thirunavukkarasu, V. & Anuradha, C.V. (2005) Taurine modifies insulin signaling enzymes in the fructose-fed insulin resistant rats. *Diabetes Metab* 31, 337–44.

1273. Narita, T., Koshimura, J., Meguro, H., *et al.* (2001) Determination of optimal protein contents for a protein restriction diet in type 2 diabetic patients with microalbuminuria. *Tohoku J Exp Med* 193, 45–55.

1274. Nathan, D.M., Buse, J.B., Davidson, M.B., *et al.* (2009) Medical management of hyperglycaemia in type 2 diabetes mellitus: a consensus algorithm for the initiation and adjustment of therapy: a consensus statement from the American Diabetes Association and the European Association for the Study of Diabetes. *Diabetologia* 52, 17–30.

1275. National Food Administration. (1986) *Food composition tables*. National Food Administration, Uppsala, Sweden.

1276. Natter, S., Granditsch, G., Reichel, G.L., *et al.* (2001) IgA cross-reactivity between a nuclear autoantigen and wheat proteins suggests molecular mimicry as a possible pathomechanism in celiac disease. *Eur J Immunol* 31, 918–28.

1277. Naughton, J.M., O'Dea, K. & Sinclair, A.J. (1986) Animal foods in traditional Australian aboriginal diets: polyunsaturated and low in fat. *Lipids* 21, 684–90.

1278. Navert, B., Sandstrom, B. & Cederblad, A. (1985) Reduction of the phytate content of bran by leavening in bread and its effect on zinc absorption in man. *Br J Nutr* 53, 47–53.

1279. Neel, J.V. (1962) Diabetes mellitus: a thrifty genotype rendered detrimental by 'progress'? *Am J Hum Genet* 14, 353–62.

1280. Neel, J.V. (1992) The thrifty genotype revisited. In: *The genetics of diabetes mellitus* (J. Kobberlong & R. Tattersall eds). Academic Press, London, pp. 283–93.

1281. Negri, E., La Vecchia, C., Pelucchi, C., Bertuzzi, M. & Tavani, A. (2003) Fiber intake and risk of nonfatal acute myocardial infarction. *Eur J Clin Nutr* 57, 464–70.

1282. Nelson, H. & Jurmain, R. (1991) *Introduction to physical anthropology*. West Publishing Co, New York.

1283. Nelson, S.M. & Fleming, R.F. (2007) The preconceptual contraception paradigm: obesity and infertility. *Hum Reprod* 22, 912–15.

1284. Ness, A., Egger, M. & Powles, J. (1999) Fruit and vegetables and ischaemic heart disease: systematic review or misleading meta-analysis? *Eur J Clin Nutr* 53, 900–904.

1285. Ness, A.R., Hughes, J., Elwood, P.C., *et al.* (2002) The long-term effect of dietary advice in men with coronary disease: follow-up of the Diet and Reinfarction trial (DART). *Eur J Clin Nutr* 56, 512–18.

1286. Nesse, R.M. & Williams, G.C. (1995) *Why we get sick. The new science of Darwinian medicine*. Times Books, New York.

1287. Neubauer, S. (2007) The failing heart– an engine out of fuel. *N Engl J Med* **356**, 1140–51.
1288. Neves, W.A., Barros, A.M. & Costa, M.A. (1999) Incidence and distribution of postcranial fractures in the prehistoric population of San Pedro de Atacama, Northern Chile. *Am J Phys Anthropol* **109**, 253–8.
1289. New, J., Cosmides, L. & Tooby, J. (2007) Category-specific attention for animals reflects ancestral priorities, not expertise. *Proc Natl Acad Sci USA* **104**, 16598–603.
1290. New, S.A. (2004) Do vegetarians have a normal bone mass? *Osteoporos Int* **15**, 679–88.
1291. New, S.A., Bolton-Smith, C., Grubb, D.A. & Reid, D.M. (1997) Nutritional influences on bone mineral density: a cross-sectional study in premenopausal women. *Am J Clin Nutr* **65**, 1831–9.
1292. New, S.A., MacDonald, H.M., Campbell, M.K., *et al.* (2004) Lower estimates of net endogenous non-carbonic acid production are positively associated with indexes of bone health in premenopausal and perimenopausal women. *Am J Clin Nutr* **79**, 131–8.
1293. Newbold, H.L. (1988) Reducing the serum cholesterol level with a diet high in animal fat. *South Med J* **81**, 61–3.
1294. Newton, J.L., Jones, D.E., Henderson, E., *et al.* (2008) Fatigue in non-alcoholic fatty liver disease (NAFLD) is significant and associates with inactivity and excessive daytime sleepiness but not with liver disease severity or insulin resistance. *Gut* **57**, 807–13.
1295. Nguyen, N.D., Frost, S.A., Center, J.R., Eisman, J.A. & Nguyen, T.V. (2007) Development of a nomogram for individualizing hip fracture risk in men and women. *Osteoporos Int* **18**, 1109–17.
1296. Nguyen, T.V., Sambrook, P.N. & Eisman, J.A. (1998) Bone loss, physical activity, and weight change in elderly women: the Dubbo Osteoporosis Epidemiology Study. *J Bone Miner Res* **13**, 1458–67.
1297. Nichols, G.A., Hillier, T.A., Erbey, J.R. & Brown, J.B. (2001) Congestive heart failure in type 2 diabetes: prevalence, incidence, and risk factors. *Diabetes Care* **24**, 1614–19.
1298. Nicklas, B.J., Cesari, M., Penninx, B.W., *et al.* (2006) Abdominal obesity is an independent risk factor for chronic heart failure in older people. *J Am Geriatr Soc* **54**, 413–20.
1299. Nicolosi, R.J., Wilson, T.A., Handelman, G., *et al.* (2002) Decreased aortic early atherosclerosis in hypercholesterolemic hamsters fed oleic acid-rich TriSun oil compared to linoleic acid-rich sunflower oil. *J Nutr Biochem* **13**, 392–402.
1300. Nicolosi, R.J., Wilson, T.A., Rogers, E.J. & Kritchevsky, D. (1998) Effects of specific fatty acids (8:0, 14:0, cis-18:1, trans-18:1) on plasma lipoproteins, early atherogenic potential, and LDL oxidative properties in the hamster. *J Lipid Res* **39**, 1972–80.
1301. Niederau, C., Strohmeyer, G. & Stremmel, W. (1994) Epidemiology, clinical spectrum and prognosis of hemochromatosis. *Adv Exp Med Biol* **356**, 293–302.
1302. Nield, L., Moore, H., Hooper, L., *et al.* (2007) Dietary advice for treatment of type 2 diabetes mellitus in adults. *Cochrane Database Syst Rev*, CD004097.
1303. Nield, L., Summerbell, C.D., Hooper, L., Whittaker, V. & Moore, H. (2008) Dietary advice for the prevention of type 2 diabetes mellitus in adults. *Cochrane Database Syst Rev*, CD005102.
1304. Nieminen, P., Mustonen, A.M., Lindstrom-Seppa, P., *et al.* (2002) Phytosterols act as endocrine and metabolic disruptors in the European polecat (Mustela putorius). *Toxicol Appl Pharmacol* **178**, 22–8.
1305. Nieschulz, O. (1967) [On the pharmacology of the active substances of betel. 1. Central effect of arecoline]. *Arzneimittelforschung* **17**, 1292–7.
1306. Nikkilä, M., Koivula, T., Niemelä, K. & Sisto, T. (1990) High density lipoprotein cholesterol and triglycerides as markers of angiographically assessed coronary artery disease. *Br Heart J* **63**, 78–81.
1307. Nilsson, M., Stenberg, M., Frid, A.H., Holst, J.J. & Bjorck, I.M. (2004) Glycemia and insulinemia in healthy subjects after lactose-equivalent meals of milk and other food proteins: the role of plasma amino acids and incretins. *Am J Clin Nutr* **80**, 1246–53.

1308. Nilsson, P.M., Nilsson, J.A., Hedblad, B., Berglund, G. & Lindgärde, F. (2002) The enigma of increased non-cancer mortality after weight loss in healthy men who are overweight or obese. *J Intern Med* **252**, 70–8.

1309. Nishikawa, A., Prokopczyk, B., Rivenson, A., Zang, E. & Hoffmann, D. (1992) A study of betel quid carcinogenesis—VIII. Carcinogenicity of 3-(methylnitrosamino)propionaldehyde in F344 rats. *Carcinogenesis* **13**, 369–72.

1310. Nishikimi, M., Fukuyama, R., Minoshima, S., Shimizu, N. & Yagi, K. (1994) Cloning and chromosomal mapping of the human nonfunctional gene for L-gulono-gamma-lactone oxidase, the enzyme for L-ascorbic acid biosynthesis missing in man. *J Biol Chem* **269**, 13685–8.

1311. Nissen, S.E. & Yock, P. (2001) Intravascular ultrasound: novel pathophysiological insights and current clinical applications. *Circulation* **103**, 604–16.

1312. Noakes, M., Foster, P.R., Keogh, J.B., *et al.* (2006) Comparison of isocaloric very low carbohydrate/high saturated fat and high carbohydrate/low saturated fat diets on body composition and cardiovascular risk. *Nutr Metab (Lond)* **3**, 7.

1313. Noble, M.I., Drake-Holland, A.J. & Vink, H. (2008) Hypothesis: arterial glycocalyx dysfunction is the first step in the atherothrombotic process. *QJM* **101**, 513–18.

1314. Nomura, A.M., Hankin, J.H., Henderson, B.E., *et al.* (2007) Dietary fiber and colorectal cancer risk: the multiethnic cohort study. *Cancer Causes Control* **18**, 753–64.

1315. Norat, T., Bingham, S., Ferrari, P., *et al.* (2005) Meat, fish, and colorectal cancer risk: the European Prospective Investigation into cancer and nutrition. *J Natl Cancer Inst* **97**, 906–16.

1316. Norat, T., Dossus, L., Rinaldi, S., *et al.* (2007) Diet, serum insulin-like growth factor-I and IGF-binding protein-3 in European women. *Eur J Clin Nutr* **61**, 91–8.

1317. Nordestgaard, B.G., Benn, M., Schnohr, P. & Tybjaerg-Hansen, A. (2007) Nonfasting triglycerides and risk of myocardial infarction, ischemic heart disease, and death in men and women. *JAMA* **298**, 299–308.

1318. Nordin, B.C. (2000) Calcium requirement is a sliding scale. *Am J Clin Nutr* **71**, 1381–3.

1319. Nordin, B.E. (1997) Calcium and osteoporosis. *Nutrition* **13**, 664–86.

1320. Nordin, B.E., Prince, R.L. & Tucker, G.R. (2008) Bone density and fracture risk. *Med J Aust* **189**, 7–8.

1321. Nordmann, A.J., Nordmann, A., Briel, M., *et al.* (2006) Effects of low-carbohydrate vs low-fat diets on weight loss and cardiovascular risk factors: a meta-analysis of randomized controlled trials. *Arch Intern Med* **166**, 285–93.

1322. Norhammar, A., Tenerz, A., Nilsson, G., *et al.* (2002) Glucose metabolism in patients with acute myocardial infarction and no previous diagnosis of diabetes mellitus: a prospective study. *Lancet* **359**, 2140–44.

1323. Normen, L., Dutta, P., Lia, A. & Andersson, H. (2000) Soy sterol esters and beta-sitostanol ester as inhibitors of cholesterol absorption in human small bowel. *Am J Clin Nutr* **71**, 908–13.

1324. Normen, L., Johnsson, M., Andersson, H., van Gameren, Y. & Dutta, P. (1999) Plant sterols in vegetables and fruits commonly consumed in Sweden. *Eur J Nutr* **38**, 84–9.

1325. Norton, T.T. & Siegwart, J.T., Jr. (1995) Animal models of emmetropization: matching axial length to the focal plane. *J Am Optom Assoc* **66**, 405–14.

1326. Norvenius, S.G. (1997) [Rachitis, English disease, punishment or curse? An old disease of new interest in Sweden]. *Läkartidningen* **94**, 122–5.

1327. Ntanios, F.Y., Jones, P.J. & Frohlich, J.J. (1998) Dietary sitostanol reduces plaque formation but not lecithin cholesterol acyl transferase activity in rabbits [In Process Citation]. *Atherosclerosis* **138**, 101–10.

1328. Nuttall, F.Q., Schweim, K., Hoover, H. & Gannon, M.C. (2006) Metabolic effect of a LoBAG30 diet in men with type 2 diabetes. *Am J Physiol Endocrinol Metab* **291**, E786–91.

1329. Nyakundi, P.M., Kinuthia, D.W. & Orinda, D.A. (1994) Clinical aspects and causes of rickets in a Kenyan population. *East Afr Med J* **71**, 536–42.

1330. O'Connell, J.F., Latz, P.K. & Barnett, P. (1983) Traditional and modern plant use among the Alyawara of central Australia. *Economic Botany* 37, 80–109.

1331. O'Dea, K. (1984) Marked improvement in carbohydrate and lipid metabolism in diabetic Australian aborigines after temporary reversion to traditional lifestyle. *Diabetes* 33, 596–603.

1332. O'Dea, K. (1992) Diabetes in Australian Aborigines: impact of the Western diet and life style. *J Intern Med* 232, 103–117.

1333. O'Dea, K. (1997) Clinical implications of the 'thrifty genotype' hypothesis: Where do we stand now? *Nutr Metab Cardiovasc Dis* 7, 281–4.

1334. O'Dea, K., Patel, M., Kubisch, D., Hopper, J. & Traianedes, K. (1993) Obesity, diabetes, and hyperlipidemia in a central Australian aboriginal community with a long history of acculturation. *Diabetes Care* 16, 1004–10.

1335. O'Dea, K., Sinclair, A.J., Niall, M. & Traianedes, K. (1986) Lean meat as part of a cholesterol-lowering diet. *Prog Lipid Res* 25, 219–20.

1336. O'Farrelly, C., Price, R., McGillivray, A.J. & Fernandes, L. (1989) IgA rheumatoid factor and IgG dietary protein antibodies are associated in rheumatoid arthritis. *Immunol Invest* 18, 753–64.

1337. O'Riordan, J.L. (2006) Rickets in the 17th century. *J Bone Miner Res* 21, 1506–10.

1338. O'Shaughnessy, K.M. & Karet, F.E. (2006) Salt handling and hypertension. *Annu Rev Nutr* 26, 343–65.

1339. Obarzanek, E., Proschan, M.A., Vollmer, W.M., *et al.* (2003) Individual blood pressure responses to changes in salt intake: results from the DASH-Sodium trial. *Hypertension* 42, 459–67.

1340. Odeleye, O.E., de Courten, M., Pettitt, D.J. & Ravussin, E. (1997) Fasting hyperinsulinemia is a predictor of increased body weight gain and obesity in Pima Indian children. *Diabetes* 46, 1341–5.

1341. Oh, K., Hu, F.B., Cho, E., *et al.* (2005) Carbohydrate intake, glycemic index, glycemic load, and dietary fiber in relation to risk of stroke in women. *Am J Epidemiol* 161, 161–9.

1342. Ohmori, T., Yatomi, Y., Wu, Y., *et al.* (2001) Wheat germ agglutinin-induced platelet activation via platelet endothelial cell adhesion molecule-1: involvement of rapid phospholipase C gamma 2 activation by Src family kinases. *Biochemistry* 40, 12992–3001.

1343. Ohtsubo, K., Takamatsu, S., Minowa, M.T., *et al.* (2005) Dietary and genetic control of glucose transporter 2 glycosylation promotes insulin secretion in suppressing diabetes. *Cell* 123, 1307–21.

1344. Ojaimi, E., Morgan, I.G., Robaei, D., *et al.* (2005) Effect of stature and other anthropometric parameters on eye size and refraction in a population-based study of Australian children. *Invest Ophthalmol Vis Sci* 46, 4424–9.

1345. Okamoto, M.M., Sumida, D.H., Carvalho, C.R., *et al.* (2004) Changes in dietary sodium consumption modulate GLUT4 gene expression and early steps of insulin signaling. *Am J Physiol Regul Integr Comp Physiol* 286, R779–85.

1346. Oki, I., Nakamura, Y., Okamura, T., *et al.* (2006) Body mass index and risk of stroke mortality among a random sample of Japanese adults: 19-year follow-up of NIPPON DATA80. *Cerebrovasc Dis* 22, 409–15.

1347. Okuwobi, B. & Strasser, T. (1972) Heart disease in Nigeria. *World Health*, 24–25.

1348. Oliveira, J.T.A., Pusztai, A. & Grant, G. (1988) Changes in organs and tissues induced by feeding of purified kidney bean (Phaseolus vulgaris) lectins. *Nutr Res* 8, 943–7.

1349. Oliver, M.F. (1989) Cigarette smoking, polyunsaturated fats, linoleic acid, and coronary heart disease [published erratum appears in *Lancet* 1989 Jun 24;1 (8652):1464]. *Lancet* i, 1241–3.

1350. Oliver, W.J., Cohen, E.L. & Neel, J.V. (1975) Blood pressure, sodium intake, and sodium related hormones in the Yanomamo Indians, a 'no-salt' culture. *Circulation* 52, 146–51.

1351. Olsen, S. (1985) *Origins of the domestic dog.* University of Arizona Press, Tucson.

1352. Olson, C.M., Rennie, D., Cook, D., *et al.* (2002) Publication bias in editorial decision making. *JAMA* **287**, 2825–8.

1353. Olsson, K.S. (1997) [Genetic screening discovers hemochromatosis. Organ damage caused by iron may be prevented]. *Läkartidningen* **94**, 3957–8.

1354. Olsson, U., Ostergren-Lunden, G. & Moses, J. (2001) Glycosaminoglycan-lipoprotein interaction. *Glycoconj J* **18**, 789–97.

1355. Omi, N., Aoi, S., Murata, K. & Ezawa, I. (1994) Evaluation of the effect of soybean milk and soybean milk peptide on bone metabolism in the rat model with ovariectomized osteoporosis. *J Nutr Sci Vitaminol (Tokyo)* **40**, 201–11.

1356. Onland-Moret, N.C., Peeters, P.H., van Gils, C.H., *et al.* (2005) Age at menarche in relation to adult height: the EPIC study. *Am J Epidemiol* **162**, 623–32.

1357. Oomen, C.M., Ocke, M.C., Feskens, E.J., *et al.* (2001) Association between trans fatty acid intake and 10-year risk of coronary heart disease in the Zutphen Elderly Study: a prospective population-based study. *Lancet* **357**, 746–51.

1358. Orban, T., Landaker, E., Ruan, Z., *et al.* (2001) High-fructose diet preserves beta-cell mass and prevents diabetes in nonobese diabetic mice: a potential role for increased insulin receptor substrate-2 expression. *Metabolism* **50**, 1369–76.

1359. Ornish, D., Brown, S.E., Scherwitz, L.W., *et al.* (1990) Can lifestyle changes reverse coronary heart disease? The Lifestyle Heart Trial [see comments]. *Lancet* **336**, 129–33.

1360. Ornish, D., Scherwitz, L.W., Billings, J.H., *et al.* (1998) Intensive lifestyle changes for reversal of coronary heart disease. *JAMA* **280**, 2001–7.

1361. Osanai, T. & Okumura, K. (2007) Therapeutic challenge to adiposity of the heart. *Circ Res* **100**, 1106–8.

1362. Ostman, E., Granfeldt, Y., Persson, L. & Bjorck, I. (2005) Vinegar supplementation lowers glucose and insulin responses and increases satiety after a bread meal in healthy subjects. *Eur J Clin Nutr* **59**, 983–8.

1363. Ostman, E.M., Liljeberg Elmstahl, H.G. & Bjorck, I.M. (2002) Barley bread containing lactic acid improves glucose tolerance at a subsequent meal in healthy men and women. *J Nutr* **132**, 1173–5.

1364. Östman, E.M., Liljeberg Elmstahl, H.G. & Bjorck, I.M. (2001) Inconsistency between glycemic and insulinemic responses to regular and fermented milk products. *Am J Clin Nutr* **74**, 96–100.

1365. Ouellet, V., Marois, J., Weisnagel, S.J. & Jacques, H. (2007) Dietary cod protein improves insulin sensitivity in insulin-resistant men and women: a randomized controlled trial. *Diabetes Care* **30**, 2816–21.

1366. Owen, O.E., Smalley, K.J., D'Alessio, D.A., Mozzoli, M.A. & Dawson, E.K. (1998) Protein, fat, and carbohydrate requirements during starvation: anaplerosis and cataplerosis]. *Am J Clin Nutr* **68**, 12–34.

1367. Ozanne, S.E. & Hales, C.N. (1999) The long-term consequences of intra-uterine protein malnutrition for glucose metabolism. *Proc Nutr Soc* **58**, 615–9.

1368. Ozkahya, M., Ok, E., Cirit, M., *et al.* (1998) Regression of left ventricular hypertrophy in haemodialysis patients by ultrafiltration and reduced salt intake without antihypertensive drugs. *Nephrol Dial Transplant* **13**, 1489–93.

1369. Page, L.B., Damon, A. & Moellering, R.J. (1974) Antecedents of cardiovascular disease in six Solomon Islands societies. *Circulation* **49**, 1132–46.

1370. Pak, C.Y., Peterson, R.D. & Poindexter, J. (2002) Prevention of spinal bone loss by potassium citrate in cases of calcium urolithiasis. *J Urol* **168**, 31–4.

1371. Palacios, C. (2006) The role of nutrients in bone health, from A to Z. *Crit Rev Food Sci Nutr* **46**, 621–8.

1372. Palinski, W. & Napoli, C. (1999) Pathophysiological events during pregnancy influence the development of atherosclerosis in humans. *Trends Cardiovasc Med* **9**, 205–14.

1373. Palmer, K., Wang, H.X., Backman, L., Winblad, B. & Fratiglioni, L. (2002) Differential evolution of cognitive impairment in nondemented older persons: results from the Kungsholmen Project. *Am J Psychiatry* **159**, 436–42.

1374. Palmer, P. (1982) Autopsies at Goroka hospital from 1978–1982: a review. *P N G Med J* **25**, 166–7.

1375. Palmquist, D.L., Doppenberg, J., Roehrig, K.L. & Kinsey, D.J. (1992) Glucose and insulin metabolism in ruminating and veal calves fed high and low fat diets. *Domest Anim Endocrinol* **9**, 233–41.

1376. Panagiotakos, D.B., Pitsavos, C., Chrysohoou, C. & Stefanadis, C. (2005) The epidemiology of type 2 diabetes mellitus in Greek adults: the ATTICA study. *Diabet Med* **22**, 1581–8.

1377. Panter-Brick, C., Layton, R.H. & Rowley-Conwy, P. (2001) *Hunter-gatherers: an interdisciplinary perspective*. Cambridge University Press, Cambridge.

1378. Paolisso, G., De Riu, S., Marrazzo, G., *et al.* (1991) Insulin resistance and hyperinsulinemia in patients with chronic congestive heart failure. *Metabolism* **40**, 972–7.

1379. Paradies, Y.C., Montoya, M.J. & Fullerton, S.M. (2007) Racialized genetics and the study of complex diseases: the thrifty genotype revisited. *Perspect Biol Med* **50**, 203–27.

1380. Parhami, F. (2003) Possible role of oxidized lipids in osteoporosis: could hyperlipidemia be a risk factor? *Prostaglandins Leukot Essent Fatty Acids* **68**, 373–8.

1381. Parhami, F., Tintut, Y., Ballard, A., Fogelman, A.M. & Demer, L.L. (2001) Leptin enhances the calcification of vascular cells: artery wall as a target of leptin. *Circ Res* **88**, 954–60.

1382. Parhami, F., Tintut, Y., Beamer, W.G., *et al.* (2001) Atherogenic high-fat diet reduces bone mineralization in mice. *J Bone Miner Res* **16**, 182–8.

1383. Parillo, M., Giacco, R., Ciardullo, A.V., Rivellese, A.A. & Riccardi, G. (1996) Does a high-carbohydrate diet have different effects in NIDDM patients treated with diet alone or hypoglycemic drugs? *Diabetes Care* **19**, 498–500.

1384. Park, H.A., Lee, J.S., Kuller, L.H. & Cauley, J.A. (2007) Effects of weight control during the menopausal transition on bone mineral density. *J Clin Endocrinol Metab* **92**, 3809–15.

1385. Park, R.G. (1968) The age distribution of common skin disorders in the Bantu of Pretoria, Transvaal. *Br J Dermatol* **80**, 758–61.

1386. Park, S.Y., Cho, Y.R., Kim, H.J., *et al.* (2005) Unraveling the temporal pattern of diet-induced insulin resistance in individual organs and cardiac dysfunction in C57BL/6 mice. *Diabetes* **54**, 3530–40.

1387. Park, S.Y., Murphy, S.P., Wilkens, L.R., *et al.* (2007) Calcium, vitamin D, and dairy product intake and prostate cancer risk: the Multiethnic Cohort Study. *Am J Epidemiol* **166**, 1259–69.

1388. Park, Y., Hunter, D.J., Spiegelman, D., *et al.* (2005) Dietary fiber intake and risk of colorectal cancer: a pooled analysis of prospective cohort studies. *JAMA* **294**, 2849–57.

1389. Park, Y., Mitrou, P.N., Kipnis, V., *et al.* (2007) Calcium, dairy foods, and risk of incident and fatal prostate cancer: the NIH-AARP Diet and Health Study. *Am J Epidemiol* **166**, 1270–79.

1390. Park, Y.K. & Yetley, E.A. (1993) Intakes and food sources of fructose in the United States. *Am J Clin Nutr* **58**, 737S–47S.

1391. Parkin, D.M. (2001) Global cancer statistics in the year 2000. *Lancet Oncol* **2**, 533–43.

1392. Parkin, D.M., Bray, F., Ferlay, J. & Pisani, P. (2005) Global cancer statistics, 2002. *CA Cancer J Clin* **55**, 74–108.

1393. Pasquali, R. (2006) Obesity, fat distribution and infertility. *Maturitas* **54**, 363–71.

1394. Patel, A., MacMahon, S., Chalmers, J., *et al.* (2008) Intensive blood glucose control and vascular outcomes in patients with type 2 diabetes. *N Engl J Med* **358**, 2560–72.

1395. Patel, B., Schutte, R., Sporns, P., *et al.* (2002) Potato glycoalkaloids adversely affect intestinal permeability and aggravate inflammatory bowel disease. *Inflamm Bowel Dis* **8**, 340–46.

1396. Patel, M.S. (1984) Diabetes, the emerging problem in Papua New Guinea [editorial]. *P N G Med J* **27**, 1–3.

1397. Paterna, S., Parrinello, G., Fasullo, S., Sarullo, F.M. & Di Pasquale, P. (2008) Normal sodium diet versus low sodium diet in compensated congestive heart failure: is sodium an old enemy or a new friend? *Clin Sci (Lond)* **114**, 221–30.

1398. Paterson, J.C., Armstrong, R. & Armstrong, E.C. (1963) Serum Lipid Levels and the Severity of Coronary and Cerebral Atherosclerosis in Adequately Nourished Men, 60 to 69 Years of Age. *Circulation* **27**, 229–36.

1399. Pathik, B. & Ram, P. (1974) Acute myocardial infarction in Fiji: a review of 300 cases. *Med J Aust* **2**, 922–4.

1400. Pattison, D.J., Symmons, D.P., Lunt, M., *et al.* (2004) Dietary risk factors for the development of inflammatory polyarthritis: evidence for a role of high level of red meat consumption. *Arthritis Rheum* **50**, 3804–12.

1401. Pawlak, D.B., Kushner, J.A. & Ludwig, D.S. (2004) Effects of dietary glycaemic index on adiposity, glucose homoeostasis, and plasma lipids in animals. *Lancet* **364**, 778–85.

1402. Pawson, I.G. (1974) Radiographic determination of excessive bone loss in Alaskan Eskimos. *Hum Biol* **46**, 369–80.

1403. Pazzanese, D., Portugal, O.P., Ramos, O.L., *et al.* (1964) Serum-lipid levels in a Brazilian Indian population. *Lancet* **2**, 615–17.

1404. Pearce, G., McGinnis, J. & Ryan, C.A. (1983) Effects of feeding a carboxypeptidase inhibitor from potatoes to newly hatched chicks. *Proc Soc Exp Biol Med* **173**, 447–53.

1405. Pearce, G., McGinnis, J. & Ryan, C.A. (1984) Nutritional studies of a carboxypeptidase inhibitor from potato tubers. *Adv Exp Med Biol* **177**, 321–32.

1406. Perantoni, A.O. (1998) Carcinogenesis. In: *The Biological Basis of Cancer* (R.G. McKinnell, R.E. Parchment, A.O. Perantoni & G.B. Pierce eds). Cambridge University Press, Cambridge, pp. 79–114.

1407. Perego, L., Pizzocri, P., Corradi, D., *et al.* (2005) Circulating leptin correlates with left ventricular mass in morbid (grade III) obesity before and after weight loss induced by bariatric surgery: a potential role for leptin in mediating human left ventricular hypertrophy. *J Clin Endocrinol Metab* **90**, 4087–93.

1408. Pereira, M.A., Jacobs, D.R., Jr., Van Horn, L., *et al.* (2002) Dairy consumption, obesity, and the insulin resistance syndrome in young adults: the CARDIA Study. *JAMA* **287**, 2081–9.

1409. Pereira, M.A., O'Reilly, E., Augustsson, K., *et al.* (2004) Dietary fiber and risk of coronary heart disease: a pooled analysis of cohort studies. *Arch Intern Med* **164**, 370–76.

1410. Perry, G.H., Dominy, N.J., Claw, K.G., *et al.* (2007) Diet and the evolution of human amylase gene copy number variation. *Nat Genet* **39**, 1256–60.

1411. Perry, I.J. & Beevers, D.G. (1992) Salt intake and stroke: a possible direct effect. *J Hum Hypertens* **6**, 23–5.

1412. Perzigian, A.J. (1973) Osteoporotic bone loss in two prehistoric Indian populations. *Am J Phys Anthropol* **39**, 87–95.

1413. Peschken, C.A. & Esdaile, J.M. (1999) Rheumatic diseases in North America's indigenous peoples. *Semin Arthritis Rheum* **28**, 368–91.

1414. Peters, U., Poole, C. & Arab, L. (2001) Does tea affect cardiovascular disease? A meta-analysis. *Am J Epidemiol* **154**, 495–503.

1415. Petersen, M., Taylor, M.A., Saris, W.H., *et al.* (2006) Randomized, multi-center trial of two hypo-energetic diets in obese subjects: high- versus low-fat content. *Int J Obes (Lond)* **30**, 552–60.

1416. Petrie, J.R., Morris, A.D., Minamisawa, K., *et al.* (1998) Dietary sodium restriction impairs insulin sensitivity in noninsulin-dependent diabetes mellitus. *J Clin Endocrinol Metab* **83**, 1552–7.

1417. Pettifor, J.M. (1994) Privational rickets: a modern perspective [editorial; comment]. *J R Soc Med* **87**, 723–5.

1418. Pfeuffer, M. & Schrezenmeir, J. (2000) Bioactive substances in milk with properties decreasing risk of cardiovascular diseases. *Br J Nutr* **84** (Suppl 1), S155–9.

1419. Pi-Sunyer, F.X. (2002) Glycemic index and disease. *Am J Clin Nutr* **76**, 290S–8S.

1420. Pihlajamaki, J., Gylling, H., Miettinen, T.A. & Laakso, M. (2004) Insulin resistance is associated with increased cholesterol synthesis and decreased cholesterol absorption in normoglycemic men. *J Lipid Res* **45**, 507–12.

1420a. Piccinini, L.A., Mackenzie, W.A., Platzer, M. & Davis, T.F. (1987) Lymphokine regulation of HLA-DR gene expression in human thyroid cell monolayers. *J Clin Endocrinol Metab* **64**, 543–8.

1421. Pirozzo, S., Summerbell, C., Cameron, C. & Glasziou, P. (2002) Advice on low-fat diets for obesity (Cochrane Review). *Cochrane Database Syst Rev* Isssue 2, Art. No. CD003640.

1422. Pirozzo, S., Summerbell, C., Cameron, C. & Glasziou, P. (2003) Should we recommend low-fat diets for obesity? *Obes Rev* **4**, 83–90.

1423. Pischon, T., Boeing, H., Hoffmann, K., *et al.* (2008) General and abdominal adiposity and risk of death in Europe. *N Engl J Med* **359**, 2105–20.

1424. Pixley, F. (1986) Epidemiology. In: *Gallstone disease and its management* (M.C. Bateson ed). MTP Press, Lancaster, pp. 1–23.

1425. Pocock, S.J., McMurray, J.J., Dobson, J., *et al.* (2008) Weight loss and mortality risk in patients with chronic heart failure in the candesartan in heart failure: assessment of reduction in mortality and morbidity (CHARM) programme. *Eur Heart J* **29**, 2641–50.

1426. Poirier, J. (2000) Apolipoprotein E and Alzheimer's disease. A role in amyloid catabolism. *Ann N Y Acad Sci* **924**, 81–90.

1427. Poirier, P., Giles, T.D., Bray, G.A., *et al.* (2006) Obesity and cardiovascular disease: pathophysiology, evaluation, and effect of weight loss: an update of the 1997 American Heart Association Scientific Statement on Obesity and Heart Disease from the Obesity Committee of the Council on Nutrition, Physical Activity, and Metabolism. *Circulation* **113**, 898–918.

1428. Poitout, V., Hagman, D., Stein, R., *et al.* (2006) Regulation of the insulin gene by glucose and fatty acids. *J Nutr* **136**, 873–6.

1429. Pollock, N.K., Laing, E.M., Baile, C.A., *et al.* (2007) Is adiposity advantageous for bone strength? A peripheral quantitative computed tomography study in late adolescent females. *Am J Clin Nutr* **86**, 1530–38.

1430. Polunin, I. (1953) The medical natural history of Malayan aborigines. *Med J Malaysia* **8**, 55–174.

1431. Popham, R.E. (1983) Variation in mortality from ischaemic heart disease in relation to alcohol and milk consumption. *Med Hypotheses* **12**, 321–9.

1432. Popper, K. (1959) *The logic of scientific discovery*. Routledge, London.

1433. Porrini, M., Santangelo, A., Crovetti, R., *et al.* (1997) Weight, protein, fat, and timing of preloads affect food intake. *Physiol Behav* **62**, 563–70.

1434. Port, S.C., Goodarzi, M.O., Boyle, N.G. & Jennrich, R.I. (2005) Blood glucose: a strong risk factor for mortality in nondiabetic patients with cardiovascular disease. *Am Heart J* **150**, 209–14.

1435. Porter, A., Ben-Josef, E., Crawford, E.D., *et al.* (2001) Advancing perspectives on prostate cancer: multihormonal influences in pathogenesis. *Mol Urol* **5**, 181–8.

1436. Potter, S.M., Baum, J.A., Teng, H., *et al.* (1998) Soy protein and isoflavones: their effects on blood lipids and bone density in postmenopausal women. *Am J Clin Nutr* **68**, 1375S–9S.

1437. Poulter, N. (1989) Blood pressure in urban and rural East Africa: the Kenyan Luo Migrant Study. In: *Ethnic factors in health and disease* (J.K. Cruickshank & D.G. Beevers eds). Wright, Oxford, pp. 61–8.

1438. Poulter, N.R., Khaw, K.T. & Sever, P.S. (1988) Higher blood pressures of urban migrants from an African low-blood pressure population are not due to selective migration. *Am J Hypertens* **1**, 143S–5S.

1439. Pour, P.M., Burnett, D. & Uchida, E. (1985) Lectin binding affinities of induced pancreatic lesions in the hamster model. *Carcinogenesis* **6**, 1775–80.

1440. Powell, B.D., Redfield, M.M., Bybee, K.A., Freeman, W.K. & Rihal, C.S. (2006) Association of obesity with left ventricular remodeling and diastolic dysfunction in patients without coronary artery disease. *Am J Cardiol* **98**, 116–20.

1441. Powell, H.A. (1956) *An analysis of present-day social structure in the Trobriand Islands.* Ph.D., University of London.

1442. Powell, H.A. (1960) Competitive leadership in Trobriand political organization. *J Royal Anthropol Inst* **90**, 118–145.

1443. Powell, H.A. (1969) Genealogy, residence and kinship in Kiriwina. *Man* **4**, 177–202.

1444. Powell, H.A. (1969) Territory, hierarchy and kinship in Kiriwina. *Man* **4**, 580–604.

1445. Power, K.A. & Thompson, L.U. (2007) Can the combination of flaxseed and its lignans with soy and its isoflavones reduce the growth stimulatory effect of soy and its isoflavones on established breast cancer? *Mol Nutr Food Res* **51**, 845–56.

1446. Prentice, A., Laskey, M.A., Shaw, J., Cole, T.J. & Fraser, D.R. (1990) Bone mineral content of Gambian and British children aged 0–36 months. *Bone Miner* **10**, 211–24.

1447. Prentice, R.L., Caan, B., Chlebowski, R.T., *et al.* (2006) Low-fat dietary pattern and risk of invasive breast cancer: the Women's Health Initiative Randomized Controlled Dietary Modification Trial. *JAMA* **295**, 629–42.

1448. Price, G.M., Uauy, R., Breeze, E., Bulpitt, C.J. & Fletcher, A.E. (2006) Weight, shape, and mortality risk in older persons: elevated waist-hip ratio, not high body mass index, is associated with a greater risk of death. *Am J Clin Nutr* **84**, 449–60.

1449. Princen, H.M., van Duyvenvoorde, W., Buytenhek, R., *et al.* (1998) No effect of consumption of green and black tea on plasma lipid and antioxidant levels and on LDL oxidation in smokers. *Arterioscler Thromb Vasc Biol* **18**, 833–41.

1450. Prior, I.A. (1974) Cardiovascular epidemiology in New Zealand and the Pacific. *N Z Med J* **80**, 245–52.

1451. Prior, I.A., Davidson, F., Salmond, C.E. & Czochanska, Z. (1981) Cholesterol, coconuts, and diet on Polynesian atolls: a natural experiment: the Pukapuka and Tokelau island studies. *Am J Clin Nutr* **34**, 1552–61.

1452. Prior, I.A., Welby, T.J., Ostbye, T., Salmond, C.E. & Stokes, Y.M. (1987) Migration and gout: the Tokelau Island migrant study. *Br Med J Clin Res Ed* **295**, 457–61.

1453. Prior, I.A.M. & Stanhope, J.M. (1980) Blood pressure patterns, salt use and migration in the Pacific. In: *Epidemiology of Arterial Blood Pressure* (H. Kesteloot & J.V. Joosens eds). Martinus Nijhoff, The Hague, pp. 243–62.

1454. Prokopczyk, B., Rivenson, A. & Hoffmann, D. (1991) A study of betel quid carcinogenesis. IX. Comparative carcinogenicity of 3-(methylnitrosamino)propionitrile and 4-(methylnitrosamino)-1-(3-pyridyl)-1-butanone upon local application to mouse skin and rat oral mucosa. *Cancer Lett* **60**, 153–7.

1455. Promislow, J.H., Goodman-Gruen, D., Slymen, D.J. & Barrett-Connor, E. (2002) Protein consumption and bone mineral density in the elderly: the Rancho Bernardo Study. *Am J Epidemiol* **155**, 636–44.

1456. Proos, L.A., Hofvander, Y. & Tuvemo, T. (1991) Menarcheal age and growth pattern of Indian girls adopted in Sweden. I. Menarcheal age. *Acta Paediatr Scand* **80**, 852–8.

1457. Psota, T.L., Gebauer, S.K. & Kris-Etherton, P. (2006) Dietary omega-3 fatty acid intake and cardiovascular risk. *Am J Cardiol* **98**, 3i–18i.

1458. Puglielli, L., Tanzi, R.E. & Kovacs, D.M. (2003) Alzheimer's disease: the cholesterol connection. *Nat Neurosci* **6**, 345–51.

1459. Purrello, F., Burnham, D.B. & Goldfine, I.D. (1983) Insulin receptor antiserum and plant lectins mimic the direct effects of insulin on nuclear envelope phosphorylation. *Science* **221**, 462–4.

1460. Pusztai, A. (1993) Dietary lectins are metabolic signals for the gut and modulate immune and hormone functions. *Eur J Clin Nutr* **47**, 691–9.

1461. Pusztai, A., Greer, F. & Grant, G. (1989) Specific uptake of dietary lectins into the systemic circulation of rats. *Biochem Soc Trans* **17**, 481–2.

1462. Qi, L., van Dam, R.M., Rexrode, K. & Hu, F.B. (2007) Heme iron from diet as a risk factor for coronary heart disease in women with type 2 diabetes. *Diabetes Care* **30**, 101–6.

1463. Qiao, Q., Pyorala, K., Pyorala, M., *et al.* (2002) Two-hour glucose is a better risk predictor for incident coronary heart disease and cardiovascular mortality than fasting glucose. *Eur Heart J* **23**, 1267.

1464. Qin, L.Q., Xu, J.Y., Tezuka, H., Wang, P.Y. & Hoshi, K. (2007) Commercial soy milk enhances the development of 7,12-dimethylbenz(a)anthracene-induced mammary tumors in rats. *In Vivo* **21**, 667–71.

1465. Raatz, S.K., Torkelson, C.J., Redmon, J.B., *et al.* (2005) Reduced glycemic index and glycemic load diets do not increase the effects of energy restriction on weight loss and insulin sensitivity in obese men and women. *J Nutr* **135**, 2387–91.

1466. Raeini-Sarjaz, M., Vanstone, C.A., Papamandjaris, A.A., Wykes, L.J. & Jones, P.J. (2001) Comparison of the effect of dietary fat restriction with that of energy restriction on human lipid metabolism. *Am J Clin Nutr* **73**, 262–7.

1467. Raisz, L.G. (2001) Pathogenesis of postmenopausal osteoporosis. *Rev Endocr Metab Disord* **2**, 5–12.

1468. Raitt, M.H., Connor, W.E., Morris, C., *et al.* (2005) Fish oil supplementation and risk of ventricular tachycardia and ventricular fibrillation in patients with implantable defibrillators: a randomized controlled trial. *JAMA* **293**, 2884–91.

1469. Ramakrishnan, U. & Yip, R. (2002) Experiences and challenges in industrialized countries: control of iron deficiency in industrialized countries. *J Nutr* **132**, 820S–4S.

1470. Ramirez-Gil, J.F., Delcayre, C., Robert, V., *et al.* (1998) In vivo left ventricular function and collagen expression in aldosterone/salt-induced hypertension. *J Cardiovasc Pharmacol* **32**, 927–34.

1471. Rand, W.M., Windham, C.T., Wyse, B.W. & Young, V.R. (1987) *Food composition data: a user's perspective.* United Nations University, Tokyo.

1472. Rank, T.C., Grappin, R. & Olson, N.F. (1985) Secondary proteolysis of cheese during ripening: a review. *J Dairy Sci* **68**, 801–5.

1473. Rasmussen, L.B., Ovesen, L., Bulow, I., *et al.* (2002) Relations between various measures of iodine intake and thyroid volume, thyroid nodularity, and serum thyroglobulin. *Am J Clin Nutr* **76**, 1069–76.

1474. Raviola, E. & Wiesel, T.N. (1985) An animal model of myopia. *N Engl J Med* **312**, 1609–15.

1475. Ravnskov, U. (1992) Cholesterol lowering trials in coronary heart disease: frequency of citation and outcome. *BMJ* **305**, 15–9.

1476. Ravnskov, U. (1998) The questionable role of saturated and polyunsaturated fatty acids in cardiovascular disease. *J Clin Epidemiol* **51**, 443–60.

1477. Rayfield, E.J., Ault, M.J., Keusch, G.T., *et al.* (1982) Infection and diabetes: the case for glucose control. *Am J Med* **72**, 439–50.

1478. Reaven, G.M. (1988) Banting lecture 1988. Role of insulin resistance in human disease. *Diabetes* **37**, 1595–607.

1479. Reaven, G.M. (2000) Diet and syndrome X. *Curr Atheroscler Rep* **2**, 503–7.

1480. Reaven, G.M. (2005) The insulin resistance syndrome: definition and dietary approaches to treatment. *Annu Rev Nutr* **25**, 391–406.

1481. Redfield, M.M., Jacobsen, S.J., Burnett, J.C., Jr., *et al.* (2003) Burden of systolic and diastolic ventricular dysfunction in the community: appreciating the scope of the heart failure epidemic. *JAMA* **289**, 194–202.

1482. Ree, G.H. (1982) Elderly ailing highlanders of Papua New Guinea. *P N G Med J* **25**, 93–6.

1483. Reed, D.M. (1990) The paradox of high risk of stroke in populations with low risk of coronary heart disease. *Am J Epidemiol* **131**, 579–88.

1484. Reed, D.M., Strong, J.P., Resch, J. & Hayashi, T. (1989) Serum lipids and lipoproteins as predictors of atherosclerosis. An autopsy study. *Arteriosclerosis* **9**, 560–64.

1485. Reed, K.E. (1997) Early hominid evolution and ecological change through the African Plio-Pleistocene. *J Hum Evol* **32**, 289–322.

1486. Reef, H. & Isaacson, C. (1962) Atherosclerosis in the Bantu. *Circulation* **25**, 66–72.

1487. Reese, D.E. (1999) Nutrient deficiencies and excesses. In: *Diseases of swine* (B.E. Straw, S. D'Allaire, W.L. Mengeling & D.J. Taylor eds). Blackwell Science, Oxford, pp. 743–55.

1488. Reeves, G.K., Pirie, K., Beral, V., *et al.* (2007) Cancer incidence and mortality in relation to body mass index in the Million Women Study: cohort study. *BMJ* **335**, 1134.

1489. Refsum, H. & Smith, A.D. (2006) Homocysteine, B vitamins, and cardiovascular disease. *N Engl J Med* **355**, 207; author reply 209–11.

1490. Reichelt, K.L. & Jensen, D. (2004) IgA antibodies against gliadin and gluten in multiple sclerosis. *Acta Neurol Scand* **110**, 239–41.

1491. Reinehr, T., de Sousa, G., Alexy, U., Kersting, M. & Andler, W. (2007) Vitamin D status and parathyroid hormone in obese children before and after weight loss. *Eur J Endocrinol* **157**, 225–32.

1492. Reitsma, S., Slaaf, D.W., Vink, H., van Zandvoort, M.A. & oude Egbrink, M.G. (2007) The endothelial glycocalyx: composition, functions, and visualization. *Pflugers Arch* **454**, 345–59.

1493. Remer, T. (2001) Influence of nutrition on acid-base balance – metabolic aspects. *Eur J Nutr* **40**, 214–20.

1494. Remer, T. & Manz, F. (1995) Potential renal acid load of foods and its influence on urine pH. *J Am Diet Assoc* **95**, 791–7.

1495. Remer, T. & Manz, F. (2001) Don't forget the acid base status when studying metabolic and clinical effects of dietary potassium depletion. *J Clin Endocrinol Metab* **86**, 5996–7.

1496. Renehan, A.G., Frystyk, J. & Flyvbjerg, A. (2006) Obesity and cancer risk: the role of the insulin-IGF axis. *Trends Endocrinol Metab* **17**, 328–36.

1497. Rennie, K.L., Coward, A. & Jebb, S.A. (2007) Estimating under-reporting of energy intake in dietary surveys using an individualised method. *Br J Nutr* **97**, 1169–76.

1498. Requejo, A.M., Navia, B., Ortega, R.M., *et al.* (1999) The age at which meat is first included in the diet affects the incidence of iron deficiency and ferropenic anaemia in a group of pre-school children from Madrid. *Int J Vitam Nutr Res* **69**, 127–31.

1499. Retnakaran, R., Cull, C.A., Thorne, K.I., Adler, A.I. & Holman, R.R. (2006) Risk factors for renal dysfunction in type 2 diabetes: U.K. Prospective Diabetes Study 74. *Diabetes* **55**, 1832–9.

1500. Rexrode, K.M., Buring, J.E. & Manson, J.E. (2001) Abdominal and total adiposity and risk of coronary heart disease in men. *Int J Obes Relat Metab Disord* **25**, 1047–56.

1501. Rich, M.W. (2000) Uric acid: is it a risk factor for cardiovascular disease? *Am J Cardiol* **85**, 1018–21.

1502. Rich-Edwards, J.W., Manson, J.E., Hennekens, C.H. & Buring, J.E. (1995) The primary prevention of coronary heart disease in women. *N Engl J Med* **332**, 1758–66.

1503. Richards, M.P. (2002) A brief review of the archaeological evidence for Palaeolithic and Neolithic subsistence. *Eur J Clin Nutr* **56**, 1270–79.

1504. Richards, M.P., Pettitt, P.B., Stiner, M.C. & Trinkaus, E. (2001) Stable isotope evidence for increasing dietary breadth in the European mid-Upper Paleolithic. *Proc Natl Acad Sci USA* **98**, 6528–32.

1505. Richardson, M., Kurowska, E.M. & Carroll, K.K. (1994) Early lesion development in the aortas of rabbits fed low-fat, cholesterol-free, semipurified casein diet. *Atherosclerosis* **107**, 165–78.

1506. Richman, E.A., Ortner, D.J. & Schulter-Ellis, F.P. (1979) Differences in intracortical bone remodeling in three aboriginal American populations: possible dietary factors. *Calcif Tissue Int* **28**, 209–14.

1507. Riemersma, R.A., Rice-Evans, C.A., Tyrrell, R.M., Clifford, M.N. & Lean, M.E. (2001) Tea flavonoids and cardiovascular health *QJM* **94**, 277–82.

1508. Rigano, R., Profumo, E., Buttari, B., *et al.* (2007) Heat shock proteins and autoimmunity in patients with carotid atherosclerosis. *Ann N Y Acad Sci* **1107**, 1–10.

1509. Rimm, E.B. (2002) Fruit and vegetables-building a solid foundation. *Am J Clin Nutr* **76**, 1–2.

1510. Rizkalla, S.W., Taghrid, L., Laromiguiere, M., *et al.* (2004) Improved plasma glucose control, whole-body glucose utilization, and lipid profile on a low-glycemic index diet in type 2 diabetic men: a randomized controlled trial. *Diabetes Care* **27**, 1866–72.

1511. Robbie-Ryan, M. & Brown, M. (2002) The role of mast cells in allergy and autoimmunity. *Curr Opin Immunol* **14**, 728–33.

1512. Roberts, C. & Manchester, K. (1997) *The archaeology of disease*. Cornell University Press, New York.

1513. Roberts, E.A. (2007) Pediatric nonalcoholic fatty liver disease (NAFLD): a 'growing' problem? *J Hepatol* **46**, 1133–42.

1514. Robertson, M.D., Bickerton, A.S., Dennis, A.L., Vidal, H. & Frayn, K.N. (2005) Insulin-sensitizing effects of dietary resistant starch and effects on skeletal muscle and adipose tissue metabolism. *Am J Clin Nutr* **82**, 559–67.

1515. Robinson, W.F. & Maxie, M.G. (1985) The cardiovascular system. In: *Pathology of domestic animals* (K.V.F. Jubb, P.C. Kennedy & N. Palmer eds). Academic Press, New York, pp. 2–83.

1516. Rocchini, A.P. (1994) The relationship of sodium sensitivity to insulin resistance. *Am J Med Sci* **307**, S75–80.

1517. Roche, A.F. (1979) Secular trends in human growth, maturation, and development. *Monogr Soc Res Child Dev* **44**, 1–120.

1518. Rockell, J.E., Williams, S.M., Taylor, R.W., *et al.* (2005) Two-year changes in bone and body composition in young children with a history of prolonged milk avoidance. *Osteoporos Int* **16**, 1016–23.

1519. Rockwood, K. & Darvesh, S. (2003) The risk of dementia in relation to statins and other lipid lowering agents. *Neurol Res* **25**, 601–4.

1520. Rode, A. & Shephard, R.J. (1995) Body fat distribution and other cardiac risk factors among circumpolar Inuit and nGanasan. *Arct Med Res* **54**, 125–33.

1521. Rodin, D.A., Bano, G., Bland, J.M., Taylor, K. & Nussey, S.S. (1998) Polycystic ovaries and associated metabolic abnormalities in Indian subcontinent Asian women. *Clin Endocrinol (Oxf)* **49**, 91–9.

1522. Roe, D.A. (1991) Rickets and osteomalacia. In: *Hunter's tropical medicine* (G.T. Strickland ed). W. B. Saunders, Philadelphia, pp. 929–32.

1523. Rogers, I., Metcalfe, C., Gunnell, D., *et al.* (2006) Insulin-like growth factor-I and growth in height, leg length, and trunk length between ages 5 and 10 years. *J Clin Endocrinol Metab* **91**, 2514–19.

1524. Rogers, W.R., Bass, R.L., 3rd, Johnson, D.E., *et al.* (1980) Atherosclerosis-related responses to cigarette smoking in the baboon. *Circulation* **61**, 1188–93.

1525. Rolland-Cachera, M.F., Deheeger, M., Maillot, M. & Bellisle, F. (2006) Early adiposity rebound: causes and consequences for obesity in children and adults. *Int J Obes (Lond)* **30** (Suppl 4), S11–17.

1526. Rolls, B.J., Drewnowski, A. & Ledikwe, J.H. (2005) Changing the energy density of the diet as a strategy for weight management. *J Am Diet Assoc* **105**, S98–103.

1527. Romero-Corral, A., Montori, V.M., Somers, V.K., *et al.* (2006) Association of bodyweight with total mortality and with cardiovascular events in coronary artery disease: a systematic review of cohort studies. *Lancet* **368**, 666–78.

1528. Romm, P.A., Green, C.E., Reagan, K. & Rackley, C. (1991) Relation of serum lipoprotein cholesterol levels to presence and severity of angiographic coronary artery disease. *Am J Cardiol* **67**, 479–83.

1529. Roper, N.A., Bilous, R.W., Kelly, W.F., Unwin, N.C. & Connolly, V.M. (2002) Cause-specific mortality in a population with diabetes: South Tees Diabetes Mortality Study. *Diabetes Care* **25**, 43–8.

1530. Ros, E. (2003) Dietary cis-monounsaturated fatty acids and metabolic control in type 2 diabetes. *Am J Clin Nutr* **78**, 617S–25S.

1531. Rosamond, W., Flegal, K., Friday, G., *et al.* (2007) Heart disease and stroke statistics – 2007 update: a report from the American Heart Association Statistics Committee and Stroke Statistics Subcommittee. *Circulation* **115**, e69–171.

1532. Rose, G. (1985) Sick individuals and sick populations. *Int J Epidemiol* **14**, 32–8.

1533. Rosell, M., Regnstrom, J., Kallner, A. & Hellenius, M.L. (1999) Serum urate determines antioxidant capacity in middle-aged men – a controlled, randomized diet and exercise intervention study. *J Intern Med* **246**, 219–26.

1534. Rosner, S.A., Akesson, A., Stampfer, M.J. & Wolk, A. (2007) Coffee consumption and risk of myocardial infarction among older Swedish women. *Am J Epidemiol* **165**, 288–93.

1535. Rossander, L., Sandberg, A.-S. & Sandström, B. (1992) The influence of dietary fibre on mineral absorption and utilisation. In: *Dietary fibre – a component of food. Nutritional function in health and disease* (T.F. Schweizer & C.A. Edwards eds), Springer, London, pp. 197–216.

1536. Rossander-Hulthén, L. & Hallberg, L. (1996) Dietary factors influencing iron absorption - an overview. In: *Iron Nutrition in Health and Disease* (L. Hallberg & N.-G. Asp eds). John Libbey, London, pp. 105–15.

1537. Roth, G.S., Ingram, D.K. & Lane, M.A. (2001) Caloric restriction in primates and relevance to humans. *Ann N Y Acad Sci* **928**, 305–15.

1538. Rothschild, B. (2002) Porotic hyperostosis as a marker of health and nutritional conditions. *Am J Human Biol* **14**, 417–18; discussion 418–20.

1539. Rothschild, B. & Martin, L. (1993) *Paleopathology: disease in the fossil record*. CRC Press, London.

1540. Rubis, B., Paszel, A., Kaczmarek, M., *et al.* (2008) Beneficial or harmful influence of phytosterols on human cells? *Br J Nutr* **100**, 1183–91.

1541. Rudel, L.L., Kelley, K., Sawyer, J.K., Shah, R. & Wilson, M.D. (1998) Dietary monounsaturated fatty acids promote aortic atherosclerosis in LDL receptor-null, human ApoB100-overexpressing transgenic mice. *Arterioscler Thromb Vasc Biol* **18**, 1818–27.

1542. Rudel, L.L., Parks, J.S., Hedrick, C.C., Thomas, M. & Williford, K. (1998) Lipoprotein and cholesterol metabolism in diet-induced coronary artery atherosclerosis in primates. Role of cholesterol and fatty acids. *Prog Lipid Res* **37**, 353–70.

1543. Rudel, L.L., Parks, J.S. & Sawyer, J.K. (1995) Compared with dietary monounsaturated and saturated fat, polyunsaturated fat protects African green monkeys from coronary artery atherosclerosis. *Arterioscler Thromb Vasc Biol* **15**, 2101–10.

1544. Ruff, C.B. (1992) Biomechanical analyses of archaeological human skeletal samples. In: *Skeletal biology of past peoples: research methods* (S.R. Saunders & A. Katzenberg eds). Wiley-Liss, New York, pp. 37–58.

1545. Rundgren, Å (1991) *Människans funktionella åldrande*. Studentlitteratur, Lund.

1546. Rushton, D.H., Dover, R., Sainsbury, A.W., *et al.* (2001) Why should women have lower reference limits for haemoglobin and ferritin concentrations than men? *BMJ* **322**, 1355–7.

1547. Russell, J.C. & Proctor, S.D. (2006) Small animal models of cardiovascular disease: tools for the study of the roles of metabolic syndrome, dyslipidemia, and atherosclerosis. *Cardiovasc Pathol* **15**, 318–30.

1548. Ryan, K.R., Patel, S.D., Stephens, L.A. & Anderton, S.M. (2007) Death, adaptation and regulation: the three pillars of immune tolerance restrict the risk of autoimmune disease caused by molecular mimicry. *J Autoimmun* **29**, 262–71.

1549. Ryden, L., Standl, E., Bartnik, M., *et al.* (2007) Guidelines on diabetes, pre-diabetes, and cardiovascular diseases: executive summary: The Task Force on Diabetes and Cardiovascular Diseases of the European Society of Cardiology (ESC) and of the European Association for the Study of Diabetes (EASD). *Eur Heart J* **28**, 88–136.

1550. Ryu, S.Y., Kim, C.-B., Nam, C.M., *et al.* (2001) Is body mass index the prognostic factor in breast cancer? A meta-analysis. *J Korean Med Sci* **16**, 610–14.

1551. Sackett, D.L., Straus, S., Richardson, W.S., Rosenberg, W. & Haynes, R.B. (2000) *Evidence-based medicine.* Churchill Livingstone, New York.

1552. Sacks, F.M., Bray, G.A., Carey, V.J., *et al.* (2009) Comparison of weight-loss diets with different compositions of fat, protein, and carbohydrates. *N Engl J Med* **360**, 859–73.

1553. Sacks, F.M., Lichtenstein, A., Van Horn, L., *et al.* (2006) Soy protein, isoflavones, and cardiovascular health: an American Heart Association Science Advisory for professionals from the Nutrition Committee. *Circulation* **113**, 1034–44.

1554. Sacks, F.M., Svetkey, L.P., Vollmer, W.M., *et al.* (2001) Effects on blood pressure of reduced dietary sodium and the Dietary Approaches to Stop Hypertension (DASH) diet. DASH-Sodium Collaborative Research Group. *N Engl J Med* **344**, 3–10.

1555. Saffran, M. (1995) Rickets. Return of an old disease. *J Am Podiatr Med Assoc* **85**, 222–5.

1556. Sakemi, T., Ikeda, Y. & Shimazu, K. (2002) Effect of soy protein added to casein diet on the development of glomerular injury in spontaneous hypercholesterolemic male Imai rats. *Am J Nephrol* **22**, 548–54.

1557. Salem, G.J., Zernicke, R.F. & Barnard, R.J. (1992) Diet-related changes in mechanical properties of rat vertebrae. *Am J Physiol* **262**, R318–21.

1558. Salmeron, J., Ascherio, A., Rimm, E.B., *et al.* (1997) Dietary fiber, glycemic load, and risk of NIDDM in men. *Diabetes Care* **20**, 545–50.

1559. Salmond, C.E., Prior, I.A. & Wessen, A.F. (1989) Blood pressure patterns and migration: a 14-year cohort study of adult Tokelauans. *Am J Epidemiol* **130**, 37–52.

1560. Salomaa, V.V., Lundberg, V., Agnarsson, U., *et al.* (1997) Fatalities from myocardial infarction in Nordic countries and Lithuania. The MONICA Investigators. *Eur Heart J* **18**, 91–8.

1561. Salvadei, L., Ricci, F. & Manzi, G. (2001) Porotic hyperostosis as a marker of health and nutritional conditions during childhood: studies at the transition between Imperial Rome and the Early Middle Ages. *Am J Human Biol* **13**, 709–17.

1562. Samelson, E.J., Cupples, L.A., Broe, K.E., *et al.* (2007) Vascular calcification in middle age and long-term risk of hip fracture: the Framingham Study. *J Bone Miner Res* **22**, 1449–54.

1563. Samelson, E.J., Hannan, M.T., Zhang, Y., *et al.* (2006) Incidence and risk factors for vertebral fracture in women and men: 25-year follow-up results from the population-based Framingham study. *J Bone Miner Res* **21**, 1207–14.

1564. Samuelson, L.C., Wiebauer, K., Snow, C.M. & Meisler, M.H. (1990) Retroviral and pseudogene insertion sites reveal the lineage of human salivary and pancreatic amylase genes from a single gene during primate evolution. *Mol Cell Biol* **10**, 2513–20.

1565. Sanchez, A. & Hubbard, R.W. (1991) Plasma amino acids and the insulin/glucagon ratio as an explanation for the dietary protein modulation of atherosclerosis. *Med Hypotheses* **36**, 27–32.

1566. Sanchez, A. & Hubbard, R.W. (1991) Plasma amino acids and the insulin/glucagon ratio as an explanation for the dietary protein modulation of atherosclerosis. *Med Hypotheses* **35**, 324–9.

1567. Sanchez-Castillo, C.P., Velazquez-Monroy, O., Berber, A., *et al.* (2003) Anthropometric cutoff points for predicting chronic diseases in the Mexican National Health Survey 2000. *Obes Res* **11**, 442–51.

1568. Sanchez-Lozada, L.G., Le, M., Segal, M. & Johnson, R.J. (2008) How safe is fructose for persons with or without diabetes? *Am J Clin Nutr* **88**, 1189–90.

1569. Sandberg, A.-S. (1996) Food processing influencing iron bioavailability. In: *Iron nutrition in health and disease* (L. Hallberg & N.-G. Asp eds). John Libbey, London, pp. 349–58.

1570. Sandberg, A.S. (1991) The effect of food processing on phytate hydrolysis and availability of iron and zinc. *Adv Exp Med Biol* **289**, 499–508.

1571. Sandberg, A.S., Hasselblad, C., Hasselblad, K. & Hulten, L. (1982) The effect of wheat bran on the absorption of minerals in the small intestine. *Br J Nutr* **48**, 185–91.

1572. Sandstead, H.H. (1992) Fiber, phytates, and mineral nutrition. *Nutr Rev* **50**, 30–31.

1573. Sandstrom, B. (1989) Food processing and trace element supply. In: *Nutritional Impact of Food Processing. Bibl Nutr Dieta* (J.C. Somogyi & H.R. Muller eds). Karger, Basel, pp. 165–72.

1574. Santosa, S., Varady, K.A., AbuMweis, S. & Jones, P.J. (2007) Physiological and therapeutic factors affecting cholesterol metabolism: does a reciprocal relationship between cholesterol absorption and synthesis really exist? *Life Sci* **80**, 505–14.

1575. Sarafidis, P.A. & Bakris, G.L. (2006) Insulin resistance, hyperinsulinemia, and hypertension: an epidemiologic approach. *J Cardiometab Syndr* **1**, 334–42; quiz 343.

1576. Saraiva, R.M., Minhas, K.M., Zheng, M., *et al.* (2007) Reduced neuronal nitric oxide synthase expression contributes to cardiac oxidative stress and nitroso-redox imbalance in ob/ob mice. *Nitric Oxide* **16**, 331–8.

1577. Saric, M., Piasek, M., Blanusa, M., Kostial, K. & Ilich, J.Z. (2005) Sodium and calcium intakes and bone mass in rats revisited. *Nutrition* **21**, 609–14.

1578. Sarwar, N., Danesh, J., Eiriksdottir, G., *et al.* (2007) Triglycerides and the risk of coronary heart disease: 10,158 incident cases among 262,525 participants in 29 Western prospective studies. *Circulation* **115**, 450–58.

1579. Sasaki, S. (2000) Alcohol and its relation to all-cause and cardiovascular mortality. *Acta Cardiol* **55**, 151–6.

1580. Sato, F., Tamura, Y., Watada, H., *et al.* (2007) Effects of diet-induced moderate weight reduction on intrahepatic and intramyocellular triglycerides and glucose metabolism in obese subjects. *J Clin Endocrinol Metab* **92**, 3326–9.

1581. Saunders, S.R. & Katzenberg, M.A. (1992) Skeletal biology of past peoples: research methods, p. 264, Wiley-Liss, New York.

1582. Sauvaget, C., Nagano, J., Hayashi, M. & Yamada, M. (2004) Animal protein, animal fat, and cholesterol intakes and risk of cerebral infarction mortality in the adult health study. *Stroke* **35**, 1531–7.

1583. Savolainen, P., Zhang, Y.P., Luo, J., Lundeberg, J. & Leitner, T. (2002) Genetic evidence for an East Asian origin of domestic dogs. *Science* **298**, 1610–13.

1584. Saw, S.M., Chua, W.H., Hong, C.Y., *et al.* (2002) Height and its relationship to refraction and biometry parameters in Singapore Chinese children. *Invest Ophthalmol Vis Sci* **43**, 1408–13.

1585. SBU. (2002) *Fetma – problem och åtgärder.* Statens beredning för medicinsk utvärdering.

1586. Schaefer, E.J., Lamon-Fava, S., Ausman, L.M., *et al.* (1997) Individual variability in lipoprotein cholesterol response to National Cholesterol Education Program Step 2 diets. *Am J Clin Nutr* **65**, 823–30.

1587. Schaefer, O. (1970) Pre- and post-natal growth acceleration and increased sugar consumption in Canadian Eskimos. *Can Med Assoc J* **103**, 1059–68.

1588. Schaefer, O. (1971) When the Eskimo comes to town. *Nutr Today* **6**, 8–16.

1589. Schaefer, O. (1981) Eskimos. In: *Western diseases: their emergence and prevention* (H.C. Trowell & D.P. Burkitt eds). Edward Arnold, London, pp. 113–28.

1590. Schatzkin, A., Lanza, E., Corle, D., *et al.* (2000) Lack of effect of a low-fat, high-fiber diet on the recurrence of colorectal adenomas. Polyp Prevention Trial Study Group. *N Engl J Med* **342**, 1149–55.

1591. Schiefenhövel, W. (1983) Die Geburt aus ethnomedizinischer Sicht. *Curare* **6**, 143–50.

1592. Schiefenhövel, W. & Bell-Krannhals, I. (1986) Wer teilt, hat Teil an der Macht: Systeme der Yams-Vergabe auf den Trobriand Inseln, Papua-Neuguinea. *Mitteilungen der Anthropologischen Gesellschaft in Wien* **116**, 19–39.

1593. Schiefenhövel, W., Schuler, J. & Pöschl, R. (1986) *Traditionelle Heilkundige — Ärztliche Persönlichkeiten im Vergleich der Kulturen und medizinischen Systeme.* Vieweg, Braunscweig u. Wiesbaden.

1594. Schmid, R., Schulte-Frohlinde, E., Schusdziarra, V., *et al.* (1992) Contribution of postprandial amino acid levels to stimulation of insulin, glucagon, and pancreatic polypeptide in humans. *Pancreas* **7**, 698–704.

1595. Schmidt, E.B., Skou, H.A., Christensen, J.H. & Dyerberg, J. (2000) N-3 fatty acids from fish and coronary artery disease: implications for public health. *Public Health Nutr* **3**, 91–8.

1596. Schmieder, R.E., Messerli, F.H., Garavaglia, G.E. & Nunez, B.D. (1988) Dietary salt intake. A determinant of cardiac involvement in essential hypertension. *Circulation* **78**, 951–6.

1597. Schoen, R.E., Tangen, C.M., Kuller, L.H., *et al.* (1999) Increased blood glucose and insulin, body size, and incident colorectal cancer. *J Natl Cancer Inst* **91**, 1147–54.

1598. Schuler, G., Hambrecht, R., Schlierf, G., *et al.* (1992) Myocardial perfusion and regression of coronary artery disease in patients on a regimen of intensive physical exercise and low fat diet. *J Am Coll Cardiol* **19**, 34–42.

1599. Schultz, M. (2001) Paleohistopathology of bone: a new approach to the study of ancient diseases. *Am J Phys Anthropol* **116** (Suppl), 106–47.

1600. Schulze, M.B., Linseisen, J., Kroke, A. & Boeing, H. (2001) Macronutrient, vitamin, and mineral intakes in the EPIC-Germany cohorts. *Ann Nutr Metab* **45**, 181–9.

1601. Schurch, M.A., Rizzoli, R., Slosman, D., *et al.* (1998) Protein supplements increase serum insulin-like growth factor-I levels and attenuate proximal femur bone loss in patients with recent hip fracture. A randomized, double-blind, placebo-controlled trial. *Ann Intern Med* **128**, 801–9.

1602. Schusdziarra, V., Henrichs, I., Holland, A., Klier, M. & Pfeiffer, E.F. (1981) Evidence for an effect of exorphins on plasma insulin and glucagon levels in dogs. *Diabetes* **30**, 362–4.

1603. Scott, F.W. (1996) Food-induced type 1 diabetes in the BB rat. *Diabetes Metab Rev* **12**, 341–59.

1604. Scott, H.D. & Laake, K. (2001) Statins for the prevention of Alzheimer's disease. *Cochrane Database Syst Rev* **4**.

1605. Scott, L.W., Kimball, K.T., Wittels, E.H., *et al.* (1991) Effects of a lean beef diet and of a chicken and fish diet on lipoprotein profiles. *Nutr Metab Cardiovasc Dis* **1**, 25–30.

1606. Scott, M.J., 3rd & Scott, A.M. (1992) Effects of anabolic-androgenic steroids on the pilosebaceous unit. *Cutis* **50**, 113–6.

1607. Scrimgeour, E.M. (1992) Prevention of fracture of the neck of the femur: evidence from developing countries of the relative unimportance of osteoporosis. *Aust N Z J Med* **22**, 85–6.

1608. Scrimgeour, E.M., McCall, M.G., Smith, D.E. & Masarei, J.R. (1989) Levels of serum cholesterol, triglyceride, HDL-cholesterol, apoproteins A-I and B, and plasma glucose, and prevalence of diastolic hypertension and cigarette smoking in Papua New Guinea highlanders. *Pathology* **21**, 46–50.

1609. Sebastian, A. (2005) Dietary protein content and the diet's net acid load: opposing effects on bone health. *Am J Clin Nutr* **82**, 921–2.

1610. Sebastian, A., Frassetto, L.A., Sellmeyer, D.E., Merriam, R.L. & Morris, R.C., Jr. (2002) Estimation of the net acid load of the diet of ancestral preagricultural Homo sapiens and their hominid ancestors. *Am J Clin Nutr* **76**, 1308–16.

1611. Sebastian, A., Harris, S.T., Ottaway, J.H., Todd, K.M. & Morris, R.C., Jr. (1994) Improved mineral balance and skeletal metabolism in postmenopausal women treated with potassium bicarbonate. *N Engl J Med* **330**, 1776–81.

1612. Seely, S. (1981) Diet and coronary disease: a survey of mortality rates and food consumption statistics of 24 countries. *Med Hypotheses* **7**, 907–18.

1613. Seftel, H.C., Keeley, K.J. & Walker, A.R.P. (1963) Characteristics of South African Bantu who have suffered from myocardial infarction. *Am J Cardiol* **12**, 149–56.

1614. Segall, J.J. (1994) Dietary lactose as a possible risk factor for ischaemic heart disease: review of epidemiology. *Int J Cardiol* **46**, 197–207.

1615. Segall, J.J. (2000) Cardiovascular disease in South Asians. *Lancet* **356**, 1853.

1616. Segall, J.J. (2002) Plausibility of dietary lactose as a coronary risk factor. *J Nutr Environ Med* **12**, 217–29.

1617. Seidell, J.C., Andres, R., Sorkin, J.D. & Muller, D.C. (1994) The sagittal waist diameter and mortality in men: the Baltimore Longitudinal Study on Aging. *Int J Obes Relat Metab Disord* **18**, 61–7.

1618. Sellmeyer, D.E., Schloetter, M. & Sebastian, A. (2002) Potassium citrate prevents increased urine calcium excretion and bone resorption induced by a high sodium chloride diet. *J Clin Endocrinol Metab* **87**, 2008–12.

1619. Sellmeyer, D.E., Stone, K.L., Sebastian, A. & Cummings, S.R. (2001) A high ratio of dietary animal to vegetable protein increases the rate of bone loss and the risk of fracture in postmenopausal women. Study of Osteoporotic Fractures Research Group. *Am J Clin Nutr* **73**, 118–22.

1620. Selvin, E., Marinopoulos, S., Berkenblit, G., *et al.* (2004) Meta-analysis: glycosylated hemoglobin and cardiovascular disease in diabetes mellitus. *Ann Intern Med* **141**, 421–31.

1621. Sennerby, U., Farahmand, B., Ahlbom, A., Ljunghall, S. & Michaelsson, K. (2007) Cardiovascular diseases and future risk of hip fracture in women. *Osteoporos Int* **18**, 1355–62.

1622. Seo, H.S., DeNardo, D.G., Jacquot, Y., *et al.* (2006) Stimulatory effect of genistein and apigenin on the growth of breast cancer cells correlates with their ability to activate ER alpha. *Breast Cancer Res Treat* **99**, 121–34.

1623. Sesso, H.D., Buring, J.E., Christen, W.G., *et al.* (2008) Vitamins E and C in the prevention of cardiovascular disease in men: the Physicians' Health Study II randomized controlled trial. *JAMA* **300**, 2123–33.

1624. Sesso, H.D., Paffenbarger, R.S., Jr., Oguma, Y. & Lee, I.M. (2003) Lack of association between tea and cardiovascular disease in college alumni. *Int J Epidemiol* **32**, 527–33.

1625. Sesti, G. (2006) Pathophysiology of insulin resistance. *Best Pract Res Clin Endocrinol Metab* **20**, 665–79.

1626. Shaffer, E.A. (2005) Epidemiology and risk factors for gallstone disease: has the paradigm changed in the 21st century? *Curr Gastroenterol Rep* **7**, 132–40.

1627. Shaffer, E.A. (2006) Gallstone disease: epidemiology of gallbladder stone disease. *Best Pract Res Clin Gastroenterol* **20**, 981–96.

1628. Shai, I., Schwarzfuchs, D., Henkin, Y., *et al.* (2008) Weight loss with a low-carbohydrate, Mediterranean, or low-fat diet. *N Engl J Med* **359**, 229–41.

1629. Shalitin, S. & Phillip, M. (2003) Role of obesity and leptin in the pubertal process and pubertal growth – a review. *Int J Obes Relat Metab Disord* **27**, 869–74.

1630. Shanik, M.H., Xu, Y., Skrha, J., *et al.* (2008) Insulin resistance and hyperinsulinemia: is hyperinsulinemia the cart or the horse? *Diabetes Care* **31** (Suppl 2), S262–8.

1631. Shaper, A. (1962) Cardiovascular studies in the Samburu tribe of northern Kenya. *Am Heart J* **63**, 437–442.

1632. Shaper, A.G. (1972) Cardiovascular disease in the tropics. IV. Coronary heart disease. *BMJ* **4**, 32–5.

1633. Shaper, A.G., Jonea, K.W., Jones, M. & Kyobe, J. (1963) Serum lipids in three nomadic tribes of Northern Kenya. *Am J Clin Nutr* **13**, 135–46.

1634. Shaper, A.G., Wright, D.H. & Kyobe, J. (1969) Blood pressure and body build in three nomadic tribes of northern Kenya. *East Afr Med J* **46**, 273–81.

1635. Shapses, S.A. & Riedt, C.S. (2006) Bone, body weight, and weight reduction: what are the concerns? *J Nutr* **136**, 1453–6.

1636. Sharan, R.N. & Wary, K.K. (1992) Study of unscheduled DNA synthesis following exposure of human cells to arecoline and extracts of betel nut in vitro. *Mutat Res* **278**, 271–6.

1637. Sharma, R. & Anker, S.D. (2002) From tissue wasting to cachexia: changes in peripheral blood flow and skeletal musculature. *Eur Heart J Suppl* **4**, D12–7.

1638. Sharma, S., Adrogue, J.V., Golfman, L., *et al.* (2004) Intramyocardial lipid accumulation in the failing human heart resembles the lipotoxic rat heart. *Faseb J* **18**, 1692–700.

1639. Shechter, M., Sharir, M., Labrador, M.J., *et al.* (2000) Oral magnesium therapy improves endothelial function in patients with coronary artery disease. *Circulation* **102**, 2353–8.

1640. Shechter, Y. (1983) Bound lectins that mimic insulin produce persistent insulin-like activities. *Endocrinology* **113**, 1921–6.

1641. Shechter, Y. & Sela, B.A. (1981) Insulin-like effects of wax bean agglutinin in rat adipocytes. *Biochem Biophys Res Commun* **98**, 367–73.

1642. Shen, W., Chen, J., Punyanitya, M., *et al.* (2007) MRI-measured bone marrow adipose tissue is inversely related to DXA-measured bone mineral in Caucasian women. *Osteoporos Int* **18**, 641–7.

1643. Shephard, R.J. & Godin, G. (1976) Energy balance of an Eskimo community. In: *Circumpolar health* (R.J. Shephard & S. Itoh eds). University of Toronto Press, Toronto, pp. 106–12.

1644. Shewry, P.R. & Halford, N.G. (2002) Cereal seed storage proteins: structures, properties and role in grain utilization. *J Exp Bot* **53**, 947–58.

1645. Shimamoto, T., Komachi, Y., Inada, H., *et al.* (1989) Trends for coronary heart disease and stroke and their risk factors in Japan. *Circulation* **79**, 503–15.

1645a. Shingu, M., Hashimoto, M., Nobunaga, M., Isayama, T., Yasutake, C. & Naono, T. (1994) Production of soluble ICAM-1 by mononuclear cells from patients with rheumatoid arthritis. *Inflammation* **18**, 23–34.

1646. Shinton, R. & Beevers, G. (1989) Meta-analysis of relation between cigarette smoking and stroke. *B M J* **298**, 789–94.

1647. Shipp, A., Lawrence, G., Gentry, R., *et al.* (2006) Acrylamide: review of toxicity data and dose-response analyses for cancer and noncancer effects. *Crit Rev Toxicol* **36**, 481–608.

1648. Shortt, C. & Flynn, A. (1990) Sodium-calcium inter-relationships with specific reference to osteoporosis. *Nutr Res Rev* **3**, 101–15.

1649. Sichieri, R., Moura, A.S., Genelhu, V., Hu, F. & Willett, W.C. (2007) An 18-mo randomized trial of a low-glycemic-index diet and weight change in Brazilian women. *Am J Clin Nutr* **86**, 707–13.

1650. Siegmund, R., Beirmann, K. & Schiefenhövel, W. (1990) Ontogenic development of time patterns in food intake – a study of German infants and preliminary data from Trobriand infants (Papua New Guinea). *J Interdiscipl Res* **21**, 246–8.

1651. Sieri, S., Krogh, V., Ferrari, P., *et al.* (2008) Dietary fat and breast cancer risk in the European Prospective Investigation into Cancer and Nutrition. *Am J Clin Nutr* **88**, 1304–12.

1652. Sikes, S.K. (1968) The disturbed habitat and its effect on the health of animal populations, with special reference to cardiovascular disease in elephants. *Proc R Soc Med* **61**, 160–61.

1653. Simoni, D. & Tolomeo, M. (2001) Retinoids, apoptosis and cancer. *Curr Pharm Des* **7**, 1823–37.

1654. Simons, L.A. (1986) Interrelationships of lipids and lipoproteins with coronary artery disease mortality in 19 countries. *Am J Cardiol* **57**, 5G–10G.

1655. Simopoulos, A.P. (2001) Evolutionary aspects of diet and essential fatty acids. *World Rev Nutr Diet* **88**, 18–27.

1656. Simopoulos, A.P. (2001) The Mediterranean diets: what is so special about the diet of Greece? The scientific evidence. *J Nutr* **131**, 3065S–73S.

1657. Simpson, H.C., Barker, K., Carter, R.D., Cassels, E. & Mann, J.I. (1982) Low dietary intake of linoleic acid predisposes to myocardial infarction. *Br Med J Clin Res Ed* **285**, 683–4.

1658. Simpson, M.D. & Norris, J.M. (2008) Mucosal immunity and type 1 diabetes: looking at the horizon beyond cow's milk. *Pediatr Diabetes* **9**, 431–3.

1659. Sinaiko, A.R., Jacobs, D.R., Jr., Steinberger, J., *et al.* (2001) Insulin resistance syndrome in childhood: associations of the euglycemic insulin clamp and fasting insulin with fatness and other risk factors. *J Pediatr* **139**, 700–707.

1660. Sinaiko, A.R., Steinberger, J., Moran, A., Prineas, R.J. & Jacobs, D.R., Jr. (2002) Relation of insulin resistance to blood pressure in childhood. *J Hypertens* **20**, 509–17.

1661. Singh, R.B., Dubnov, G., Niaz, M.A., *et al.* (2002) Effect of an Indo-Mediterranean diet on progression of coronary artery disease in high risk patients (Indo-Mediterranean Diet Heart Study): a randomised single-blind trial. *Lancet* **360**, 1455–61.

1662. Singh, R.B., Rastogi, S.S., Verma, R., *et al.* (1992) Randomised controlled trial of cardioprotective diet in patients with recent acute myocardial infarction: results of one year follow up. *BMJ* **304**, 1015–9.

1663. Singh-Manoux, A. & Marmot, M. (2005) High blood pressure was associated with cognitive function in middle-age in the Whitehall II study. *J Clin Epidemiol* **58**, 1308–15.

1664. Sinitskaya, N., Gourmelen, S., Schuster-Klein, C., *et al.* (2007) Increasing the fat-to-carbohydrate ratio in a high-fat diet prevents the development of obesity but not a prediabetic state in rats. *Clin Sci (Lond)* **113**, 417–25.

1665. Sinnett, P. (1977) *The people of Murapin*. EW Classey Ltd, Oxford.

1666. Sinnett, P. & Buck, L. (1974) Coronary heart disease in Papua New Guinea: present and future. *P N G Med J* **17**, 242–7.

1667. Sinnett, P.F., Kevau, I.H. & Tyson, D. (1992) Social change and the emergence of degenerative cardiovascular disease in Papua New Guinea. In: *Human biology in Papua New Guinea. The small cosmos* (R.D. Attenborough & M.P. Alpers eds). Clarendon Press, Oxford, pp. 373–86.

1668. Sinnett, P.F. & Whyte, H.M. (1973) Epidemiological studies in a highland population of New Guinea: environment, culture, and health status. *Human Ecology* **1**, 245–77.

1669. Sinnett, P.F. & Whyte, H.M. (1973) Epidemiological studies in a total highland population, Tukisenta, New Guinea. Cardiovascular disease and relevant clinical, electrocardiographic, radiological and biochemical findings. *J Chronic Dis* **26**, 265–90.

1670. Sjögren, P., Rosell, M., Skoglund-Andersson, C., *et al.* (2004) Milk-derived fatty acids are associated with a more favorable LDL particle size distribution in healthy men. *J Nutr* **134**, 1729–35.

1671. Sjolander, A., Magnusson, K.E. & Latkovic, S. (1984) The effect of concanavalin A and wheat germ agglutinin on the ultrastructure and permeability of rat intestine. A possible model for an intestinal allergic reaction. *Int Arch Allergy Appl Immunol* **75**, 230–36.

1671a. Sjolander, A., Magnusson, K.E. & Latkovic, S. (1986) Morphological changes of rat small intestine after short-time exposure to concanavalin A or wheat germ agglutinin. *Cell Struct Funct* **11**, 285–93.

1672. Sjolin, J., Hjort, G., Friman, G. & Hambraeus, L. (1987) Urinary excretion of 1-methylhistidine: a qualitative indicator of exogenous 3-methylhistidine and intake of meats from various sources. *Metabolism* **36**, 1175–84.

1673. Sjostrom, L., Narbro, K., Sjostrom, C.D., *et al.* (2007) Effects of bariatric surgery on mortality in Swedish obese subjects. *N Engl J Med* **357**, 741–52.

1674. Skeller, E. (1954) Anthropological and ophthalmological studies on the Angmagssalik Eskimos. *Meddelelser om Grønland* **107**, 167–211.

1675. Skog, K., Augustsson, K., Steineck, G., Stenberg, M. & Jagerstad, M. (1997) Polar and non-polar heterocyclic amines in cooked fish and meat products and their corresponding pan residues. *Food Chem Toxicol* **35**, 555–65.

1676. Sköldstam, L. (2002) Reumatoid artrit, kost och evolutionsmedicin. *Medikament*, 68–72.

1677. Sköldstam, L., Hagfors, L. & Johansson, G. (2002) Reumatoid artrit och kretensisk medelhavskost. *Svensk Rehabilitering*, 45–51.

1678. Sköldstam, L., Larsson, L. & Lindström, F.D. (1979) Effect of fasting and lactovegetarian diet on rheumatoid arthritis. *Scand J Rheumatol* **8**, 249–55.

1679. Skorupa, D.A., Dervisefendic, A., Zwiener, J. & Pletcher, S.D. (2008) Dietary composition specifies consumption, obesity, and lifespan in Drosophila melanogaster. *Aging Cell* **7**, 478–90.

1680. Skov, A.R., Haulrik, N., Toubro, S., Molgaard, C. & Astrup, A. (2002) Effect of protein intake on bone mineralization during weight loss: a 6-month trial. *Obes Res* **10**, 432–8.

1681. Skov, A.R., Toubro, S., Ronn, B., Holm, L. & Astrup, A. (1999) Randomized trial on protein vs carbohydrate in ad libitum fat reduced diet for the treatment of obesity. *Int J Obes Relat Metab Disord* **23**, 528–36.

1682. Skyler, J.S., Bergenstal, R., Bonow, R.O., *et al.* (2009) Intensive glycemic control and the prevention of cardiovascular events: implications of the ACCORD, ADVANCE, and VA diabetes trials: a position statement of the American Diabetes Association and a scientific statement of the American College of Cardiology Foundation and the American Heart Association. *Diabetes Care* **32**, 187–92.

1683. Slavin, J.L., Martini, M.C., Jacobs, D.R., Jr. & Marquart, L. (1999) Plausible mechanisms for the protectiveness of whole grains. *Am J Clin Nutr* **70**, 459S–63S.

1684. Smedman, A.E., Gustafsson, I.B., Berglund, L.G. & Vessby, B.O. (1999) Pentadecanoic acid in serum as a marker for intake of milk fat: relations between intake of milk fat and metabolic risk factors. *Am J Clin Nutr* **69**, 22–9.

1685. Smith, E.O. (1999) Evolution, substance abuse, and addiction. In: *Evolutionary Medicine* (W.R. Trevathan, E.O. Smith & J.J. McKenna eds). Oxford University Press, Oxford, pp. 375–405.

1686. Smith, J. & Godlee, F. (2005) Investigating allegations of scientific misconduct. *BMJ* **331**, 245–6.

1687. Smith, P.G. & Day, N.E. (1984) The design of case-control studies: the influence of confounding and interaction effects. *Int J Epidemiol* **13**, 356–65.

1688. Smith, S.C., Jr., Blair, S.N., Bonow, R.O., *et al.* (2001) AHA/ACC Scientific Statement: AHA/ACC guidelines for preventing heart attack and death in patients with atherosclerotic cardiovascular disease: 2001 update: a statement for healthcare professionals from the American Heart Association and the American College of Cardiology. *Circulation* **104**, 1577–9.

1689. Smith-Warner, S.A. & Stampfer, M.J. (2007) Fat intake and breast cancer revisited. *J Natl Cancer Inst* **99**, 418–9.

1690. Smithard, A., Glazebrook, C. & Williams, H.C. (2001) Acne prevalence, knowledge about acne and psychological morbidity in mid-adolescence: a community-based study. *Br J Dermatol* **145**, 274–9.

1691. Snijder, M.B., van Dam, R.M., Visser, M., *et al.* (2005) Adiposity in relation to vitamin D status and parathyroid hormone levels: a population-based study in older men and women. *J Clin Endocrinol Metab* **90**, 4119–23.

1692. Snowdon, D.A., Kemper, S.J., Mortimer, J.A., *et al.* (1996) Linguistic ability in early life and cognitive function and Alzheimer's disease in late life. Findings from the Nun Study. *JAMA* **275**, 528–32.

1693. Sofi, A., Conti, A.A., Gori, A.M., *et al.* (2007) Coffee consumption and risk of coronary heart disease: a meta-analysis. *Nutr Metab Cardiovasc Dis* **17**, 209–23.

1694. Sofi, F., Cesari, F., Abbate, R., Gensini, G.F. & Casini, A. (2008) Adherence to Mediterranean diet and health status: meta-analysis. *BMJ* **337**, a1344.

1695. Soh, N.L. & Brand-Miller, J. (1999) The glycaemic index of potatoes: the effect of variety, cooking method and maturity. *Eur J Clin Nutr* **53**, 249–54.

1696. Solberg, L.A. & McGarry, P.A. (1972) Cerebral atherosclerosis in Negroes and Caucasians. *Atherosclerosis* **16**, 141–54.

1697. Solomon, L. (1979) Bone density in ageing Caucasian and African populations. *Lancet* **2**, 1326–30.

1698. Somers, K. (1974) Cardiology in Papua New Guinea. *P N G Med J* 17, 235–41.
1699. Song, Y., Manson, J.E., Cook, N.R., *et al.* (2005) Dietary magnesium intake and risk of cardiovascular disease among women. *Am J Cardiol* 96, 1135–41.
1700. Sorensen, T.I., Rissanen, A., Korkeila, M. & Kaprio, J. (2005) Intention to lose weight, weight changes, and 18-y mortality in overweight individuals without co-morbidities. *PLoS Med* 2, e171.
1701. Spady, D.K. (1999) Dietary fatty acids and atherosclerosis regression. *Br J Nutr* 82, 337–8.
1702. Spielman, R.S., Fajans, S.S., Neel, J.V., *et al.* (1982) Glucose tolerance in two unacculturated Indian tribes of Brazil. *Diabetologia* 23, 90–3.
1703. Spivey Fox, M.R. & Tao, S.-H. (1989) Antinutritive effects of phytate and other phosphorylated derivatives. In: *Nutritional toxicology*, Vol. 3 (J.N. Hathcock ed). Academic Press, New York, pp. 59–96.
1704. Spoelstra-de Man, A.M., Brouwer, C.B., Stehouwer, C.D. & Smulders, Y.M. (2001) Rapid progression of albumin excretion is an independent predictor of cardiovascular mortality in patients with type 2 diabetes and microalbuminuria. *Diabetes Care* 24, 2097–101.
1705. Stabler, S.P. & Allen, R.H. (2004) Vitamin B12 deficiency as a worldwide problem. *Annu Rev Nutr* 24, 299–326.
1706. Stambolian, D., Ibay, G., Reider, L., *et al.* (2006) Genome-wide scan of additional Jewish families confirms linkage of a myopia susceptibility locus to chromosome 22q12. *Mol Vis* 12, 1499–505.
1707. Stamler, J., Wentworth, D. & Neaton, J.D. (1986) Is relationship between serum cholesterol and risk of premature death from coronary heart disease continuous and graded? Findings in 356,222 primary screenees of the Multiple Risk Factor Intervention Trial (MRFIT). *JAMA* 256, 2823–8.
1708. Stampfer, M.J., Sacks, F.M., Salvini, S., Willett, W.C. & Hennekens, C.H. (1991) A prospective study of cholesterol, apolipoproteins, and the risk of myocardial infarction [see comments]. *N Engl J Med* 325, 373–81.
1709. Stanford, C.B. (1999) *The hunting apes. Meat eating and the origins of human behaviour.* Princeton University Press, Princeton.
1710. Stanford, C.B., Wallis, J., Matama, H. & Goodall, J. (1994) Patterns of predation by chimpanzees on red colobus monkeys in Gombe National Park, 1982–1991. *Am J Phys Anthropol* 94, 213–28.
1711. Stanhope, J.M. (1968) Blood pressures of the Tinam-Aigram people, near Simbai, Madang District. *P N G Med J* 11, 60–1.
1712. Stanhope, J.M. (1969) Mortality and population growth: Losuia area, Kiriwina, Trobriand Islands. *Papua New Guinea Med J* 12, 42–48.
1713. Stanhope, J.M., Sampson, V.M. & Prior, I.A. (1981) The Tokelau Island Migrant Study: serum lipid concentration in two environments. *J Chronic Dis* 34, 45–55.
1714. Stanner, S.A., Hughes, J., Kelly, C.N. & Buttriss, J. (2004) A review of the epidemiological evidence for the 'antioxidant hypothesis'. *Public Health Nutr* 7, 407–22.
1715. Stary, H.C. (2000) Lipid and macrophage accumulations in arteries of children and the development of atherosclerosis. *Am J Clin Nutr* 72, 1297S–306S.
1716. Stearns, S.C. (1999) *Evolution in health and disease.* Oxford University Press, Oxford.
1717. Stegmayr, B., Asplund, K., Kuulasmaa, K., *et al.* (1997) Stroke incidence and mortality correlated to stroke risk factors in the WHO MONICA Project. An ecological study of 18 populations. *Stroke* 28, 1367–74.
1718. Stehbens, W.E. (2001) Coronary heart disease, hypercholesterolemia, and atherosclerosis. I. False premises. *Exp Mol Pathol* 70, 103–19.
1719. Steinberg, D. & Witztum, J.L. (2002) Is the oxidative modification hypothesis relevant to human atherosclerosis? Do the antioxidant trials conducted to date refute the hypothesis? *Circulation* 105, 2107–11.
1720. Steiner, P.E. (1946) Necropsies on Okinawans. Anantomic and pathologic observations. *Arch Pathol* 42, 359–80.

1721. Stender, S., Dyerberg, J. & Astrup, A. (2006) High levels of industrially produced trans fat in popular fast foods. *N Engl J Med* **354**, 1650–52.

1722. Stenvinkel, P. (2001) Inflammatory and atherosclerotic interactions in the depleted uremic patient. *Blood Purif* **19**, 53–61.

1723. Sterne, J.A. & Egger, M. (2001) Funnel plots for detecting bias in meta-analysis: guidelines on choice of axis. *J Clin Epidemiol* **54**, 1046–55.

1724. Stevens, J., Cai, J., Pamuk, E.R., *et al.* (1998) The effect of age on the association between body-mass index and mortality. *N Engl J Med* **338**, 1–7.

1725. Stewart, S., MacIntyre, K., Hole, D.J., Capewell, S. & McMurray, J.J. (2001) More 'malignant' than cancer? Five-year survival following a first admission for heart failure. *Eur J Heart Fail* **3**, 315–22.

1726. Stich, H.F., Mathew, B., Sankaranarayanan, R. & Nair, M.K. (1991) Remission of oral precancerous lesions of tobacco/areca nut chewers following administration of beta-carotene or vitamin A, and maintenance of the protective effect. *Cancer Detect Prev* **15**, 93–8.

1727. Stills, H.F., Jr., Bullock, B.C. & Clarkson, T.B. (1983) Increased atherosclerosis and glomerulonephritis in cynomolgus monkeys (Macaca fascicularis) given injections of BSA over an extended period of time. *Am J Pathol* **113**, 222–34.

1728. Stipanuk, M.H. (1999) Homocysteine, cysteine, and taurine. In: *Modern nutrition in health and disease* (M.E. Shils, J.A. Olson, M. Shike & A.C. Ross eds). Lippincott Williams & Wilkins, Philadelphia, PA, pp. 543–58.

1729. Stoll, B.A. (2002) Upper abdominal obesity, insulin resistance and breast cancer risk. *Int J Obes Relat Metab Disord* **26**, 747–53.

1730. Stout, L.C. & Bohorquez, F. (1974) Significance of intimal arterial changes in non-human vertebrates. *Med Clin North Am* **58**, 245–55.

1731. Stout, R.W. & Vallance-Owen, J. (1969) Insulin and atheroma. *Lancet* **1**, 1078–80.

1732. Stout, S.D. (1992) Methods of determining age at death using bone microstructure. In: *Skeletal biology of past peoples: research methods* (S.R. Saunders & A. Katzenberg eds). Wiley-Liss, New York, pp. 21–35.

1733. Stranges, S., Marshall, J.R., Natarajan, R., *et al.* (2007) Effects of long-term selenium supplementation on the incidence of type 2 diabetes: a randomized trial. *Ann Intern Med* **147**, 217–23.

1734. Stratton, I.M., Adler, A.I., Neil, H.A., *et al.* (2000) Association of glycaemia with macrovascular and microvascular complications of type 2 diabetes (UKPDS 35): prospective observational study. *BMJ* **321**, 405–12.

1735. Streppel, M.T., Ocke, M.C., Boshuizen, H.C., Kok, F.J. & Kromhout, D. (2008) Dietary fiber intake in relation to coronary heart disease and all-cause mortality over 40 y: the Zutphen Study. *Am J Clin Nutr* **88**, 1119–25.

1736. Strickland, S.S. & Ulijaszek, S.J. (1993) Body mass index, ageing and differential reported morbidity in rural Sarawak. *Eur J Clin Nutr* **47**, 9–19.

1737. Stringer, C. (2003) Human evolution: out of Ethiopia. *Nature* **423**, 692–3, 695.

1738. Stuart-Macadam, P. (1992) Porotic hyperostosis: a new perspective. *Am J Phys Anthropol* **87**, 39–47.

1739. Stuart-Macadam, P.L. (1989) Nutritional deficiency diseases: a survey of scurvy, rickets, and iron-deficiency anemia. In: *Reconstruction of life from the human skeleton* (M.Y. Işcan & K.A.R. Kennedy eds). Wiley-Liss, New York, pp. 201–22.

1740. Sugiishi, M. & Takatsu, F. (1993) Cigarette smoking is a major risk factor for coronary spasm. *Circulation* **87**, 76–9.

1741. Sugimoto, K., Fujimura, A., Takasaki, I., *et al.* (1998) Effects of renin-angiotensin system blockade and dietary salt intake on left ventricular hypertrophy in Dahl salt-sensitive rats. *Hypertens Res* **21**, 163–8.

1742. Sullivan, M., Karlsson, J., Sjostrom, L., *et al.* (1993) Swedish obese subjects (SOS)–an intervention study of obesity. Baseline evaluation of health and psychosocial functioning in the first 1743 subjects examined. *Int J Obes Relat Metab Disord* **17**, 503–12.

1743. Summerbell, C.D., Cameron, C. & Glasziou, P.P. (2008) WITHDRAWN: advice on low-fat diets for obesity. *Cochrane Database Syst Rev*, CD003640.

1744. Summers, L.K., Fielding, B.A., Bradshaw, H.A., *et al.* (2002) Substituting dietary saturated fat with polyunsaturated fat changes abdominal fat distribution and improves insulin sensitivity. *Diabetologia* **45**, 369–77.

1745. Sun, S.Y. & Lotan, R. (2002) Retinoids and their receptors in cancer development and chemoprevention. *Crit Rev Oncol Hematol* **41**, 41–55.

1746. Sundqvist, K. & Grafstrom, R.C. (1992) Effects of areca nut on growth, differentiation and formation of DNA damage in cultured human buccal epithelial cells. *Int J Cancer* **52**, 305–10.

1747. Surmacz, E. (2007) Obesity hormone leptin: a new target in breast cancer? *Breast Cancer Res* **9**, 301.

1748. Suzuki, M., Yamamoto, D., Suzuki, T., *et al.* (2006) High fat and high fructose diet induced intracranial atherosclerosis and enhanced vasoconstrictor responses in non-human primate. *Life Sci* **80**, 200–204.

1749. Svanberg, U. & Sandberg, A.-S. (1989) Improved iron availability in weaning foods using germination and fermentation. In: *Nutrient availability: chemical and biological aspects* (D.A.T. Southgate, I.T. Johnson & G.R. Fenwick eds). Cambridge University Press, Cambridge, pp. 179–81.

1750. Svensson, M. & Eriksson, J.W. (2006) Insulin resistance in diabetic nephropathy–cause or consequence? *Diabetes Metab Res Rev* **22**, 401–10.

1751. Swerdlow, A.J., Higgins, C.D., Adlard, P. & Preece, M.A. (2002) Risk of cancer in patients treated with human pituitary growth hormone in the UK, 1959–85: a cohort study. *Lancet* **360**, 273–7.

1752. Swinburn, B.A., Nyomba, B.L., Saad, M.F., *et al.* (1991) Insulin resistance associated with lower rates of weight gain in Pima Indians. *J Clin Invest* **88**, 168–73.

1753. Szczech, R., Hering, D. & Narkiewicz, K. (2004) Smoking and cardiovascular risk: new mechanisms and further evidence for a 'guilty' verdict. *J Hypertens* **22**, 31–4.

1754. Szczepaniak, L.S., Victor, R.G., Orci, L. & Unger, R.H. (2007) Forgotten but not gone: the rediscovery of fatty heart, the most common unrecognized disease in America. *Circ Res* **101**, 759–67.

1755. Szulc, P., Munoz, F., Marchand, F. & Delmas, P.D. (2001) Semiquantitative evaluation of prevalent vertebral deformities in men and their relationship with osteoporosis: the MINOS study. *Osteoporos Int* **12**, 302–10.

1756. Tabas, I., Williams, K.J. & Boren, J. (2007) Subendothelial lipoprotein retention as the initiating process in atherosclerosis: update and therapeutic implications. *Circulation* **116**, 1832–44.

1757. Takahashi, E. (1966) Growth and environmental factors in Japan. *Hum Biol* **38**, 112–30.

1758. Takishita, S., Fukiyama, K., Eto, T., *et al.* (1996) Blood pressure and its regulation in spontaneously hypertensive rats bred on the lowest sodium diet for normal growth. *Hypertension* **27**, 90–95.

1759. Taleb, S., Herbin, O., Ait-Oufella, H., *et al.* (2007) Defective leptin/leptin receptor signaling improves regulatory T cell immune response and protects mice from atherosclerosis. *Arterioscler Thromb Vasc Biol* **27**, 2691–8.

1760. Tallman, M.S., Nabhan, C., Feusner, J.H. & Rowe, J.M. (2002) Acute promyelocytic leukemia: evolving therapeutic strategies. *Blood* **99**, 759–67.

1761. Tanaka, H., Tanaka, Y., Hayashi, M., *et al.* (1982) Secular trends in mortality for cerebrovascular diseases in Japan, 1960 to 1979. *Stroke* **13**, 574–81.

1762. Tang, B.M., Eslick, G.D., Nowson, C., Smith, C. & Bensoussan, A. (2007) Use of calcium or calcium in combination with vitamin D supplementation to prevent fractures and bone loss in people aged 50 years and older: a meta-analysis. *Lancet* **370**, 657–66.

1763. Tanne, D., Koren-Morag, N., Graff, E. & Goldbourt, U. (2001) Blood lipids and first-ever ischemic stroke/transient ischemic attack in the Bezafibrate Infarction Prevention (BIP) Registry: high triglycerides constitute an independent risk factor. *Circulation* **104**, 2892–7.

1764. Tanner, J.M., Hayashi, T., Preece, M.A. & Cameron, N. (1982) Increase in length of leg relative to trunk in Japanese children and adults from 1957 to 1977: comparison with British and with Japanese Americans. *Ann Hum Biol* **9**, 411–23.

1765. Tapp, D.C., Wortham, W.G., Addison, J.F., *et al.* (1989) Food restriction retards body growth and prevents end-stage renal pathology in remnant kidneys of rats regardless of protein intake. *Lab Invest* **60**, 184–95.

1766. Taskinen, M.R. (2003) LDL-cholesterol, HDL-cholesterol or triglycerides – which is the culprit? *Diabetes Res Clin Pract* **61** (Suppl 1), S19–26.

1767. Tavani, A., Gallus, S., Bosetti, C., *et al.* (2006) Dietary iron intake and risk of non-fatal acute myocardial infarction. *Public Health Nutr* **9**, 480–84.

1768. Taylor, C.B. & Ho, K.J. (1971) Studies on the Masai. *Am J Clin Nutr* **24**, 1291–3.

1769. Taylor, R., Badcock, J., King, H., *et al.* (1992) Dietary intake, exercise, obesity and non-communicable disease in rural and urban populations of three Pacific Island countries. *J Am Coll Nutr* **11**, 283–93.

1770. Taylor, R., Bennett, P., Uili, R., *et al.* (1987) Hypertension and indicators of coronary heart disease in Wallis Polynesians: an urban-rural comparison. *Eur J Epidemiol* **3**, 247–56.

1771. Taylor, R. & Thoma, K. (1985) Mortality patterns in the modernized Pacific Island nation of Nauru. *Am J Public Health* **75**, 149–55.

1772. Teede, H.J., Dalais, F.S., Kotsopoulos, D., *et al.* (2001) Dietary soy has both beneficial and potentially adverse cardiovascular effects: a placebo-controlled study in men and postmenopausal women. *J Clin Endocrinol Metab* **86**, 3053–60.

1773. Teikari, J.M. (1987) Myopia and stature. *Acta Ophthalmol (Copenh)* **65**, 673–6.

1774. Tejada, C., Strong, J.P., Montenegro, M.R., Restrepo, C. & Solberg, L.A. (1968) Distribution of coronary and aortic atherosclerosis by geographic location, race, and sex. *Lab Invest* **18**, 509–26.

1775. Tengstrand, B., Cederholm, T., Soderqvist, A. & Tidermark, J. (2007) Effects of protein-rich supplementation and nandrolone on bone tissue after a hip fracture. *Clin Nutr* **26**, 460–65.

1776. Terént, A. & Breig-Åsberg, E. (1994) Epidemiological perspectives of body position and arm level in blood pressure measurement. *Blood Pressure* **3**, 156–63.

1777. Teschemacher, H., Koch, G. & Brantl, V. (1997) Milk protein-derived opioid receptor ligands. *Biopolymers* **43**, 99–117.

1778. Thacher, S.M., Vasudevan, J. & Chandraratna, R.A. (2000) Therapeutic applications for ligands of retinoid receptors. *Curr Pharm Des* **6**, 25–58.

1779. Thane, C.W., Stephen, A.M. & Jebb, S.A. (2009) Whole grains and adiposity: little association among British adults. *Eur J Clin Nutr* **63**, 229–37.

1780. Theuwissen, E. & Mensink, R.P. (2008) Water-soluble dietary fibers and cardiovascular disease. *Physiol Behav* **94**, 285–92.

1781. Thiboutot, D. (2001) Hormones and acne: pathophysiology, clinical evaluation, and therapies. *Semin Cutan Med Surg* **20**, 144–53.

1782. Thirsk, J. (1990) *Chapters from the Agrarian History of England and Wales.* Cambridge University Press, Cambridge.

1783. Thomas, D. & Elliott, E.J. (2009) Low glycaemic index, or low glycaemic load, diets for diabetes mellitus. *Cochrane Database Syst Rev*, CD006296.

1784. Thomas, D.E., Elliott, E. & Baur, L. (2007) Low glycaemic index or low glycaemic load diets for overweight and obesity. *Cochrane Database Syst Rev*, CD005105.

1785. Thomas, D.M., Udagawa, N., Hards, D.K., *et al.* (1998) Insulin receptor expression in primary and cultured osteoclast-like cells. *Bone* **23**, 181–6.

1786. Thomas, M.K., Lloyd-Jones, D.M., Thadhani, R.I., *et al.* (1998) Hypovitaminosis D in medical inpatients. *N Engl J Med* 338, 777–83.
1787. Thomas, S.J. & MacLennan, R. (1992) Slaked lime and betel nut cancer in Papua New Guinea. *Lancet* ii, 577–8.
1788. Thomas, W., Davies, J., O'Nea, l.R. & Dimakulangan, A. (1960) Incidence of myocardial infarction correlated with venous and pulmonary thrombosis and embolism. A geographic study based on autopsies in Uganda, East Africa and St Louis, USA. *Am J Cardiol* 5, 41–47.
1789. Thompson, D.D. & Gunness, H.M. (1981) Bone mineral-osteon analysis of Yupik-Inupiaq skeletons. *Am J Phys Anthropol* 55, 1–7.
1790. Thorburn, A.W., Brand, J.C., O'Dea, K., Spargo, R.M. & Truswell, A.S. (1987) Plasma glucose and insulin responses to starchy foods in Australian aborigines: a population now at high risk of diabetes. *Am J Clin Nutr* 46, 282–5.
1791. Thorburn, A.W., Brand, J.C. & Truswell, A.S. (1987) Slowly digested and absorbed carbohydrate in traditional bushfoods: a protective factor against diabetes? *Am J Clin Nutr* 45, 98–106.
1792. Thorogood, M., Mann, J., Appleby, P. & McPherson, K. (1994) Risk of death from cancer and ischaemic heart disease in meat and non- meat eaters [see comments]. *BMJ* 308, 1667–70.
1793. Thorsdottir, I., Birgisdottir, B.E., Johannsdottir, I.M., *et al.* (2000) Different beta-casein fractions in Icelandic versus Scandinavian cow's milk may influence diabetogenicity of cow's milk in infancy and explain low incidence of insulin-dependent diabetes mellitus in Iceland. *Pediatrics* 106, 719–24.
1794. Thorvaldsen, P., Davidsen, M., Bronnum-Hansen, H. & Schroll, M. (1999) Stable stroke occurrence despite incidence reduction in an aging population: stroke trends in the danish monitoring trends and determinants in cardiovascular disease (MONICA) population. *Stroke* 30, 2529–34.
1795. Thouez, J.P., Ekoé, J.M., Foggin, P.M., *et al.* (1990) Obesity, hypertension, hyperuricemia and diabetes mellitus among the Cree and Inuit of Northern Cuébec. *Arct Med Res* 49, 180–88.
1796. Thrailkill, K.M., Lumpkin, C.K., Jr., Bunn, R.C., Kemp, S.F. & Fowlkes, J.L. (2005) Is insulin an anabolic agent in bone? Dissecting the diabetic bone for clues. *Am J Physiol Endocrinol Metab* 289, E735–45.
1797. Tinker, L.F., Bonds, D.E., Margolis, K.L., *et al.* (2008) Low-fat dietary pattern and risk of treated diabetes mellitus in postmenopausal women: the Women's Health Initiative randomized controlled dietary modification trial. *Arch Intern Med* 168, 1500–511.
1798. Tkatch, L., Rapin, C.H., Rizzoli, R., *et al.* (1992) Benefits of oral protein supplementation in elderly patients with fracture of the proximal femur. *J Am Coll Nutr* 11, 519–25.
1799. Toal, C.B. & Leenen, F.H. (1987) Dietary sodium restriction, blood pressure and sympathetic activity in spontaneously hypertensive rats. *J Hypertens* 5, 107–13.
1800. Tobian, L. (1986) High-potassium diets markedly protect against stroke deaths and kidney disease in hypertensive rats, an echo from prehistoric days. *J Hypertens Suppl* 4, S67–76.
1801. Tobian, L., Lange, J.M., Ulm, K.M., Wold, L.J. & Iwai, J. (1984) Potassium prevents death from strokes in hypertensive rats without lowering blood pressure. *J Hypertens Suppl* 2, S363–6.
1802. Tomobe, K., Philbrick, D.J., Ogborn, M.R., Takahashi, H. & Holub, B.J. (1998) Effect of dietary soy protein and genistein on disease progression in mice with polycystic kidney disease. *Am J Kidney Dis* 31, 55–61.
1803. Tonetti, D.A., Zhang, Y., Zhao, H., Lim, S.B. & Constantinou, A.I. (2007) The effect of the phytoestrogens genistein, daidzein, and equol on the growth of tamoxifen-resistant T47D/PKC alpha. *Nutr Cancer* 58, 222–9.
1804. Tovar, A.R., Torre-Villalvazo, I., Ochoa, M., *et al.* (2005) Soy protein reduces hepatic lipotoxicity in hyperinsulinemic obese Zucker fa/fa rats. *J Lipid Res* 46, 1823–32.

1805. Tran, T.T., Naigamwalla, D., Oprescu, A.I., *et al.* (2006) Hyperinsulinemia, but not other factors associated with insulin resistance, acutely enhances colorectal epithelial proliferation in vivo. *Endocrinology* **147**, 1830–37.

1806. Travers, S.H., Jeffers, B.W. & Eckel, R.H. (2002) Insulin resistance during puberty and future fat accumulation. *J Clin Endocrinol Metab* **87**, 3814–8.

1807. Travers, S.H., Labarta, J.I., Gargosky, S.E., *et al.* (1998) Insulin-like growth factor binding protein-I levels are strongly associated with insulin sensitivity and obesity in early pubertal children. *J Clin Endocrinol Metab* **83**, 1935–9.

1808. Tremblay, F., Lavigne, C., Jacques, H. & Marette, A. (2003) Dietary cod protein restores insulin-induced activation of phosphatidylinositol 3-kinase/Akt and GLUT4 translocation to the T-tubules in skeletal muscle of high-fat-fed obese rats. *Diabetes* **52**, 29–37.

1809. Trevathan, W.R., Smith, E.O. & McKenna, J.J. (1999) *Evolutionary medicine.* Oxford University Press, Oxford.

1810. Trichopoulou, A., Toupadaki, N., Tzonou, A., *et al.* (1993) The macronutrient composition of the Greek diet: estimates derived from six case-control studies. *Eur J Clin Nutr* **47**, 549–58.

1811. Troilo, D. & Wallman, J. (1991) The regulation of eye growth and refractive state: an experimental study of emmetropization. *Vision Res* **31**, 1237–50.

1812. Trowell, H.C. (1960) *Non-infective diseases in Africa.* Edward Arnold Ltd, London.

1813. Trowell, H.C. (1981) Hypertension, obesity diabetes mellitus and coronary heart disease. In: *Western diseases: their emergence and prevention* (H.C. Trowell & D.P. Burkitt eds). Edward Arnold, London, pp. 3–32.

1814. Trowell, H.C. & Burkitt, D.P. (1981) *Western diseases: their emergence and prevention.* Harvard University Press, Cambridge, Mass.

1815. Trujillo, J., Ramirez, V., Perez, J., *et al.* (2005) Renal protection by a soy diet in obese Zucker rats is associated with restoration of nitric oxide generation. *Am J Physiol Renal Physiol* **288**, F108–16.

1816. Truswell, A.S. (2002) Cereal grains and coronary heart disease. *Eur J Clin Nutr* **56**, 1–14.

1817. Truswell, A.S. & Hansen, J.D.L. (1976) Medical research among the !Kung. In: *Kalahari Hunter-gatherers* (R.B. Lee & I. DeVore eds). Harvard University Press, Cambridge, Mass, pp. 166–95.

1818. Truswell, A.S., Kennelly, B.M., Hansen, J.D. & Lee, R.B. (1972) Blood pressures of Kung bushmen in Northern Botswana. *Am Heart J* **84**, 5–12.

1819. Truswell, A.S. & Mann, J.I. (1972) Epidemiology of serum lipids in Southern Africa. *Atherosclerosis* **16**, 15–29.

1820. Tsimikas, S., Aikawa, M., Miller, F.J., Jr., *et al.* (2007) Increased plasma oxidized phospholipid:apolipoprotein B-100 ratio with concomitant depletion of oxidized phospholipids from atherosclerotic lesions after dietary lipid-lowering: a potential biomarker of early atherosclerosis regression. *Arterioscler Thromb Vasc Biol* **27**, 175–81.

1821. Tsui, H., Razavi, R., Chan, Y., Yantha, J. & Dosch, H.M. (2007) 'Sensing' autoimmunity in type 1 diabetes. *Trends Mol Med* **13**, 405–13.

1822. Tucker, K.L., Hannan, M.T., Chen, H., *et al.* (1999) Potassium, magnesium, and fruit and vegetable intakes are associated with greater bone mineral density in elderly men and women. *Am J Clin Nutr* **69**, 727–36.

1823. Tunstall-Pedoe, H. (1998) Nuts to you (. . .and you, and you). Eating nuts may be beneficial- though it is unclear why. *BMJ* **317**, 1332–3.

1824. Tuohimaa, P., Tenkanen, L., Syvala, H., *et al.* (2007) Interaction of factors related to the metabolic syndrome and vitamin D on risk of prostate cancer. *Cancer Epidemiol Biomarkers Prev* **16**, 302–7.

1825. Tuomainen, T.P., Kontula, K., Nyyssonen, K., *et al.* (1999) Increased risk of acute myocardial infarction in carriers of the hemochromatosis gene Cys282Tyr mutation : a prospective cohort study in men in eastern Finland. *Circulation* **100**, 1274–9.

1826. Tuomainen, T.P., Punnonen, K., Nyyssonen, K. & Salonen, J.T. (1998) Association between body iron stores and the risk of acute myocardial infarction in men. *Circulation* **97**, 1461–6.

1827. Tuomilehto, J., Jousilahti, P., Rastenyte, D., *et al.* (2001) Urinary sodium excretion and cardiovascular mortality in Finland: a prospective study. *Lancet* **357**, 848–51.

1828. Tuomilehto, J., Lindstrom, J., Eriksson, J.G., *et al.* (2001) Prevention of type 2 diabetes mellitus by changes in lifestyle among subjects with impaired glucose tolerance. *N Engl J Med* **344**, 1343–50.

1829. Tuttle, K.R. (2005) Renal manifestations of the metabolic syndrome. *Nephrol Dial Transplant* **20**, 861–4.

1830. Tuttle, K.R., Shuler, L.A., Packard, D.P., *et al.* (2008) Comparison of low-fat versus Mediterranean-style dietary intervention after first myocardial infarction (from The Heart Institute of Spokane Diet Intervention and Evaluation Trial). *Am J Cardiol* **101**, 1523–30.

1831. Tuzcu, E.M., Kapadia, S.R., Tutar, E., *et al.* (2001) High prevalence of coronary atherosclerosis in asymptomatic teenagers and young adults: evidence from intravascular ultrasound. *Circulation* **103**, 2705–10.

1831a. Udey, M.C., Chaplin, D.D., Wedner, H.J. & Parker, C.W. (1980) Early activation events in lectin stimulated human lymphocytes: evidence that wheat germ agglutinin and mitogenic lectins cause similar early changes in lymphocyte metabolism. *J Immunol* **125**, 1544–50.

1832. Uenishi, K., Ishida, H., Toba, Y., *et al.* (2007) Milk basic protein increases bone mineral density and improves bone metabolism in healthy young women. *Osteoporos Int* **18**, 385–90.

1833. Ueshima, H., Zhang, X.H. & Choudhury, S.R. (2000) Epidemiology of hypertension in China and Japan. *J Hum Hypertens* **14**, 765–9.

1834. UK Prospective Diabetes Study Group (1998) Intensive blood-glucose control with sulphonylureas or insulin compared with conventional treatment and risk of complications in patients with type 2 diabetes (UKPDS 33). UK Prospective Diabetes Study (UKPDS) Group. *Lancet* **352**, 837–53.

1835. Ulijaszek, S.J. (1991) Human dietary change. *Philos Trans R Soc Lond B Biol Sci* **334**, 271–8; discussion 278–9.

1836. Ulijaszek, S.J. & Strickland, S.S. (1993) *Nutritional anthropology: prospects and perspectives*. Smith-Gordon, London.

1837. Unger, R.H. (2002) Lipotoxic diseases. *Annu Rev Med* **53**, 319–36.

1838. Unger, R.H. (2003) Lipid overload and overflow: metabolic trauma and the metabolic syndrome. *Trends Endocrinol Metab* **14**, 398–403.

1839. Unger, R.H. (2003) Minireview: weapons of lean body mass destruction: the role of ectopic lipids in the metabolic syndrome. *Endocrinology* **144**, 5159–65.

1840. Unger, R.H. (2005) Longevity, lipotoxicity and leptin: the adipocyte defense against feasting and famine. *Biochimie* **87**, 57–64.

1841. Unger, R.H., Zhou, Y.T. & Orci, L. (1999) Regulation of fatty acid homeostasis in cells: novel role of leptin. *Proc Natl Acad Sci USA* **96**, 2327–32.

1842. Utzschneider, K.M. & Kahn, S.E. (2006) Review: the role of insulin resistance in nonalcoholic fatty liver disease. *J Clin Endocrinol Metab* **91**, 4753–61.

1843. Uusitupa, M.I. (1994) Fructose in the diabetic diet. *Am J Clin Nutr* **59**, 753S–7S.

1844. Vaarala, O., Atkinson, M.A. & Neu, J. (2008) The 'perfect storm' for type 1 diabetes: the complex interplay between intestinal microbiota, gut permeability, and mucosal immunity. *Diabetes* **57**, 2555–62.

1845. Vacaresse, N., Vieira, O., Robbesyn, F., *et al.* (2001) Phenolic antioxidants trolox and caffeic acid modulate the oxidized LDL- induced EGF-receptor activation. *Br J Pharmacol* **132**, 1777–88.

1846. Vague, J. (1956) The degree of masculine differentiation of obesities: a factor determining predisposition to diabetes, atherosclerosis, gout, and uric calculous disease. *Am J Clin Nutr* **4**, 20–34.

1847. van Berge-Henegouwen, G.P. & Mulder, C.J. (1993) Pioneer in the gluten free diet: Willem-Karel Dicke 1905–1962, over 50 years of gluten free diet. *Gut* **34**, 1473–5.

1848. Van Damme, E.J.M., Peumans, W.J., Pusztai, A. & Bardocz, S. (1998) *Handbook of plant lectins: properties and biomedical applications.* John Wiley, New York.

1849. van de Vijver, L.P., van den Bosch, L.M., van den Brandt, P.A. & Goldbohm, R.A. (2009) Whole-grain consumption, dietary fibre intake and body mass index in the Netherlands cohort study. *Eur J Clin Nutr* **63**, 31–8.

1850. van den Berg, B.M., Nieuwdorp, M., Stroes, E.S. & Vink, H. (2006) Glycocalyx and endothelial (dys) function: from mice to men. *Pharmacol Rep* **58** (Suppl), 75–80.

1850a. van den Bourne, B.E., Kijkmans, B.A., de Rooij, H.H., le Cessie, S. & Verweij, C.L. (1997) Chloroquine and hydroxychloroquine equally affect tumor necrosis factor-alpha, interleukin-6, and interferon-gamma production by peripheral blood mononuclear cells. *J Rheumatol* **24**, 55–60.

1851. van den Brandt, P.A. & Goldbohm, R.A. (2006) Nutrition in the prevention of gastrointestinal cancer. *Best Pract Res Clin Gastroenterol* **20**, 589–603.

1852. van der A, D.l., Peeters, P.H., Grobbee, D.E., *et al.* (2006) HFE mutations and risk of coronary heart disease in middle-aged women. *Eur J Clin Invest* **36**, 682–90.

1853. van der Wielen, R.P., Lowik, M.R., van den Berg, H., *et al.* (1995) Serum vitamin D concentrations among elderly people in Europe. *Lancet* **346**, 207–10.

1854. van Haeften, T.W., Pimenta, W., Mitrakou, A., *et al.* (2002) Disturbances in beta-cell function in impaired fasting glycemia. *Diabetes* **51** (Suppl 1), S265–70.

1855. Van Teeffelen, J.W., Brands, J., Stroes, E.S. & Vink, H. (2007) Endothelial glycocalyx: sweet shield of blood vessels. *Trends Cardiovasc Med* **17**, 101–5.

1856. Vanderjagt, D.J., Freiberger, C., Vu, H.T., *et al.* (2000) The trypsin inhibitor content of 61 wild edible plant foods of Niger. *Plant Foods Hum Nutr* **55**, 335–46.

1857. Vasankari, T.J. & Vasankari, T.M. (2006) Effect of dietary fructose on lipid metabolism, body weight and glucose tolerance in humans. *Scand J Food Nutr* **50**, 55–63.

1858. Velican, C. & Velican, D. (1980) Incidence, topography and light-microscopic feature of coronary atherosclerotic plaques in adults 26–35 years old. *Atherosclerosis* **35**, 111–22.

1859. Velican, D. & Velican, C. (1979) Study of fibrous plaques occurring in the coronary arteries of children. *Atherosclerosis* **33**, 201–5.

1860. Velican, D. & Velican, C. (1980) Atherosclerotic involvement of the coronary arteries of adolescents and young adults. *Atherosclerosis* **36**, 449–60.

1861. Verdery, R.B. & Walford, R.L. (1998) Changes in plasma lipids and lipoproteins in humans during a 2-year period of dietary restriction in Biosphere 2. *Arch Intern Med* **158**, 900–906.

1862. Verhave, J.C., Hillege, H.L., Burgerhof, J.G., *et al.* (2005) The association between atherosclerotic risk factors and renal function in the general population. *Kidney Int* **67**, 1967–73.

1863. Verlee, D.L. (1968) Ophthalmic survey in the Solomon Islands. *Am J Ophthalmol* **66**, 304–19.

1864. Vescini, F., Buffa, A., La Manna, G., *et al.* (2005) Long-term potassium citrate therapy and bone mineral density in idiopathic calcium stone formers. *J Endocrinol Invest* **28**, 218–22.

1865. Vescovo, G., Ravara, B., Gobbo, V., *et al.* (2002) L-Carnitine: a potential treatment for blocking apoptosis and preventing skeletal muscle myopathy in heart failure. *Am J Physiol Cell Physiol* **283**, C802–10.

1866. Vessby, B., Unsitupa, M., Hermansen, K., *et al.* (2001) Substituting dietary saturated for monounsaturated fat impairs insulin sensitivity in healthy men and women: The KANWU Study. *Diabetologia* **44**, 312–9.

1867. Villareal, D.T., Banks, M., Sinacore, D.R., Siener, C. & Klein, S. (2006) Effect of weight loss and exercise on frailty in obese older adults. *Arch Intern Med* **166**, 860–66.

1868. Villarreal, M.G., Ohlsson, J., Abrahamsson, M., Sjostrom, A. & Sjostrand, J. (2000) Myopisation: the refractive tendency in teenagers. Prevalence of myopia among young teenagers in Sweden. *Acta Ophthalmol Scand* **78**, 177–81.

1869. Villegas, J.C. & Broadwell, R.D. (1993) Transcytosis of protein through the mammalian cerebral epithelium and endothelium. II. Adsorptive transcytosis of WGA-HRP and the blood-brain and brain-blood barriers. *J Neurocytol* **22**, 67–80.

1870. Vines, A.P. (1970) *An epidemiological sample survey of the highlands, mainland and island regions of the Territory of Papua and New Guinea*. Department of Public Health, Territory of Papua and New Guinea, Port Moresby.

1871. Vint, F.W. (1937) Postmortem findings in the natives of Kenya. *East Afr Med J* **13**, 332–40.

1872. Visscher, T.L., Seidell, J.C., Molarius, A., *et al.* (2001) A comparison of body mass index, waist-hip ratio and waist circumference as predictors of all-cause mortality among the elderly: the Rotterdam study. *Int J Obes Relat Metab Disord* **25**, 1730–35.

1873. Visser, J., Brugman, S., Klatter, F., *et al.* (2003) Short-term dietary adjustment with a hydrolyzed casein-based diet postpones diabetes development in the diabetes-prone BB rat. *Metabolism* **52**, 333–7.

1874. Vlachopoulos, C., Alexopoulos, N., Dima, I., *et al.* (2006) Acute effect of black and green tea on aortic stiffness and wave reflections. *J Am Coll Nutr* **25**, 216–23.

1875. Volek, J.S., Phinney, S.D., Forsythe, C.E., *et al.* (2009) Carbohydrate restriction has a more favorable impact on the metabolic syndrome than a low fat diet. *Lipids* **44**, 297–309.

1876. Volek, J.S., Sharman, M.J. & Forsythe, C.E. (2005) Modification of lipoproteins by very low-carbohydrate diets. *J Nutr* **135**, 1339–42.

1877. Vollmer, W.M., Sacks, F.M., Ard, J., *et al.* (2001) Effects of diet and sodium intake on blood pressure: subgroup analysis of the DASH-sodium trial. *Ann Intern Med* **135**, 1019–28.

1878. von Haehling, S., Horwich, T.B., Fonarow, G.C. & Anker, S.D. (2007) Tipping the scale: heart failure, body mass index, and prognosis. *Circulation* **116**, 588–90.

1879. Vormann, J. & Daniel, H. (2001) The role of nutrition in human acid-base homeostasis. *Eur J Nutr* **40**, 187–8.

1880. Vorster, H.H., Benade, A.J., Barnard, H.C., *et al.* (1992) Egg intake does not change plasma lipoprotein and coagulation profiles. *Am J Clin Nutr* **55**, 400–410.

1881. Vrba, E.S., Denton, G.H., Partridge, T.C. & Burckle, L.H. (1996) *Paleoclimate and Evolution, with Emphasis on Human Origins*. Yale University Press, New Haven.

1882. Vuguin, P., Saenger, P. & Dimartino-Nardi, J. (2001) Fasting glucose insulin ratio: a useful measure of insulin resistance in girls with premature adrenarche. *J Clin Endocrinol Metab* **86**, 4618–21.

1883. Wagner, J.D., Cefalu, W.T., Anthony, M.S., *et al.* (1997) Dietary soy protein and estrogen replacement therapy improve cardiovascular risk factors and decrease aortic cholesteryl ester content in ovariectomized cynomolgus monkeys. *Metabolism* **46**, 698–705.

1884. Wagner, J.D., Zhang, L., Greaves, K.A., Shadoan, M.K. & Schwenke, D.C. (2000) Soy protein reduces the arterial low-density lipoprotein (LDL) concentration and delivery of LDL cholesterol to the arteries of diabetic and nondiabetic male cynomolgus monkeys. *Metabolism* **49**, 1188–96.

1885. Wainwright, S.A., Marshall, L.M., Ensrud, K.E., *et al.* (2005) Hip fracture in women without osteoporosis. *J Clin Endocrinol Metab* **90**, 2787–93.

1886. Wakai, K., Date, C., Fukui, M., *et al.* (2007) Dietary fiber and risk of colorectal cancer in the Japan collaborative cohort study. *Cancer Epidemiol Biomarkers Prev* **16**, 668–75.

1887. Wald, D., Wald, N.J., Morris, J.K. & Law, M. (2006) Folic acid, homocysteine, and cardiovascular disease: judging causality in the face of inconclusive evidence. *BMJ* **333**, 1114–17.

1888. Walker, A.R. (1975) The epidemiological emergence of ischemic arterial diseases. *Am Heart J* **89**, 133–6.

1889. Walker, A.R.P. (1963) Mortality from coronary heart disease and from cerebral vascular disease in the different racial populations in South Africa. *South Afr Med J* **37**, 1155–9.

1890. Walker, A.R.P. (1964) Overweight and hypertension in emerging populations. *Am Heart J* **68**, 581–5.

1891. Walkingshaw, R. (1964) Control of progressive myopia through modification of diet. *Paper pres. The First International Conference on Myopia*, Chicago.

1892. Wallach, S., Feinblatt, J.D., Carstens, J.H., Jr. & Avioli, L.V. (1992) The bone 'quality' problem. *Calcif Tissue Int* **51**, 169–72.

1893. Walldius, G., Jungner, I., Holme, I., *et al.* (2001) High apolipoprotein B, low apolipoprotein A-I, and improvement in the prediction of fatal myocardial infarction (AMORIS study): a prospective study. *Lancet* **358**, 2026–33.

1894. Wallington, M. (1986) Cancer in Papua New Guinea, 1985. *P N G Med J* **29**, 333–6.

1895. Wallman, J. (1990) Myopia and the control of eye growth. Introduction. *Ciba Found Symp* **155**, 1–4.

1896. Wang, B., Yang, L., Wang, Z. & Zheng, H. (2007) Amyolid precursor protein mediates presynaptic localization and activity of the high-affinity choline transporter. *Proc Natl Acad Sci USA* **104**, 14140–5.

1897. Wang, J., Ruotsalainen, S., Moilanen, L., *et al.* (2008) The metabolic syndrome predicts incident stroke: a 14-year follow-up study in elderly people in Finland. *Stroke* **39**, 1078–83.

1898. Wang, Q., Yu, L.G., Campbell, B.J., Milton, J.D. & Rhodes, J.M. (1998) Identification of intact peanut lectin in peripheral venous blood. *Lancet* **352**, 1831–2.

1899. Wang, X., Qin, X., Demirtas, H., *et al.* (2007) Efficacy of folic acid supplementation in stroke prevention: a meta-analysis. *Lancet* **369**, 1876–82.

1900. Wang, X.Y., Bergdahl, K., Heijbel, A., Liljebris, C. & Bleasdale, J.E. (2001) Analysis of in vitro interactions of protein tyrosine phosphatase 1B with insulin receptors. *Mol Cell Endocrinol* **173**, 109–20.

1901. Wang, Y., McCullough, M.L., Stevens, V.L., *et al.* (2007) Nested case-control study of energy regulation candidate gene single nucleotide polymorphisms and breast cancer. *Anticancer Res* **27**, 589–93.

1902. Wannamethee, S.G. (2001) Serum uric acid is not an independent risk factor for coronary heart disease. *Curr Hypertens Rep* **3**, 190–6.

1903. Wannamethee, S.G., Shaper, A.G. & Lennon, L. (2005) Reasons for intentional weight loss, unintentional weight loss, and mortality in older men. *Arch Intern Med* **165**, 1035–40.

1904. Warensjö, E., Jansson, J.H., Berglund, L., *et al.* (2004) Estimated intake of milk fat is negatively associated with cardiovascular risk factors and does not increase the risk of a first acute myocardial infarction. A prospective case–control study. *Br J Nutr* **91**, 635–42.

1905. Waring, W.S., Webb, D.J. & Maxwell, S.R. (2001) Systemic uric acid administration increases serum antioxidant capacity in healthy volunteers. *J Cardiovasc Pharmacol* **38**, 365–71.

1906. Wasmuth, H.E. & Kolb, H. (2000) Cow's milk and immune-mediated diabetes. *Proc Nutr Soc* **59**, 573–9.

1907. Watkins, M.L., Rasmussen, S.A., Honein, M.A., Botto, L.D. & Moore, C.A. (2003) Maternal obesity and risk for birth defects. *Pediatrics* **111**, 1152–8.

1908. Watts, G.F., Ahmed, W., Quiney, J., *et al.* (1988) Effective lipid lowering diets including lean meat. *Br Med J (Clin Res Ed)* **296**, 235–7.

1909. Watts, G.F., Lewis, B., Brunt, J.N., *et al.* (1992) Effects on coronary artery disease of lipid-lowering diet, or diet plus cholestyramine, in the St Thomas' Atherosclerosis Regression Study (STARS) [see comments]. *Lancet* **339**, 563–9.

1910. Webb, S. (1995) Palaeopathology of Aboriginal Australians. Health and disease across a hunter-gatherer continent. Cambridge University Press, Cambridge.

1911. Weggemans, R.M., Zock, P.L. & Katan, M.B. (2001) Dietary cholesterol from eggs increases the ratio of total cholesterol to high-density lipoprotein cholesterol in humans: a meta-analysis. *Am J Clin Nutr* **73**, 885–91.

1912. Wei, M., Gaskill, S.P., Haffner, S.M. & Stern, M.P. (1997) Waist circumference as the best predictor of noninsulin dependent diabetes mellitus (NIDDM) compared to body mass index, waist/hip ratio and other anthropometric measurements in Mexican Americans – a 7-year prospective study. *Obes Res* **5**, 16–23.

1913. Weickert, M.O., Mohlig, M., Schofl, C., *et al.* (2006) Cereal fiber improves whole-body insulin sensitivity in overweight and obese women. *Diabetes Care* **29**, 775–80.

1914. Weih, M., Wiltfang, J. & Kornhuber, J. (2007) Non-pharmacologic prevention of Alzheimer's disease: nutritional and life-style risk factors. *J Neural Transm* **114**, 1187–97.

1915. Weikert, C., Walter, D., Hoffmann, K., *et al.* (2005) The relation between dietary protein, calcium and bone health in women: results from the EPIC-Potsdam cohort. *Ann Nutr Metab* **49**, 312–8.

1916. Weinbaum, S., Tarbell, J.M. & Damiano, E.R. (2007) The structure and function of the endothelial glycocalyx layer. *Annu Rev Biomed Eng* **9**, 121–67.

1917. Weinberg, J.M. (2006) Lipotoxicity. *Kidney Int* **70**, 1560–6.

1918. Weinehall, L., Hellsten, G., Boman, K., *et al.* (2001) Can a sustainable community intervention reduce the health gap? – 10-year evaluation of a Swedish community intervention program for the prevention of cardiovascular disease. *Scand J Public Health* **56** (Suppl), 59–68.

1919. Weiner, A.B. (1976) *Women of value, men of renown.* University of Texas Press, Austin.

1920. Weiner, A.B. (1988) *The Trobrianders of Papua New Guinea.* Holt, Rinehart and Winston, New York.

1921. Weinsier, R.L. & Krumdieck, C.L. (2000) Dairy foods and bone health: examination of the evidence. *Am J Clin Nutr* **72**, 681–9.

1922. Weir, M.R. & Fink, J.C. (2005) Salt intake and progression of chronic kidney disease: an overlooked modifiable exposure? A commentary. *Am J Kidney Dis* **45**, 176–88.

1923. Welborn, T.A., Dhaliwal, S.S. & Bennett, S.A. (2003) Waist-hip ratio is the dominant risk factor predicting cardiovascular death in Australia. *Med J Aust* **179**, 580–85.

1924. Welch, A.A., Bingham, S.A., Reeve, J. & Khaw, K.T. (2007) More acidic dietary acid-base load is associated with reduced calcaneal broadband ultrasound attenuation in women but not in men: results from the EPIC-Norfolk cohort study. *Am J Clin Nutr* **85**, 1134–41.

1925. Welsh, C.J., Hanglow, A.C., Conn, P., Barker, T.H. & Coombs, R.R. (1985) Early rheumatoid-like synovial lesions in rabbits drinking cow's milk. I. Joint pathology. *Int Arch Allergy Appl Immunol* **78**, 145–51.

1926. West, C.E., Sullivan, D.R., Katan, M.B., Halferkamps, I.L. & van der Torre, H.W. (1990) Boys from populations with high-carbohydrate intake have higher fasting triglyceride levels than boys from populations with high-fat intake. *Am J Epidemiol* **131**, 271–82.

1927. Westerbacka, J., Lammi, K., Hakkinen, A.M., *et al.* (2005) Dietary fat content modifies liver fat in overweight nondiabetic subjects. *J Clin Endocrinol Metab* **90**, 2804–9.

1927a. Weetman, A.P., Volkman, D.J., Burman, K.D., Gerrard, T.L. & Fauci, A.S. (1985) The in vitro regulation of human thyrocyte HLA-DR antigen expression. *J Clin Endocrinol Metab* **61**, 817–24.

1928. Whelton, P.K., He, J., Cutler, J.A., *et al.* (1997) Effects of oral potassium on blood pressure. Meta-analysis of randomized controlled clinical trials. *JAMA* **277**, 1624–32.

1929. Whelton, S.P., Hyre, A.D., Pedersen, B., *et al.* (2005) Effect of dietary fiber intake on blood pressure: a meta-analysis of randomized, controlled clinical trials. *J Hypertens* **23**, 475–81.

1930. White, C. (2005) Suspected research fraud: difficulties of getting at the truth. *BMJ* **331**, 281–8.

1931. Whitehead, C.C. & Fleming, R.H. (2000) Osteoporosis in cage layers. *Poult Sci* **79**, 1033–41.

1932. Whitelaw, D.C., O'Kane, M., Wales, J.K. & Barth, J.H. (2001) Risk factors for coronary heart disease in obese non-diabetic subjects. *Int J Obes Relat Metab Disord* **25**, 1042–6.

1933. Whitlock, G., Lewington, S., Sherliker, P., *et al.* (2009) Body-mass index and cause-specific mortality in 900 000 adults: collaborative analyses of 57 prospective studies. *Lancet* **373**, 1083–96.

1934. Whitney, J.C. (1975) The spontaneous cardiovascular diseases of animals. In: *The pathology of the heart* (A. Pomerance & M.J. Davies eds). Blackwell, Oxford, pp. 579–610.

1935. Whorton, J. (2000) Civilisation and the colon: constipation as the 'disease of diseases'. *BMJ* **321**, 1586–9.

1936. Whorton, J.C. (2000) *Inner Hygiene – constipation and the pursuit of health in modern society*. Oxford University Press, Oxford.

1937. Whyte, H. (1958) Body fat and blood pressure of natives in New Guinea: Reflections on essential hypertension. *Aust Ann Med* **7**, 36–46.

1938. Wick, G., Knoflach, M. & Xu, Q. (2004) Autoimmune and inflammatory mechanisms in atherosclerosis. *Annu Rev Immunol* **22**, 361–403.

1939. Wijayasinghe, M.S., Smith, N.E. & Baldwin, R.L. (1984) Growth, health, and blood glucose concentrations of calves fed high-glucose or high-fat milk replacers. *J Dairy Sci* **67**, 2949–56.

1940. Wild, R.A. (2002) Polycystic ovary syndrome: a risk for coronary artery disease? *Am J Obstet Gynecol* **186**, 35–43.

1941. Wild, S.H., Roglic, G., Green, A., Sicree, R. & King, H. (2004) Global prevalence of diabetes: estimates for the year 2000 and projections for 2030: response to rathman and giani. *Diabetes Care* **27**, 2569–70.

1942. Wiley, A.S. (2005) Does milk make children grow? Relationships between milk consumption and height in NHANES 1999–2002. *Am J Hum Biol* **17**, 425–41.

1943. Wilhelmsen, L. (1981) Risk factors for disease according to population studies in Göteborg, Sweden. In: *Medical aspects of mortality statistics, Skandia International Symposium 1980* (J. Waldenström, T. Larsson & L. N. eds). Almqvist & Wiksell International, Stockholm, pp. 73–85.

1944. Wilhelmsen, L. (1988) Coronary heart disease: epidemiology of smoking and intervention studies of smoking. *Am Heart J* **115**, 242–9.

1945. Wilhelmsen, L., Rosengren, A., Eriksson, H. & Lappas, G. (2001) Heart failure in the general population of men – morbidity, risk factors and prognosis. *J Intern Med* **249**, 253–61.

1946. Will, J.M., Johnson, J.V. & White, A.L. (1992) Nutrition of the dog. *J Vet Med* **1**, 1–15.

1947. Williams, A.J., Baker, F. & Walls, J. (1987) Effect of varying quantity and quality of dietary protein intake in experimental renal disease in rats. *Nephron* **46**, 83–90.

1948. Williams, B., Poulter, N.R., Brown, M.J., *et al.* (2004) Guidelines for management of hypertension: report of the fourth working party of the British Hypertension Society, 2004-BHS IV. *J Hum Hypertens* **18**, 139–85.

1949. Williams, E.A., Perkins, S.N., Smith, N.C., Hursting, S.D. & Lane, M.A. (2007) Carbohydrate versus energy restriction: effects on weight loss, body composition and metabolism. *Ann Nutr Metab* **51**, 232–43.

1950. Williamson, C.S., Foster, R.K., Stanner, S.A. & Buttriss, J.L. (2005) Red meat in the diet. *Nutr Bull* **30**, 323–355.

1951. Wilson, M.E. (1998) Premature elevation in serum insulin-like growth factor-I advances first ovulation in rhesus monkeys. *J Endocrinol* **158**, 247–57.

1952. Wilson, P.W., Abbott, R.D. & Castelli, W.P. (1988) High density lipoprotein cholesterol and mortality. The Framingham Heart Study. *Arteriosclerosis* **8**, 737–41.

1953. Wilson, T.A., Nicolosi, R.J., Marchello, M.J. & Kritchevsky, D. (2000) Consumption of ground bison does not increase early atherosclerosis development in hypercholesterolemic hamsters. *Nutr Res* **20**, 707–19.

1954. Winer, S., Astsaturov, I., Cheung, R.K., *et al.* (2001) T cells of multiple sclerosis patients target a common environmental peptide that causes encephalitis in mice. *J Immunol* **166**, 4751–6.

1955. Winter, Y., Rohrmann, S., Linseisen, J., *et al.* (2008) Contribution of obesity and abdominal fat mass to risk of stroke and transient ischemic attacks. *Stroke* **39**, 3145–51.

1956. Winzenberg, T., Shaw, K., Fryer, J. & Jones, G. (2006) Effects of calcium supplementation on bone density in healthy children: meta-analysis of randomised controlled trials. *BMJ* **333**, 775–80.

1957. Winzenberg, T.M., Shaw, K., Fryer, J. & Jones, G. (2006) Calcium supplementation for improving bone mineral density in children. *Cochrane Database Syst Rev*, CD005119.

1958. Wolever, T.M. (2002) American diabetes association evidence-based nutrition principles and recommendations are not based on evidence. *Diabetes Care* 25, 1263–4.

1959. Wolever, T.M., Campbell, J.E., Geleva, D. & Anderson, G.H. (2004) High-fiber cereal reduces postprandial insulin responses in hyperinsulinemic but not normoinsulinemic subjects. *Diabetes Care* 27, 1281–5.

1960. Wolever, T.M., Gibbs, A.L., Mehling, C., *et al.* (2008) The Canadian Trial of Carbohydrates in Diabetes (CCD), a 1-y controlled trial of low-glycemic-index dietary carbohydrate in type 2 diabetes: no effect on glycated hemoglobin but reduction in C-reactive protein. *Am J Clin Nutr* 87, 114–25.

1961. Wolever, T.M., Jenkins, D.J., Ocana, A.M., Rao, V.A. & Collier, G.R. (1988) Second-meal effect: low-glycemic-index foods eaten at dinner improve subsequent breakfast glycemic response. *Am J Clin Nutr* 48, 1041–7.

1962. Wolf, G., Hamann, A., Han, D.C., *et al.* (1999) Leptin stimulates proliferation and TGF-beta expression in renal glomerular endothelial cells: potential role in glomerulosclerosis [see comments]. *Kidney Int* 56, 860–72.

1963. Wolfe, B.M. & Piche, L.A. (1999) Replacement of carbohydrate by protein in a conventional-fat diet reduces cholesterol and triglyceride concentrations in healthy normolipidemic subjects. *Clin Invest Med* 22, 140–48.

1964. Wolk, A., Mantzoros, C.S., Andersson, S.O., *et al.* (1998) Insulin-like growth factor 1 and prostate cancer risk: a population-based, case-control study. *J Natl Cancer Inst* 90, 911–15.

1965. Wolpowitz, D. & Gilchrest, B.A. (2006) The vitamin D questions: how much do you need and how should you get it? *J Am Acad Dermatol* 54, 301–17.

1966. Wong, W.W., Copeland, K.C., Hergenroeder, A.C., *et al.* (1999) Serum concentrations of insulin, insulin-like growth factor-I and insulin-like growth factor binding proteins are different between white and African American girls. *J Pediatr* 135, 296–300.

1967. World health Organization/Food and Agriculture Organization (2003) *Diet, nutrition and the prevention of chronic diseases: WHO Technical Report Series 916*, World Health Organization, Geneva.

1968. Worthman, C.M. (1999) Evolutionary aspects on the onset of puberty. In: *Evolutionary medicine* (W.R. Trevathan, E.O. Smith & J.J. McKenna eds). Oxford University Press, Oxford, pp. 135–63.

1969. Wortmann, R.L. (2002) Gout and hyperuricemia. *Curr Opin Rheumatol* 14, 281–6.

1970. Wortsman, J., Matsuoka, L.Y., Chen, T.C., Lu, Z. & Holick, M.F. (2000) Decreased bioavailability of vitamin D in obesity. *Am J Clin Nutr* 72, 690–93.

1971. Wrangham, R. & Conklin-Brittain, N. (2003) 'Cooking as a biological trait'. *Comp Biochem Physiol A Mol Integr Physiol* 136, 35–46.

1972. Wrangham, R.W., Holland Jones, J., Laden, G., Pilbeam, D. & Conklin-Brittain, N.L. (1999) The raw and the stolen. Cooking and the ecology of human origins. *Current Anthropol* 40, 567–94.

1973. Writers of Nordic Nutrition Recommendations. (2004) *Nordic nutrition recommendations*. Nordic Council of Ministers, Copenhagen.

1974. Wu, K., Kim, H.T., Rodriquez, J.L., *et al.* (2002) Suppression of mammary tumorigenesis in transgenic mice by the RXR-selective retinoid, LGD1069. *Cancer Epidemiol Biomarkers Prev* 11, 467–74.

1975. Wu, K.K., Wu, T.J., Chin, J., *et al.* (2005) Increased hypercholesterolemia and atherosclerosis in mice lacking both ApoE and leptin receptor. *Atherosclerosis* 181, 251–9.

1976. Wynne-Edwards, K.E. (2001) Evolutionary biology of plant defenses against herbivory and their predictive implications for endocrine disruptor susceptibility in vertebrates. *Environ Health Perspect* 109, 443–8.

1977. Xu, W., Qiu, C., Winblad, B. & Fratiglioni, L. (2007) The effect of borderline diabetes on the risk of dementia and Alzheimer's disease. *Diabetes* **56**, 211–16.

1978. Yamamoto, M., Yamaguchi, T., Yamauchi, M., Kaji, H. & Sugimoto, T. (2009) Diabetic patients have an increased risk of vertebral fractures independent of BMD or diabetic complications. *J Bone Miner Res* **24**, 702–9.

1979. Yamaoka, K. & Tango, T. (2005) Efficacy of lifestyle education to prevent type 2 diabetes: a meta-analysis of randomized controlled trials. *Diabetes Care* **28**, 2780–86.

1980. Yamori, Y., Horie, R., Nara, Y., *et al.* (1984) Dietary prevention of hypertension in animal models and its applicability to human. *Ann Clin Res* **43**, 28–31.

1981. Yancy, W.S., Jr., Foy, M., Chalecki, A.M., Vernon, M.C. & Westman, E.C. (2005) A low-carbohydrate, ketogenic diet to treat type 2 diabetes. *Nutr Metab (Lond)* **2**, 34.

1982. Yang, R. & Barouch, L.A. (2007) Leptin signaling and obesity: cardiovascular consequences. *Circ Res* **101**, 545–59.

1983. Yellayi, S., Naaz, A., Szewczykowski, M.A., *et al.* (2002) The phytoestrogen genistein induces thymic and immune changes: a human health concern? *Proc Natl Acad Sci USA* **99**, 7616–21.

1984. Yesner, D.R. (1981) Degenerative and traumatic pathologies of the Aleut vertebral column. *Arch Calif Chirop Assoc* **5**, 45–57.

1985. Yeung, G.S. & Zlotkin, S.H. (2000) Efficacy of meat and iron-fortified commercial cereal to prevent iron depletion in cow milk-fed infants 6 to 12 months of age: a randomized controlled trial. *Can J Public Health* **91**, 263–7.

1986. Yevdokimova, N.Y. & Yefimov, A.S. (2001) Effects of wheat germ agglutinin and concanavalin A on the accumulation of glycosaminoglycans in pericellular matrix of human dermal fibroblasts. A comparison with insulin. *Acta Biochim Pol* **48**, 563–72.

1987. Yip, R. & Ramakrishnan, U. (2002) Experiences and challenges in developing countries. *J Nutr* **132**, 827S–30S.

1988. Yoon, G.A. & Hwang, H.J. (2006) Effect of soy protein/animal protein ratio on calcium metabolism of the rat. *Nutrition* **22**, 414–8.

1989. Yoshikawa, H., Kotaru, M., Tanaka, C., Ikeuchi, T. & Kawabata, M. (1999) Characterization of kintoki bean (Phaseolus vulgaris) alpha-amylase inhibitor: inhibitory activities against human salivary and porcine pancreatic alpha-amylases and activity changes by proteolytic digestion. *J Nutr Sci Vitaminol (Tokyo)* **45**, 797–802.

1990. Young, D.B. & Ma, G. (1999) Vascular protective effects of potassium. *Semin Nephrol* **19**, 477–86.

1991. Young, F.A., Beattle, R. & Newby, F.J. (1954) The Pullman study: a visual survey of Pullman school children. *Am J Opt* **31**, 111.

1992. Young, S.E., Mainous, A.G., 3rd & Carnemolla, M. (2006) Hyperinsulinemia and cognitive decline in a middle-aged cohort. *Diabetes Care* **29**, 2688–93.

1993. Young, V.R. & Pellett, P.L. (1994) Plant proteins in relation to human protein and amino acid nutrition. *Am J Clin Nutr* **59**, 1203S–12S.

1994. Yu, H.C., Burrell, L.M., Black, M.J., *et al.* (1998) Salt induces myocardial and renal fibrosis in normotensive and hypertensive rats. *Circulation* **98**, 2621–8.

1995. Yusuf, S., Hawken, S., Ounpuu, S., *et al.* (2005) Obesity and the risk of myocardial infarction in 27,000 participants from 52 countries: a case-control study. *Lancet* **366**, 1640–9.

1996. Zachara, N.E. & Hart, G.W. (2004) O-GlcNAc modification: a nutritional sensor that modulates proteasome function. *Trends Cell Biol* **14**, 218–21.

1997. Zahnley, J.C. (1984) Stability of enzyme inhibitors and lectins in foods and the influence of specific binding interactions. *Adv Exp Med Biol* **177**, 333–65.

1998. Zangarelli, A., Chanseaume, E., Morio, B., *et al.* (2006) Synergistic effects of caloric restriction with maintained protein intake on skeletal muscle performance in 21-month-old rats: a mitochondria-mediated pathway. *Faseb J* **20**, 2439–50.

1999. Zanoni, G., Navone, R., Lunardi, C., *et al.* (2006) In celiac disease, a subset of autoantibodies against transglutaminase binds toll-like receptor 4 and induces activation of monocytes. *PLoS Med* 3, e358.

2000. Zargar, A.H., Ahmad, S., Masoodi, S.R., *et al.* (2007) Vitamin D status in apparently healthy adults in Kashmir Valley of Indian subcontinent. *Postgrad Med J* 83, 713–16.

2001. Zarraga, I.G. & Schwarz, E.R. (2006) Impact of dietary patterns and interventions on cardiovascular health. *Circulation* 114, 961–73.

2002. Zernicke, R.F., Salem, G.J., Barnard, R.J. & Schramm, E. (1995) Long-term, high-fat-sucrose diet alters rat femoral neck and vertebral morphology, bone mineral content, and mechanical properties. *Bone* 16, 25–31.

2003. Zhang, F., Chen, Y., Heiman, M. & Dimarchi, R. (2005) Leptin: structure, function and biology. *Vitam Horm* 71, 345–72.

2004. Zhang, J., Sasaki, S., Amano, K. & Kesteloot, H. (1999) Fish consumption and mortality from all causes, ischemic heart disease, and stroke: an ecological study. *Prev Med* 28, 520–29.

2005. Ziegler, E. (1967) Secular changes in the stature of adults and the secular trend of the modern sugar consumption. *Z Kinderheilkd* 99, 146–66.

2006. Ziegler, E. (1969) Height and weight of British men. *Lancet* 1, 1318.

2007. Ziegler, J.L. (1991) Malignant disease. In: *Hunter's tropical medicine* (G.T. Strickland ed). W. B. Saunders, Philadelphia, pp. 103–14.

2008. Zimmet, P. (1979) Epidemiology of diabetes and its macrovascular manifestations in Pacific populations: the medical effects of social progress. *Diabetes Care* 2, 144–53.

2009. Zimmet, P. (1982) Type 2 (non-insulin-dependent) diabetes–an epidemiological overview. *Diabetologia* 22, 399–411.

2010. Zimmet, P., Jackson, L. & Whitehouse, S. (1980) Blood pressure studies in two Pacific populations with varying degrees of modernisation. *N Z Med J* 91, 249–52.

2011. Zimmet, P.Z. (1993) Hyperinsulinemia – how innocent a bystander? *Diabetes Care* 3, 56–70.

2012. Zimmet, P.Z. Taylor, R., Jackson, L., *et al.* (1980) Blood pressure studies in rural and urban Western Samoa. *Med J Aust* 2, 202–5.

2013. Zohary, D. & Hopf, M. (1973) Domestication of Pulses in the Old World: legumes were companions of wheat and barley when agriculture began in the Near East. *Science* 182, 887–894.

2014. Colman R.J., Anderson R.M., Johnson S.C., Kastman E.K., Kosmatka K.J., Beasley T.M., Allison D.B., Cruzen C., Simmons H.A., Kemnitz J.W. & Weindruch R. (2009) Caloric restriction delays disease onset and mortality in rhesus monkeys. *Science* 325, 201–4.

2015. Brinkworth, G.D., Noakes, M., Buckley, J.D., Keogh, J.B. & Clifton, P.M. (2009) Long-term effects of a very-low-carbohydrate weight loss diet compared with an isocaloric low-fat diet after 12 mo. *Am J Clin Nutr* 90, 23–32.

2016. Mozaffarian, D. & Rimm, E.B. (2006) Fish intake, contaminants, and human health: evaluating the risks and the benefits. *JAMA* 296, 1885–99.

2017. Wang, C., Harris, W.S., Chung, M., *et al.* (2006) n-3 fatty acids from fish or fish-oil supplements, but not alpha-linolenic acid, benefit cardiovascular disease outcomes in primary- and secondary-prevention studies: a systematic review. *Am J Clin Nutr* 84, 5–17.

2018. Frassetto, L.A., Schloetter, M., Mietus-Synder, M., Morris, R.C., Jr. & Sebastian, A. (2009) Metabolic and physiologic improvements from consuming a paleolithic, hunter-gatherer type diet. *Eur J Clin Nutr* 63, 947–55.

2019. Kirk, J.K., Graves, D.E., Craven, T.E., Lipkin, E.W., Austin, M. & Margolis, K.L. (2008) Restricted-carbohydrate diets in patients with type 2 diabetes: a meta-analysis. *J Am Diet Assoc* 108, 91–100.

2020. Kodama, S., Saito, K., Tanaka, S., *et al.* (2009) Influence of fat and carbohydrate proportions on the metabolic profile in patients with type 2 diabetes: a meta-analysis. *Diabetes Care* 32, 959–65.

2021. Davis, N.J., Tomuta, N., Schechter, C., Isasi, C.R., Segal-Isaacson, C.J., Stein, D., Zonszein, J. & Wylie-Rosett, J. (2009) Comparative study of the effects of a 1-year dietary intervention of a low-carbohydrate diet versus a low-fat diet on weight and glycemic control in type 2 diabetes. *Diabetes Care* **32**, 1147–52.

2022. Kirk, J.K., Graves, D.E., Craven, T.E., Lipkin, E.W., Austin, M. & Margolis, K.L. (2008) Restricted-carbohydrate diets in patients with type 2 diabetes: a meta-analysis. *J Am Diet Assoc* **108**, 91–100.

2023. Kodama, S., Saito, K., Tanaka, S., *et al.* (2009) Influence of fat and carbohydrate proportions on the metabolic profile in patients with type 2 diabetes: a meta-analysis. *Diabetes Care* **32**, 959–65.

2024. Davis, N.J., Tomuta, N., Schechter, C., Isasi, C.R., Segal-Isaacson, C.J., Stein, D., Zonszein, J. & Wylie-Rosett, J. (2009) Comparative study of the effects of a 1-year dietary intervention of a low-carbohydrate diet versus a low-fat diet on weight and glycemic control in type 2 diabetes. *Diabetes Care* **32**, 1147–52.

2025. Pan, Y, Guo, L.L. & Jin, H.M. (2008) Low-protein diet for diabetic nephropathy: a meta-analysis of randomized controlled trials. *Am J Clin Nutr* **88**, 660–6.

2026. Österdahl, M., Kocturk, T., Koochek, A. & Wändell, P.E. (2008) Effects of a short-term intervention with a paleolithic diet in healthy volunteers. *Eur J Clin Nutr* **62**, 682–5.

2027. Brinkworth, G.D., Noakes, M., Buckley, J.D., Keogh, J.B. & Clifton, P.M. (2009) Long-term effects of a very-low-carbohydrate weight loss diet compared with an isocaloric low-fat diet after 12 mo. *Am J Clin Nutr* **90**, 23–32.

2028. Andersson, A., Tengblad, S., Karlstrom, B. Kamal-Eldin, A. Landberg, R. Basu, S. Aman, P. & Vessby, B. (2007) Whole-grain foods do not affect insulin sensitivity or markers of lipid peroxidation and inflammation in healthy, moderately overweight subjects. *J Nutr* **137**, 1401–7.

2029. He, J., Ogden., L.G., Bazzano, L.A., Vupputuri, S., Loria, C. & Whelton, P.K. (2001) Risk factors for congestive heart failure in US men and women: NHANES I epidemiologic follow-up study. *Arch Intern Med* **161**, 996–1002.

2030. Kenchaiah, S., Evans, J.C., Levy, D., Wilson, P.W., Benjamin, E.J., Larson, M.G., Kannel, W.B. & Vasan, R.S. (2002) Obesity and the risk of heart failure. *N Engl J Med* **347**, 305–13.

2031. Sahu, M., Bhatia, V., Aggarwal, A., Rawat, V., Saxena, P., Pandey, A. & Das, V. (2009) Vitamin D deficiency in rural girls and pregnant women despite abundant sunshine in northern India. *Clin Endocrinol (Oxf)* **70**, 680–4.

2032. Pentti, K., Tuppurainen, M.T., Honkanen, R., Sandini, L., Kroger, H., Alhava, E. & Saarikoski, S. (2009) Use of calcium supplements and the risk of coronary heart disease in 52-62-year-old women: the kuopio osteoporosis risk factor and prevention study. *Maturitas* **63**, 73–8.

2033. Mojibian, M., Chakir, H., Lefebvre, D.E., Crookshank, J. A., Sonier, B., Keely, E. & Scott, F.W. (2009) Diabetes-specific HLA-DR-restricted proinflammatory T-cell response to wheat polypeptides in tissue transglutaminase antibody-negative patients with type 1 diabetes. *Diabetes* **58**, 1789–96.

2034. Streppel, M.T., Arends, L.R., van't Veer, P., Grobbee, D.E. & Geleijnse, J.M. (2005) Dietary fiber and blood pressure: a meta- analysis of randomized placebo-controlled trials. *Arch Intern Med* **165**, 150–6.

Index (*see also* Glossary)

α-linolenic acid, 45, 65–6
β-casein A1, 26, 73, 93, 98, 130, 154, 214
β-casomorphin-7, 130, 154
β-cellulin, 98

Aborigines, Australian, 31, 111, 126, *see also* hunter-gatherers
acid-base balance, 52, 200–201
acne, 143, *149–51*
acrylamide, 55
ageing, normal versus Western, 11, 39, 62, 90, 93, 196
alcohol
  in ancestral diets, 33–4
  and cancer, 188
  and hypertension, 161–3
  and ischaemic heart disease, 71–2
  and osteoporosis, 203
allergy, 41, 211, 229
American Heart Association, viii, 64, 74, 83, 124
amylase, salivary, 28, 32
amylopectin, 108, 112
angina pectoris, 57–8, 62–3, 66–7, 73–4, 82, *see also* ischaemic heart disease
angiotensin-converting enzyme (ACE) inhibitors, 165, 219
angiotensin receptor blockers, 165, 219
'animal' proteins, *see* proteins, animal
antioxidants, 14, 29, 55, 81, 82, 98, 190
apolipoproteins B and A1, 175–6
Arctic, 33, 40, 57, 136, 185, 195, 225, *see also* Eskimo
ascorbic acid, *see* vitamin C
Asian Indians, 73, 147, 151, 206

atherosclerosis
  and autoimmunity, 215
  carotid, 85, 96, 98, 146
  and dementia, 183
  and diet, 94–101
  and dyslipidaemia, 166, 170, 175
  and heart failure, 179
  and insulin resistance, 141–3
  and ischaemic heart disease, 57
  and osteoporosis, 202
  prevalence
    in animals, 93–4, 148
    in humans, 26, 64, 88, 90, 92–3, 170
  regression, 94–5, 175
  and stroke, 87
Atkins diet, 27–8, 133, 178, *see also* carbohydrates
atrial fibrillation, 85
asthma, 125
autoimmune disease, 8, 100, *210–15*
'autointoxication', 22
autopsy studies, 26, 57–8, 63, 72, 92–3, 125

Banting, William, 27, 131–3
barley, 7, 53, 92, 207
beans, *see also* plant lectins; proteins, soya
  in ancestral diets, 31
  and endocrine disruption, 191, 218, 227
  nutritional characteristics, 36, 40–41, 50, 52–4, 201, 209–10
  and sarcopenia, 155
betel chewing, 150, 185–6
bioactive substances, 1, 5, 7, 17, 31–2, 52, 54–5, 229, *see also* phytochemicals

birds, 70, 97, 99, 101, 110, 131
birth defects, 126
blood pressure, *see also* hypertension
  'normal', 11–12, 93
  in traditional populations, 157–9
blood sugar, *see* diabetes; glucose tolerance;
    hyperglycaemia
body weight, *see* overweight/obesity;
    underweight; weight loss
bone
  density, *see* osteoporosis
  fossil, *see* Palaeolithic skeletons
breathing difficulties, 125, 143, 178
Brillat-Savarin, Anthelme, 27
Burkitt, Denis, 22
Bushmen, 31, 58, 84, 158, 208

calcium, *see* minerals
calorie restriction, *see* energy restriction
cancer, *see also* myeloma; leukaemia; lymphoma
  and diet, 13, 22, 24, 26, 55, 90, 185, 187–92
  and insulin resistance, 143–4, 151
  metastatic, 186–7, 190, 192
  and overweight/obesity, 122, 124
  prevalence, 8–9, 150, 185–7
  types
    breast, 9–10, 124, 143, 151, 185–91
    cervix, 186
    colorectal, 9, 124, 151, 185, 188–91
    kidney, 124, 191
    liver, 54, 186, 188
    oral, 185
    ovarian, 124, 186
    pancreatic, 124, 188
    prostate, 82, 150–51, 185–6, 190–91
    sarcoma, 187
    skeletal, 186–7
    stomach, 9, 186
carbohydrates
  in ancestral diets, 32, 49–51
  and diabetes type 2, 108–9, 112–13
  and dyslipidaemia, 178
  food sources, 20, 32, 42, 49–51
  glycaemic index (GI)
    in ancestral diets, 49–50
    determinants, 112
    and diabetes types type 2, 105, 108
    of fruit, 115
    and insulin resistance, 153
    and ischaemic heart disease, 76–8
    and overweight, 130
    problem of use, 15
  and insulin resistance, 136–7, 153–4
  and ischaemic heart disease, 76–8
  and liver steatosis, 153
  'low carbohydrate' diets, 20, 27–8, 77, 112,
    178

and overweight, 129–30
starch
  in ancestral diets, 32, 51, 55
  and health, 27, 28, 78, 97, 108, 112–13,
    129
sugars, *see also* fructose; lactose; sucrose
  in ancestral diets, 31–2, 49, 50–52
  and health, 78, 97, 108–9, 115, 128, 145,
    153
carnitine, 181
carnivore connection hypothesis, 136–7
casein
  and atherosclerosis, 93, 97–8
  and breast cancer, 188
  and diabetes type 2, 108–10, 114
  and diabetes type 1, 214
  and dyslipidaemia, 178
  and growth, 146
  and insulin resistance, 153–4
  and ischaemic heart disease, 26, 73
  and osteoporosis, 202
  and overweight, 130
  versus soya protein, 83, 114, 178, 202
cassava, 54, 218
cereals
  and atherosclerosis, 99–101
  and diabetes type 2, 110, 112, 115,
    154–5
  nutritional characteristics, 34–7, 38–41, 49,
    51–5, 100
  and osteoporosis, 199, 201
  and overweight, 131
  and rickets, 206–10
  whole grains 131, 154
    and colorectal cancer, 189–90
    and confounding, 23, 190
    and ischaemic heart disease, 79–81
    and plant lectins, *see* plant lectins
cheese
  and ischaemic heart disease, 72–3
  and osteoporosis, 201
childhood, 56, 62, 130, 142, 145–8, 151, 198,
    204–6, 208–9, 214, 217
China, 27, 84, 89, 120, 125, 151, 166, 194
chloride, 37, 52, 201
cholesterol
  blood, *see* dyslipidaemia
  dietary, 42, 48–9, 75–6, 97
cobalamin, *see* vitamins, B$_{12}$
Cochrane reviews
  calcium supplementation and bone density in
    children, 198
  dietary prevention of diabetes type 2,
    104
  glycaemic index in diabetes type 2, 112
  glycaemic index or load and obesity, 130
  low-fat diets and obesity, 129

magnesium and hypertension, 165
omega-3 fats and cancer, 26
omega-3 fats and cardiovascular disease, 26, 65
potassium and hypertension, 165
total/saturated fat and cardiovascular disease, 74
vitamin A, C or E, or selenium and cardiovascular disease, 82
vitamin D and osteoporosis, 197
weight reduction for primary prevention of stroke, 124
coconut, 44–5, 58–9, 71, 97, 167, 170
coeliac disease, *see* gluten intolerance
coffee, 81–2, 166
compromises, 229
confounding
    and antioxidants, 14, 190
    and dairy products, 139
    and fibre, 23, 80, 190
    and fish, 66
    and weight loss, 122, 129
    and fruit and vegetables, 68
    and meat, 69, 189, 213
    and Mediterranean-like diets, 64
    and nuts, 70
    and tea, 81
    and wine, 14
cooking, 32, 41, 46, 52–3, 55, 99, 189
coronary heart disease, *see* ischaemic heart disease
C-reactive protein, 24, 70, 126
Crete, 22, 25–6, 64, 104
cyanogenic glycosides, 5, 54, 218

dairy food, *see* milk
DART trial, 26, 65–7, 80
Darwin, Charles, 1
DASH trial, 73, 162–5
death
    causes, 8–11
    premature, 5, 8, 23, 83, 119–22, 178, 190
    sudden, 8, 11, 58, 59, 62, 65, 66, 67, 70, 74, 76, 198
dementia, 8–10, 59, 90, *183–4*
diabetes
    in natural selection, 3, 135–9
    type 2
        and dementia, 184
        and diet, 27, 104–15, 219
        and heart failure, 179–80
        and ischaemic heart disease, 101–2
        and kidney failure, 152
        mechanisms, 101–2, 104, 124, 135–40
        prevalence, 26, 102–4, 154
        and osteoporosis, 202–3

and prostatic hyperplasia, 149
    and stroke, 85, 87–8
    type 1, 113, 114, 202, *213–4*
diagenesis, 186, 195
dietary assessment, 13–15
dietary guidelines
    old and new concepts, 21–9
    methodological problems, 13–21
diet-induced thermogenesis, *see* energy
docosahexaenoic acid, 45
dogs, 24, 94, 108, 135, 148, 150, 152, 154, 190
drinking, *see* fluid
drug treatment, *see* medication
dyslipidaemia, 105, 111–12, 166–78

Eaton, Boyd, vii, xi
eggs, 30, 33, 47, 49, 76, 95, 125, 177, 201
elderly
    health status in the West, 11, 27, 39, 90, 93, 126, 151, 196
    importance in hunter-gatherer societies, 6
    prevalence in traditional populations, 56–7, 59–62
endocrine disruption, 53, 128, 145, 147, 151, 155, 191, 225, 227
endothelium, 75–6, 81, 91–2, 97, 142, 166
energy
    density of foods, 30, 33, 43, 49, 51, 76, 112, 128–9, 228
    intake, 13, 15, 31–3, 52, 76
    restriction, 23–5, 76, 98, 107, 113, 115, 128–9, 152, 177, 189, 224
    thermodynamics, 25, 128–9
epidermal growth factor (EGF), 98–9, 155
Eskimo, 26, 65, 96, 125, 145, 167, 194–7, 201, 213
ethnicity
    and adult lactose tolerance, 3, 73, 138
    and impact of urbanisation, 135–9, 147–8, 151, 161
evolution, 1–7
exercise, *see* physical activity

famine, 59, 135–7, 139, 145
fat, abdominal, *see* overweight/obesity, abdominal
fats, dietary
    and atherosclerosis, 96–7
    and cancer, 189, 191
    cholesterol, *see* cholesterol, dietary
    and diabetes type 2, 107–8, 112–13
    and dyslipidaemia, 176
    fatty acids
        monounsaturated
            in ancestral diets, 45, 48
            and atherosclerosis, 96–7
            and diabetes type 2, 112

fats, dietary (*Cont.*)
    and dyslipidaemia, 178
    and insulin sensitivity, 152
    and ischaemic heart disease, 74
  omega-3
    and atherosclerosis, 96
    and blood pressure, 166
    in ancestral diets, 45–8
    and ischaemic heart disease, 18, 65–7
    requirements, 45
  omega-6, 42, 45–8, 71, 74–5, 96, 100, 213
  saturated
    in ancestral diets, 45
    and atherosclerosis, 95–6
    and diabetes, 112–13
    and dyslipidaemia, 167, 170, 176, 178
    and insulin resistance, 152
    and ischaemic heart disease, 18, 22–3,
      59, 64, 74–5
  trans, 22, 48, 75, 105, 112, 176
  total
    and atherosclerosis, 95–7
    and cancer, 187, 189, 191
    and diabetes type 2, 107–8, 112–13
    and dyslipidaemia, 176
    in ancestral diets, 42–5, 47
    and insulin resistance, 152
    and ischaemic heart disease, 22–3,
      74–5
    and osteoporosis, 202
    and overweight, 129–30
    and stroke, 90
  fatty foods
    fatty ancestral foods, 31, 33, 42–5, 47
    margarine, 44, 46, 48
    olive oil, 25, 46
    rapeseed oil, 26, 46
  and insulin resistance, 152–3
  and ischaemic heart disease, 65–7, 73–6
  and liver steatosis, 153
  'low fat' diets, 20, 22–3, 107, 129
  and overweight, 129–30
  and stroke, 90
fatty liver, *see* liver steatosis
fermentation, 34, 39, 98, 112, 206–7
fertility, 5, 20, 53, 126, 135, 139, 151
fibre, dietary
  in ancestral diets, 52
  and cancer, 187, 189–90
  as health trend, 22–3
  cereal, 19, 22–3, 80, 110, 154
  and diabetes type 2, 105, 110–12, 115
  and dyslipidaemia, 176–7
  and hypertension, 166
  and ischaemic heart disease, 80–81
  soluble, 58, 71, 74, 95, 115, 176–7

Finland, 57, 78, 89, 105, 120–21, 175, 194,
    213, 217
fire, 32
fish
  in ancestral diets, 33
  and ischaemic heart disease, 65–7
  nutritional characteristics, 35–6, 38–40, 46–9,
    51, 217–18
  and stroke, 90
flavonoids, 53, 218, 227
fluid
  restriction in heart failure, 182
  mineral water, 228
  soft drinks, 17, 24, 78, 128, 139, 198,
    226
  water, 24, 34–5, 43–4, 49, 51, 228
folate, *see* vitamins
France, 27, 64, 72, 120, 135, 170, 194, 205,
    207, 214
fructose
  in ancestral diets, 49, 51, 109
  and atherosclerosis, 97
  and diabetes type 2, 108–9, 115
  and insulin resistance, 153
  and ischaemic heart disease, 78
fruit
  in ancestral diets, 30–34
  and diabetes type 2, 109, 115
  and hypertension, 162–3
  and insulin resistance, 153
  and ischaemic heart disease, 58, 67–8
  nutritional characteristics, 35–6, 38–40,
    50–52
  and stroke, 89

galactosylation, 97–8, 153
gallstones, 28, 125
genetic
  adaptation to 'new' diets, 3, 5–7, 17, 94,
    136–9, 206
  variation and modern disease, 12–13, 63, 92,
    104, 144, 147, 184, 211, 214, 216
genistein, 18, 191, 227, *see also* phytoestrogens
gliadin, *see* gluten
glucose
  blood/plasma, *see* diabetes; glycaemic index;
    hyperglycaemia
  dietary, *see* carbohydrates
  tolerance, *see also* diabetes; hyperglycaemia
    and dementia, 183
    and diabetes type 2, 101–2, 104–10
    and dyslipidaemia, 175
    and insulin resistance, 133, 138–40, 152
    and osteoporosis, 202
    and salt-sensitive hypertension, 165
    and stroke, 87

gluten
  and ataxia, 212
  and atherosclerosis, 99–100
  and diabetes type 1, 214
  and insulin release, 154
  and intestinal permeability, 210
  intake, 42, 131
  intolerance (coeliac disease), 12, 211–12
  and leptin binding, 100
  and multiple sclerosis, 214
  and rheumatoid arthritis, 213
glycaemic index, *see* carbohydrates
glycocalyx, 91, 98–9, 211
glycosylation, 52, 99–100, 109, 131, 202, 210
goitre, 36, 38, 54, 217–18, 227
gout, 142–3
grains, *see* cereals
Greece, 25, 46, 64, 87, 104, 120, 151, 194, 204,
      see also Crete
growth
  body, 116, 144–7, 187–8, 193
  tissue, 99, 143–52

haemochromatosis, 83, 208, *216–17*
HDL cholesterol, 71, 94, 101, 167, 170–71,
      173–8, *see also* dyslipidaemia
heart disease, *see* heart failure; ischaemic heart
      disease
heart failure, 8, 10, 16, 74, 101–2, 142–3,
      178–83
height, *see* stature
heredity, *see* genetics
heterocyclic amines, 189
homocysteine, 82, 90, 99, 184
honey, 31–2, 49–51
hunter-gatherers
  contemporary
    blood lipids, 167
    blood pressure, 156–8, 165
    BMI, 115, 134
    cancer, 185
    food access, 135–6
    food habits, 31–3, 35, 37, 40, 46, 48, 52
    glucose metabolism, 102, 111, 133
    iron status, 208
    myopia, 148
    puberty, 147
    sudden death, 58
    urate, 143
  Palaeolithic, *see* Palaeolithic
hyperglycaemia, 77, 87, 101–2, *see also*
      diabetes; glucose tolerance
hyperinsulinaemia
  and atherosclerosis, 142
  and diabetes, 108, 188
  and enhanced tissue growth, 143–4

  and insulin resistance, 139
  and ischaemic heart disease, 77
  and milk, 110
  and overweight, 130
  and osteoporosis, 202
hypertension
  definitions, 11–12, 156–7
  and diet, 161–6
  and drug treatment, 10, 219
  mechanisms, 133, 135, 155, 157, 165
  prevalence, 26, 157–60
  and stroke, 85–8, 161
hypotension, 219

Iceland, 73, 194, 214
industry funding, 17
infertility, *see* fertility
inflammation, 41, 70, 81, 92, 126, 142, 149,
      212–13, 215
insects (as food), 5, 33, 39–40, 43
insulin-like growth factor-1 (IGF-1), 130,
      143–7, 149, 151, 155
insulin resistance
  associated abnormalities,
    acne, 149–50
    atherosclerosis, 142
    benign prostatic hyperplasia, 149–50
    cancer, 151, 188–90
    cardiovascular disease, 142
    dementia, 184
    diabetes type 2, 140
    early puberty, 147
    enhanced tissue growth, 143–51
    gout, 142
    hypertension, 165
    increased stature, 144–7
    infertility, 151
    kidney failure, 152
    lipotoxicity, 141–2, 152
    liver steatosis, 141–2
    metabolic syndrome, 140
    myopia, 147–8
    obstructive sleep apnoea, 143
    osteoporosis, 202–3
  and diet, 152–6
  mechanisms, 133, 135–9, 141–2, 152–5
  prevalence, 133–5
intestinal permeability, 99, 210–11, 214–15
iodine, *see* minerals
iron, *see* minerals
ischaemic heart disease
  and diabetes type 2, 101–2
  and diet, 21–9, 63–84, 95
  and dyslipidaemia, 166, 174–6, 179–80
  and insulin resistance, 142–3
  and osteoporosis, 202

ischaemic heart disease (*Cont.*)
  and overweight, 123
  prevalence, 57–63
Italy, 25, 81, 83, 87, 120, 125, 135, 194, 213

Japan, 25, 27, 46, 57, 67, 84, 87, 89, 90, 93,
    120, 124, 145–6, 167, 175, 191, 194,
    202, 213–4
Jenkins, David, 177
Jüptner, Horst, 62–3, 85, 150, 179, 186, 193

Kenya, 22, 86, 161
Kellogg, John Harvey, xii, 71
Keys, Ancel, 64
kidneys
  and abdominal obesity, 126
  and calcium excretion, 196, 199–200,
    205
  cancer, 124, 188
  and diabetes, 102, 113–15
  failure, 152
  and lipotoxicity, 140, 154
  and pyrrolizidine alkaloids, 54
  and salt intake, 165
Kitava studies
  acne, 149–50
  blood pressure, 134, 157–60
  cancer, 185
  carbohydrate intake, 78
  dementia, 183
  diabetes type 2, 102–3
  diet
    carbohydrate, 78, 178
    food access, 116, 135
    food items, 58–9, 78
    protein, 146
    salt, 159
    saturated fat, 59, 167, 178
  electrocardiography (ECG), 62, 179
  haemostatic variables, 134
  heart failure, 179
  insulin, serum, 133–4
  ischaemic heart disease, 58–63
  leptin, 134, 141
  lipids, blood, 134, 167–73, 175–6
  Lp(a), 134
  osteoporosis, 193–4
  overweight, 116–19, 134
  physical activity, 84
  plasminogen activator inhibitor-1, 112,
    134
  smoking, 84
  stature, 146
  stroke, 85
  'underweight', 116–17
  urate, serum, 143

lactose, 138, 153, 190, 198
  in ancestral diets, 50–51
  and atherosclerotic disease, 73, 97–8
  and diabetes, 138
  and insulin resistance, 109, 153
  tolerance, 6, 12, 138, 198
LDL cholesterol, 94, 101, 167, 170, 175–8, 202,
    see also dyslipidaemia
lectins, *see* plant lectins
leptin, 92, 100, 128, 131, 133, 141, 146–7, 183,
    202
leukaemia, 124, 143
lifespan
  and calorie restriction, 24
  in traditional populations, 56–7, 59–62
Lifestyle Heart Trial, 95
lipids
  blood, *see* dyslipidaemia
  dietary, *see* fats
  intracellular, *see* lipotoxicity
lipotoxicity, 141–2, 152, 154–5, 179
liver
  cancer, *see* cancer
  as food, 49
  metabolism, 41, 75, 98, 136, 173, 177
  steatosis, 125, 141–2, 153–4
'low-carbohydrate' diets, *see* carbohydrates
lymphoma, 22, 124, 186
Lyon Diet Heart Trial, 18, 24, 26, 64, 67
lysine, 41, 181

macronutrients, *see* alcohol; carbohydrates; fats;
    proteins
magnesium, *see* minerals
malnutrition, 59, 113, 116, 139, 182, 191, 203,
    see also sarcopenia; underweight;
    weight loss
Masai, 98, 167, 170
meat
  in ancestral diets, 30, 32–4
  and atherosclerosis, 97
  and cancer, 187–9
  domestic, 35, 44–8, 51
  and dyslipidaemia, 177
  and haemochromatosis, 216
  and hypertension, 166
  and iron deficiency, 209
  and ischaemic heart disease, 68–70, 73, 76
  nutritional characteristics, 36, 38–49, 51, 139
  and osteoporosis, 201
  poultry, 37, 43, 45, 47–8, 70, 189
  red, 29, 70, 73, 166, 177, 188–9
  and rheumatoid arthritis, 213
  wild, 5, 40–41, 44
media, 14, 21
medication, 10–11, 77, 102, 156, 181–3, 219

Mediterranean(-like) diets
  and atherosclerosis, 97
  and diabetes type 2, 104, 106, 110
  and dyslipidaemia, 170
  as health trend, 25
  and ischaemic heart disease, 64–5
  and rheumatoid arthritis, 213
  and stroke, 87
menarche, *see* puberty
metabolic syndrome, 140, *see also* diabetes, type
      2; dyslipidaemia; hypertension;
      overweight/obesity, abdominal
micronutrients, *see* minerals, vitamins
milk, *see also* proteins, milk
  and atherosclerosis, 92–3, 97–8
  and calcium, 37
  and confounding, 14
  and diabetes type 2, 109–10, 114,
      138–9
  and diabetes type 1, 213–14
  and dyslipidaemia, 170, 178
  and insulin resistance, 145–6, 153–4
  and ischaemic heart disease, 72–3
  and the Masai, 98, 170
  in natural selection, 5–7
  and osteoporosis, 196, 198, 201, 203
  and overweight, 130
  and prostate cancer, 190
minerals
  calcium
    absorption, 54, 196, 199
    content in food, 35, 37
    depletion, 199–201
    supplementation, 197–8
  iodine, 36, 38, 54, 217–18
  iron
    absorption, 36, 54, 71, 209–10, 216
    deficiency, 208–10
    and ischaemic heart disease, 83
    overload, *see* haemochromatosis
  magnesium, 18, 35–6, 54, 71, 83, 99–100,
      166, 200
  potassium, 35–7, 52, 83, 89–90, 99–100, 165,
      201
  selenium, 27, 36, 82, 98, 100, 190
  zinc, 35–6, 54, 71, 99–100
molecular mimicry, 211, 214
mortality, *see* death
mutagens, 192
myeloma, 124, 186–7
myocardial infarction, 8, 10–12, 57–8, 62–5, *see*
      also ischaemic heart disease
myopia, 2, 143, *147–8*

National Health and Nutrition Examination
      Surveys, 68, 79, 89, 119, 180

natural
  food, 5, 20, 52, 192
  habitat, 94, 96, 110
  selection, 1–3, 6, 36, 89, 138, 148, 218
nitrate, 189
non-alcoholic fatty liver disease (NAFLD), *see*
      liver steatosis
non-thrifty genotype hypothesis, 137–8
'normality', 11–12, 91, 93, 107, 115, 116, 134,
      146, 156–7, 161, 179
Nurses' Health Study, 15, 68, 77
nutrigenomics, 13
nuts
  intake, 30, 33
  and ischaemic heart disease, 70–71
  nutritional composition, 35, 38, 40–46, 48, 51

oats, 7, 24, 52, 54, 66, 92, 177, 206–7
obesity, *see* overweight/obesity
obstructive sleep apnoea, 125, 143
oils, *see* fats, fatty foods
osteoarthritis, 126, 213
osteology, *see* Palaeolithic skeletons
osteoporosis, 8, 13, *192–204*, 207
overweight/obesity
  abdominal, *see also* insulin resistance
    and diet, 126–33
    potential consequences, 121–6, 179, 187,
        189, 202
    prevalence, 115–19
  definitions, 116
  and diet, 79, 126–31, 135–9
  potential consequences
    breathing difficulties, 125
    cancer, 124, 188
    diabetes type 2, 105, 140
    gallstones, 125
    gout, 142
    heart failure, 179–80
    hypertension, 162
    infertility, 126, 151
    inflammation, 126
    ischaemic heart disease, 123
    kidney disease, 126
    liver steatosis, 141–2
    metabolic syndrome, 140
    osteoarthritis, 126
    pregnancy complications, 126
    premature death, 119–22
    stroke, 88, 124
  prevalence, 115–20

Palaeolithic
  diet, 209, 212–13, 215–20
    as assumed to have been originally eaten,
        30–55, 136–7, 192

Palaeolithic (*Cont.*)
  in clinical trials, 57, 106–7, 109, 111–13,
    126–8, 131, 146, 152
  as compared with other dietary models, 64,
    79, 95, 105, 163, 178, 196, 212–13
  as eaten by modern hunter-gatherers,
    30–35, 37, 40, 70, 111, 135
  nutritional characteristics, 34–55, 78, 82,
    99, 105, 113, 115, 128, 137, 192, 209
  as recommended here, 57, 90, 111, 114,
    147, 149, 203, 208, 215, 219, 227–30
  Era, 29–34, 56
  lifespan, 56
  skeletons, 31, 56, 186, 194–6, 204, 208–9,
    213
Papua New Guinea, 21, 56, 58, 85–7, 120, 143,
    186, 193, *see also* Kitava studies
peanut, 33, 71, 99, 229
peripheral arterial disease, 74, 101
persistent organic pollutants, 155
Pima Indians, 104, 116, 125, 136–8, 213
pregnancy, 62, 94, 139, 151, 186, 208, 217–18,
    227, *see also* fertility
physical activity
  and health, 57, 84, 111, 156, 161–2, 188, 192
  in non-Western populations, 52, 135, 173
Physicians' Health Study, 70
phytate, 54, 71
  and iron deficiency, 209
  and osteoporosis, 199
  and rickets, 206–7
phytochemicals, 5, 7, 33, 52, 110, 131, 221
phytoestrogen, 20, 53, 191, 227
phytosterols, *see* plant sterols
plant foods, 31–4, 49, 201
plant lectins, 52–3
  and atherosclerosis, 99–100
  and autoimmune disease, 210–15
  and glucose metabolism, 155
  and intestinal permeability, 99, 210–11, 214
  peanut, 99
  and vascular permeabilty, 211, 214
  wheat, 99–100, 155, 211–12, 212, 214
plant sterols
  and dyslipidaemia, 177
  and ischaemic heart disease, 76
polycyclic aromatic hydrocarbons, 189, 192
polycystic ovary syndrome, 151
potassium, *see* minerals
potato, 7, 37, 44, 50–3, 76, 92, 201, 211
primates, non-human, 24, 31–3, 76, 97–8, 135,
    147, 152, 163, 208
prostate
  benign hyperplasia, 149–50
  cancer, *see* cancer
protease inhibitors, 5, 41, 53, 215, 226

proteins
  'animal', 114
  cereal, *see* gluten; plant lectins
  meat, 41, 97, 130, 154, 166
  milk
    and atherosclerosis, 97–8
    and breast cancer, 188
    in cheese, 72
    and diabetes type 2, 109, 114
    and growth, 145–6,
    and insulin release, 110, 154
    and insulin resistance, 153–4
    and ischaemic heart disease, 73
    and overweight, 130
    and osteoporosis, 201–2
    and rheumatoid arthritis, 212–14
  plant, 41, 52–3, 97
  soya
    and atherosclerosis, 97
    and cancer, 188, 191
    and diabetes type 1, 214
    and diabetes type 2, 114
    and dyslipidaemia, 154
    and insulin resistance, 154
    and ischaemic heart disease, 83
    and osteoporosis, 201–2
  total
    in ancestral diets, 40–41
    and diabetes type 2, 113–14
    and hypertension, 165–6
    and insulin resistance, 136–7, 139
    and myopia, 148
    and osteoporosis, 201, 203
    and overweight, 129
    and sarcopenia, 25
    and stature, 145
    and stroke, 90
puberty, 144–5, 147–8, 188
pyrrolizidine alkaloids, 54

renal disease, *see* kidneys
renin-angiotensin system, 79, 155–6, 182, *see
    also* angiotensin-converting enzyme
    inhibitors
retinoid receptors, 142–4, 147–9, 151
rickets, *204–7*
root vegetables, 7, 32, 36, 38–41, 49, 51–2, 58,
    76, 201, 228
ruminants, 7, 48, 75, 224
rye, 7, 44, 52–3, 207, 212

salt, dietary
  in ancestral diets, 36–7
  and ACE inhibitor treatment, 219
  and diabetes, 114–15
  and heart failure, 180–82

and hypertension, 26–7, 159, 163–5
and insulin resistance, 155
and iodine, 38, 217–18
and ischaemic heart disease, 78–9
and osteoporosis, 199–201
and rickets, 207
sensitivity, 155, 165
and stroke, 89–90
variation, 15
San, *see* Bushmen
sarcopenia, 25, 122, 155, 182, *see also*
    malnutriton; underweight; weight loss
satiation, satiety, 24, 34, 76, 80, 100, 105, 113,
    128–31, 141, 227, 247
Schiefenhövel, Wulf, 58, 62, 85, 147, 150, 179,
    193
seeds, 7, 30–31, 52–4, 99–101, 110–11
selenium, *see* minerals
Seven Countries Study, 22, 25, 69, 84
shellfish, 30, 33, 36, 38–40, 45, 51, 111, 137,
    177, 218
Sippy diet, 72
smoking, 15, 57, 83–5, 88–9, 94, 161, 175, 180,
    192
sodium, *see* salt
soft drinks, 78, 109, 128, 139
soya, *see* proteins, soya
Spain, 25, 104, 120, 194
starch, *see* carbohydrates
sterols, *see* plant sterols
stature, 116, 143–51, 187–8, 193
stroke
    and atherosclerosis, 87
    and blood pressure, 87, 161
    and BMI, 124
    and diet, 89–90, 218
    and diabetes, 85, 87–9, 101–2
    incidence, 8, 10, 62, 85–8
    risk factors, 85, 88, 142–3, 176, 217
    and waist circumference, 88, 135
sucrose, 25, 51, 78, 97, 145, 148, 153
sudden (cardiac) death, *see* death, sudden
sugars, *see* carbohydrates; lactose; sucrose
sunlight, 35, 39, 194, 192, 196–7, 206
sweet potato, 54, 58, 218

taurine, 99–100, 109, 139
tea, 54, 81, 210
thermodynamics, *see* energy
THIS-DIET trial, 65
threonine, 41
thrifty genotype hypothesis, 135–9
thrifty phenotype hypothesis, 139
thyroid, 38, 186, 217–18, 227
TIA/minor stroke, 85
Tokelau Island Migrant Study, 119, 143

tomato, 42, 229
tooth, 31–2
trace elements, *see* minerals
trans fats, *see* fats
triacylglycerols, *see* triglycerides
triglycerides
    intracellular, *see* lipid droplets; lipotoxicity
    serum, 111–12, 115, 167, 172–3, 176–8,
        see also dyslipidaemia
Trobriand Islands, *see* Kitava Studies
Trowell, Hugh, 22, 86, 184, 185
tubers, *see* root vegetables

Uganda, 22, 57–8, 86, 104, 125, 185
underweight, 116, 182, 196, 203, *see also*
    malnutrition
urate, 142–3
urbanisation, 12, 63, 104, 124–5, 135–6, 148,
    159–61, 170–75, 204
urinary retention, 149

vegan diets, *see* vegetarian diets
vegetables
    in ancestral diets, 5, 30
    and ischaemic heart disease, 63–4, 66–8, 73
    nutritional composition, 34–6, 38–43,
        50–52
    and osteoporosis, 201
    and stroke, 89–90
vegetarian diets
    and atherosclerosis, 95
    and cancer, 187, 189
    and dyslipidaemia, 177
    in human evolution, 30
    and ischaemic heart disease, 68–9
    and nutrient deficiencies
        minerals, 199, 208
        amino acids, 41
        iodine, 217
        iron, 210
        taurine, 139
        vitamin B_{12}, 39, 82
        vitamin D, 196
    and osteoporosis, 201
    and rheumatoid arthritis, 213
vitamins
    A, 27, 36, 39, 82, 98, 166, 188
    B_6, 36, 39, 82, 90, 99–100
    B_{12}, 36, 39, 82, 90, 99–100, 208
    C, 27, 36–8, 65, 67, 82, 98, 100, 166, 190,
        208–9, 216
    D, 36, 39, 100, 196–7, 204–6
    E, 27, 36, 39, 82, 98, 166, 190
    and ischaemic heart disease, 82
    K, 39, 219
    folate, 34, 36,39, 82, 90, 99–100, 184

waist circumference, *see* overweight/obesity,
    abdominal
warfarin, 219–20
weight loss, *see also* energy restriction;
    overweight/obesity; underweight
  and blood pressure, 162
  and diabetes prevention,
    105–7
  and diet, 128–31
  and fertility, 151
  and gallstones, 125
  and mortality, 76, 121–23
  and osteoporosis, 196,
    203
Westernisation *see* urbanisation

wheat
  health effects, *see* cereals; fibre; gluten; plant
    lectins
  intake in traditional populations, 19, 31
whey protein, 110, 130, 146, 154, 188
whole grains, *see* cereals
wine, 14, 26, 28–9, 33, 64, 71–2, *see also*
    alcohol
Women's Health Initiative Dietary Modification
    Trial, 22, 75, 107, 189

yam, 58, 191
Yanomamo Indians, 37, 79, 155, 158

zinc, *see* minerals